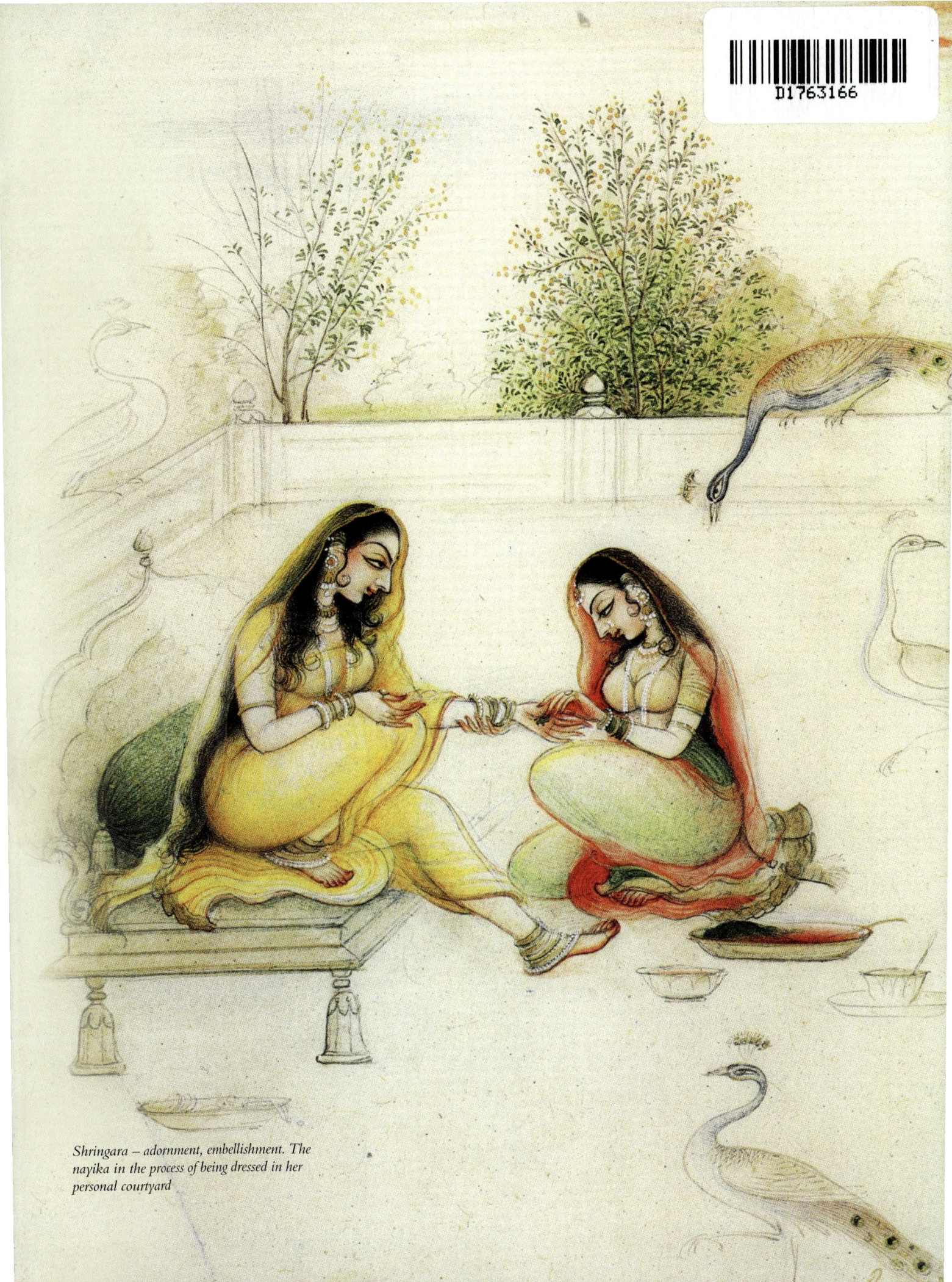

Shringara – adornment, embellishment. The nayika in the process of being dressed in her personal courtyard

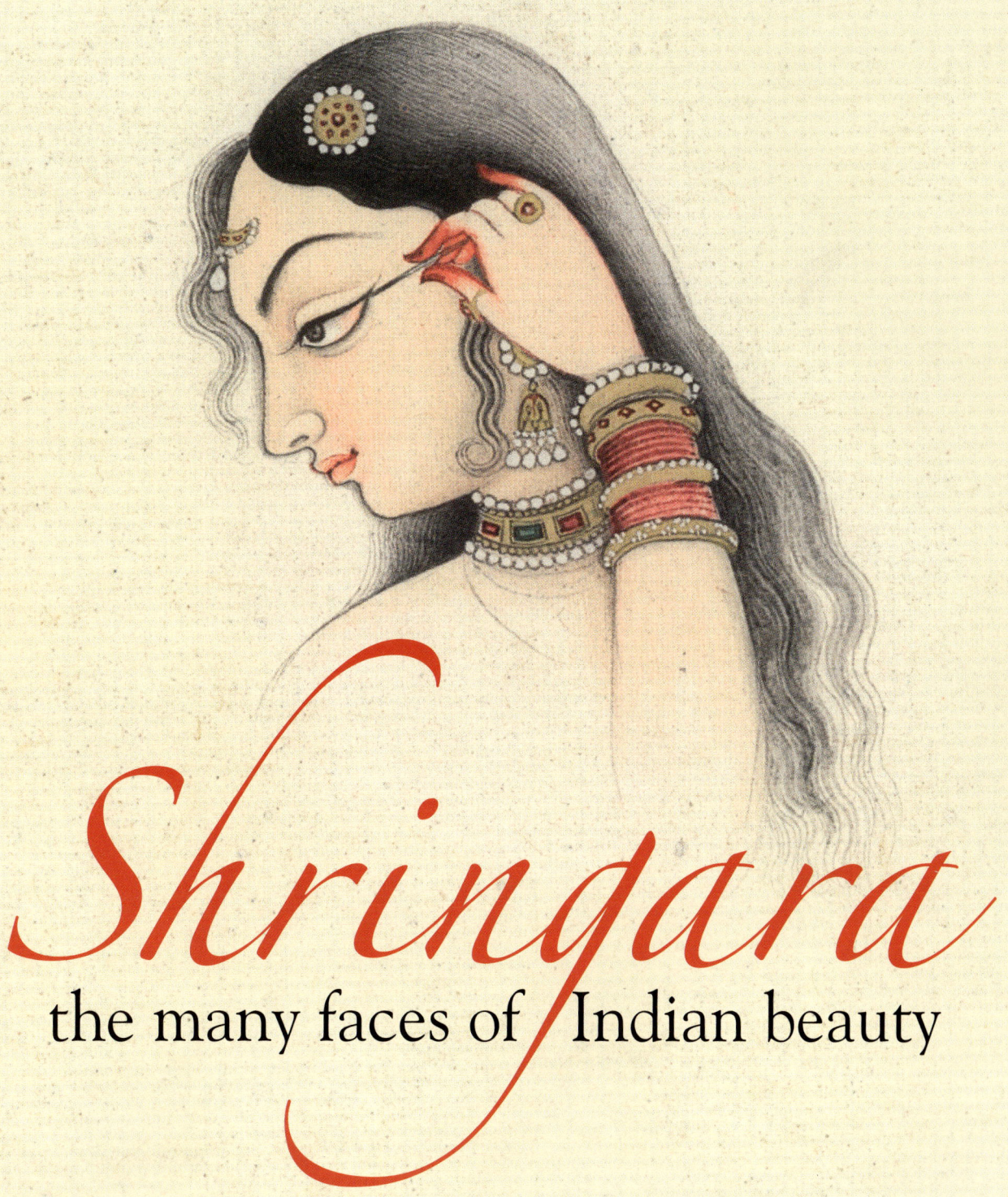

Shringara
the many faces of Indian beauty

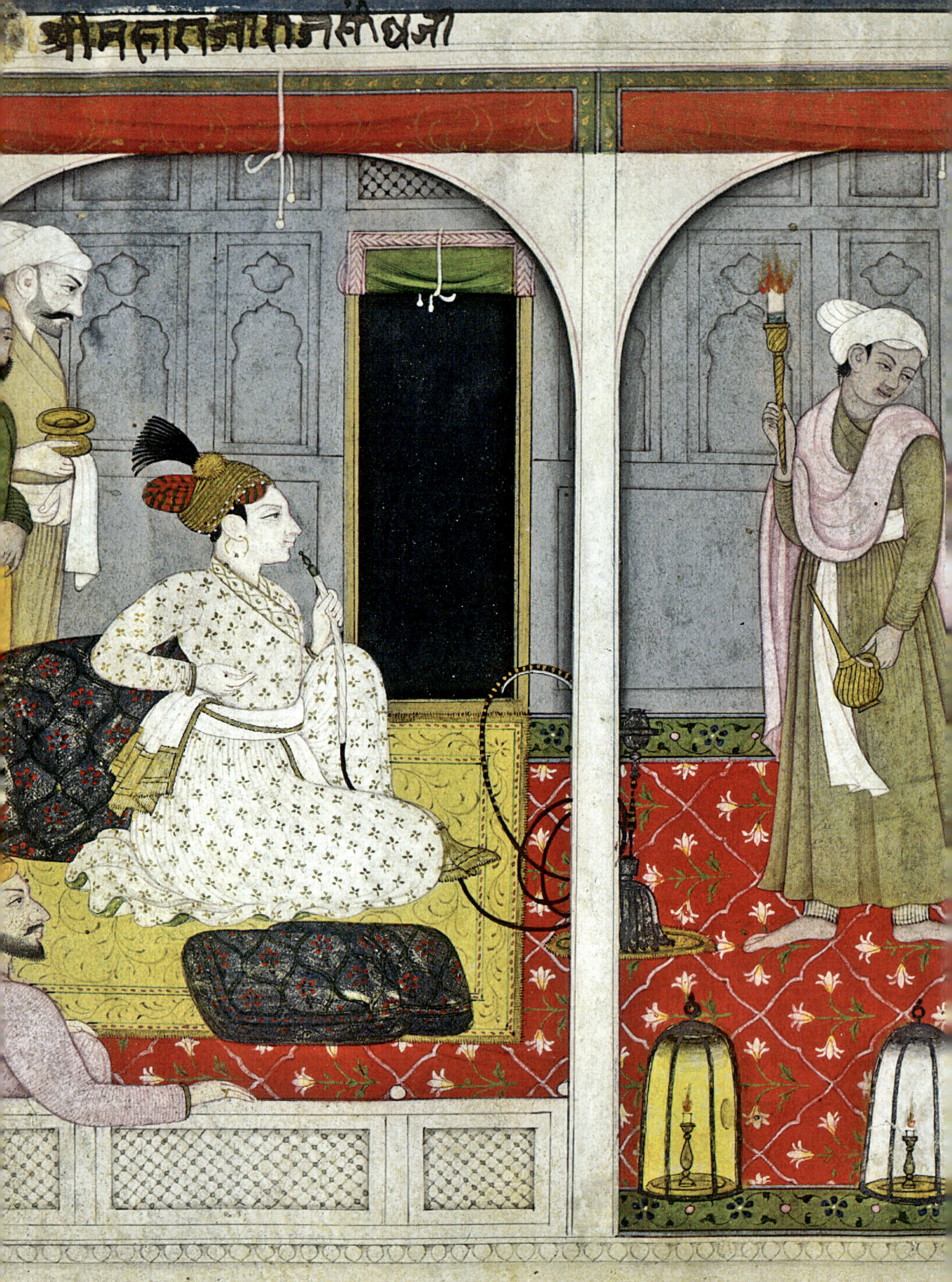

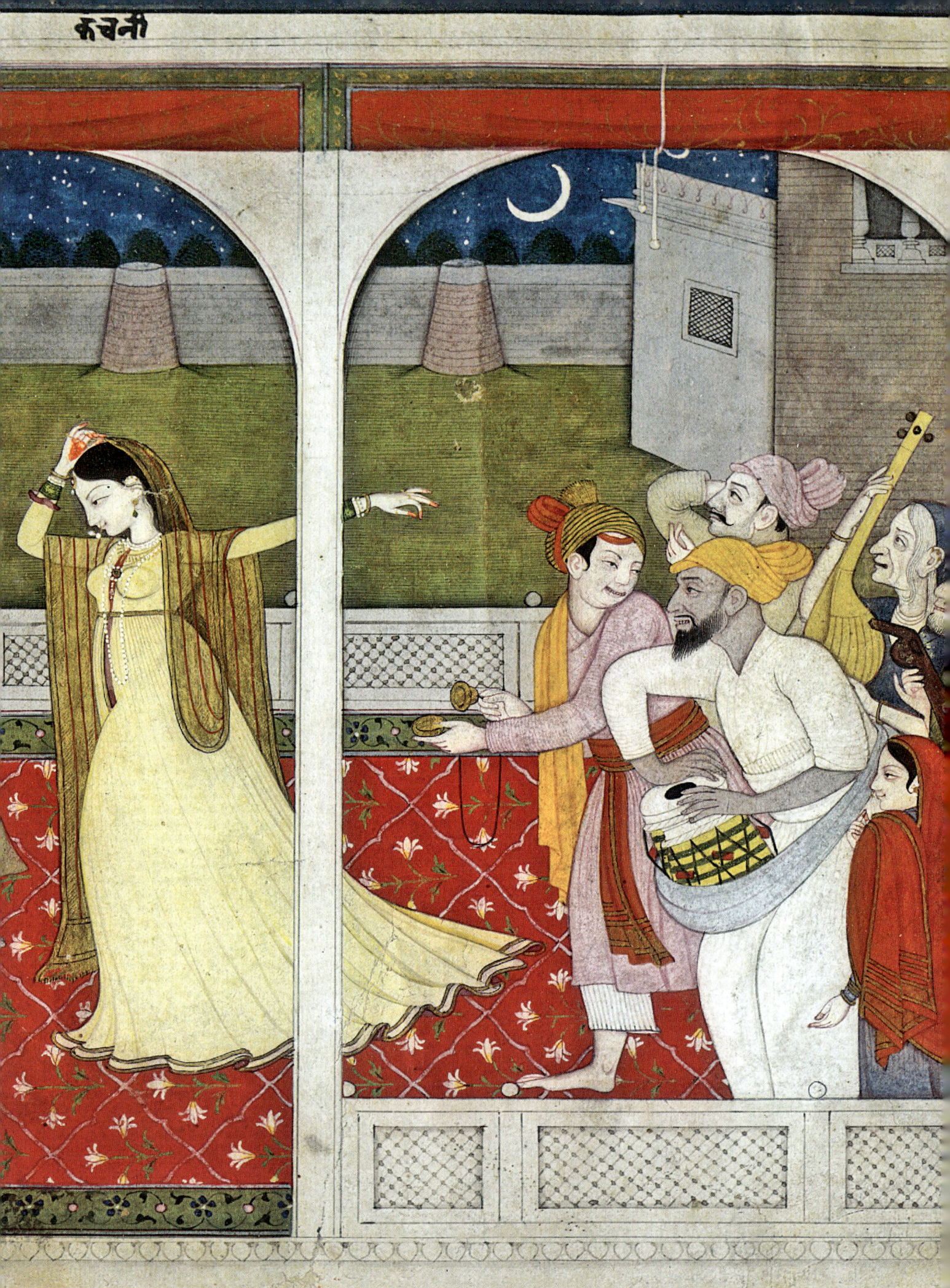

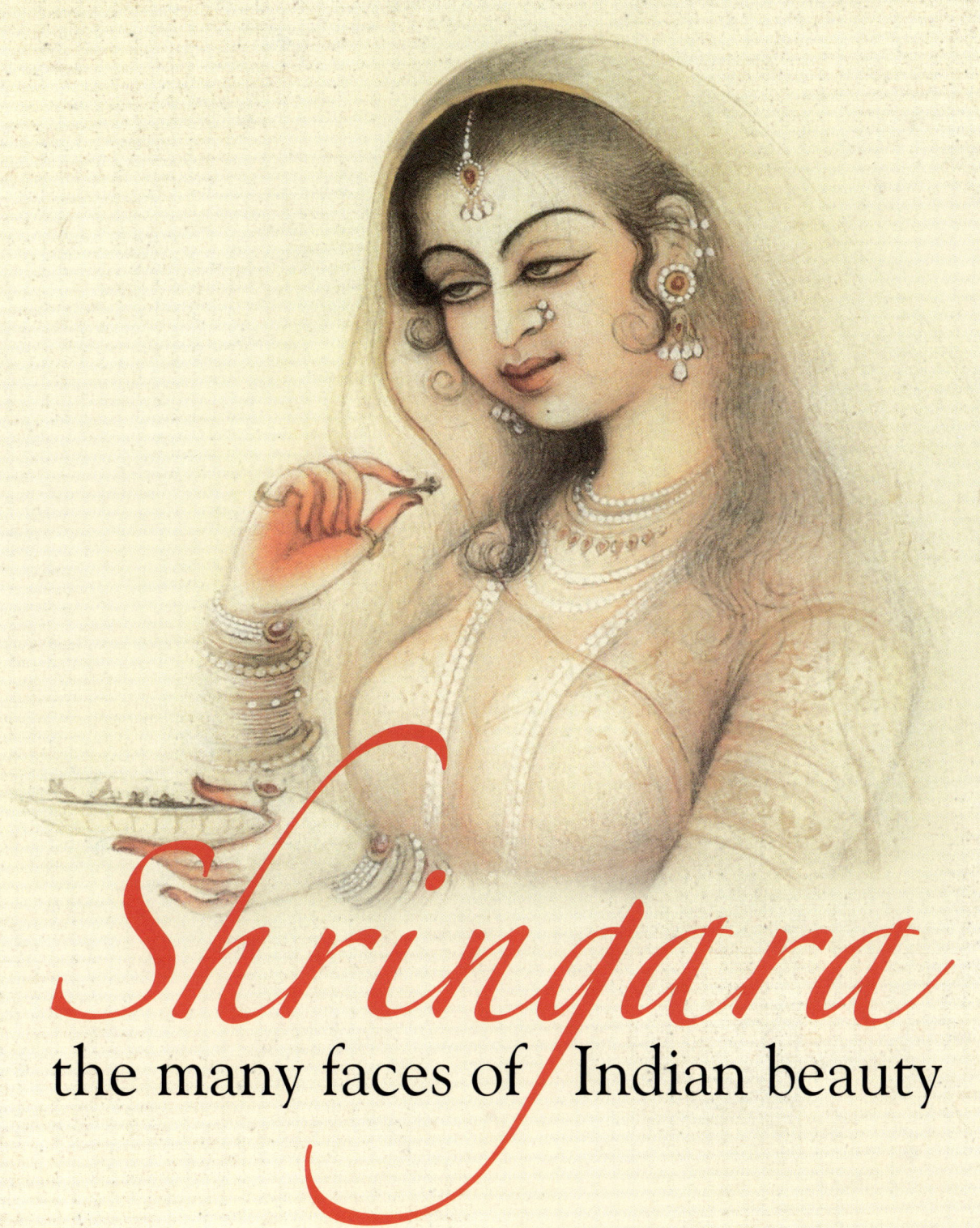

Shringara

the many faces of Indian beauty

Alka Pande

Rupa & Co

Copyright © Alka Pande 2011

Published in 2011 by
Rupa Publications India Pvt Ltd.
7/16, Ansari Road, Daryaganj,
New Delhi 110 002

Sales Centres:
Allahabad Bengaluru Chennai
Hyderabad Jaipur Kathmandu Kolkata
Mumbai

All rights reserved.
No part of this publication may be reproduced,
stored in a retrieval system, or transmitted,
in any form or by any means, electronic,
mechanical, photocopying, recording or otherwise,
without the prior permission of the publishers.

The author asserts the moral right to be
identified as the author of this work.

Cover and book design: Peali Dutta Gupta
E-mail: *pealiduttagupta@pealidezine.com*

Printed in India by Lustra Print Process
B-249, Naraina Industrial Area, Phase-I, New Delhi-110 028.

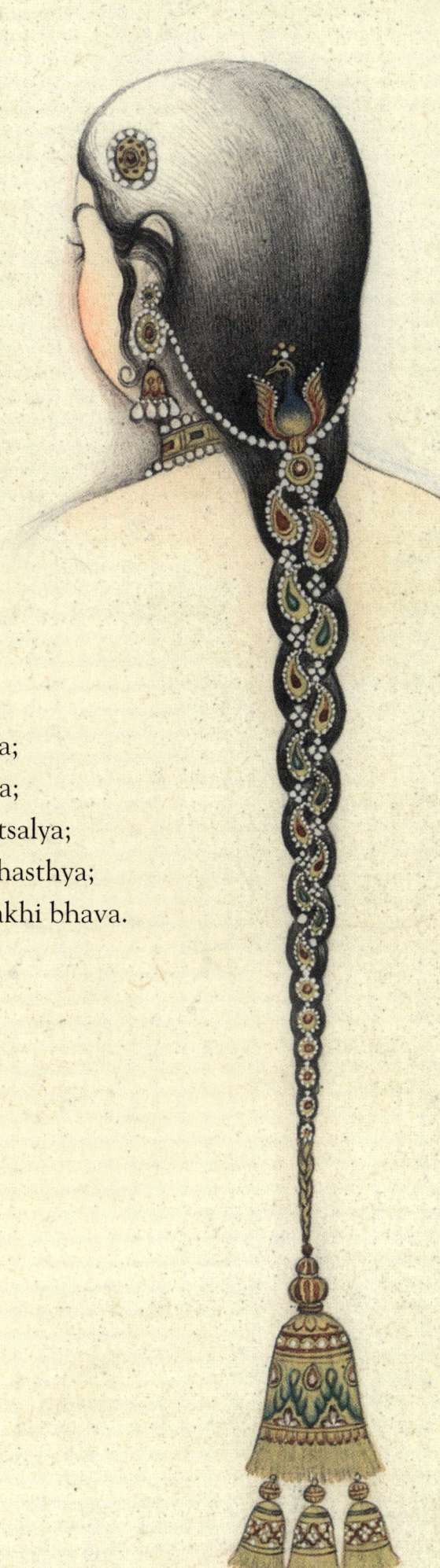

Dedication

To my mother who taught me beauty through svara;
To my father who taught me beauty through karma;
To my daughter who taught me beauty through vatsalya;
To my husband who taught me beauty through grihasthya;
To all my friends who taught me beauty through sakhi bhava.

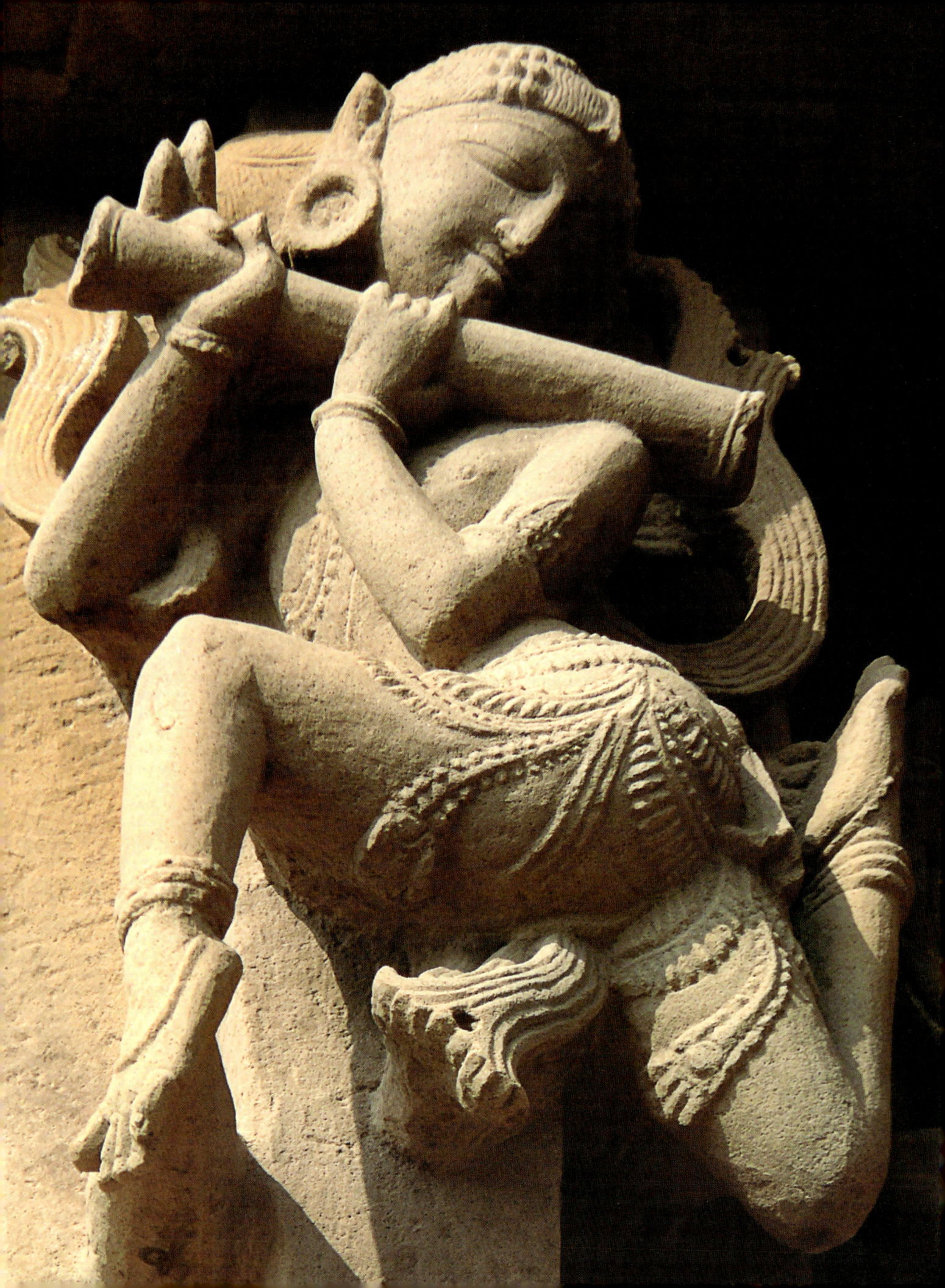

Contents

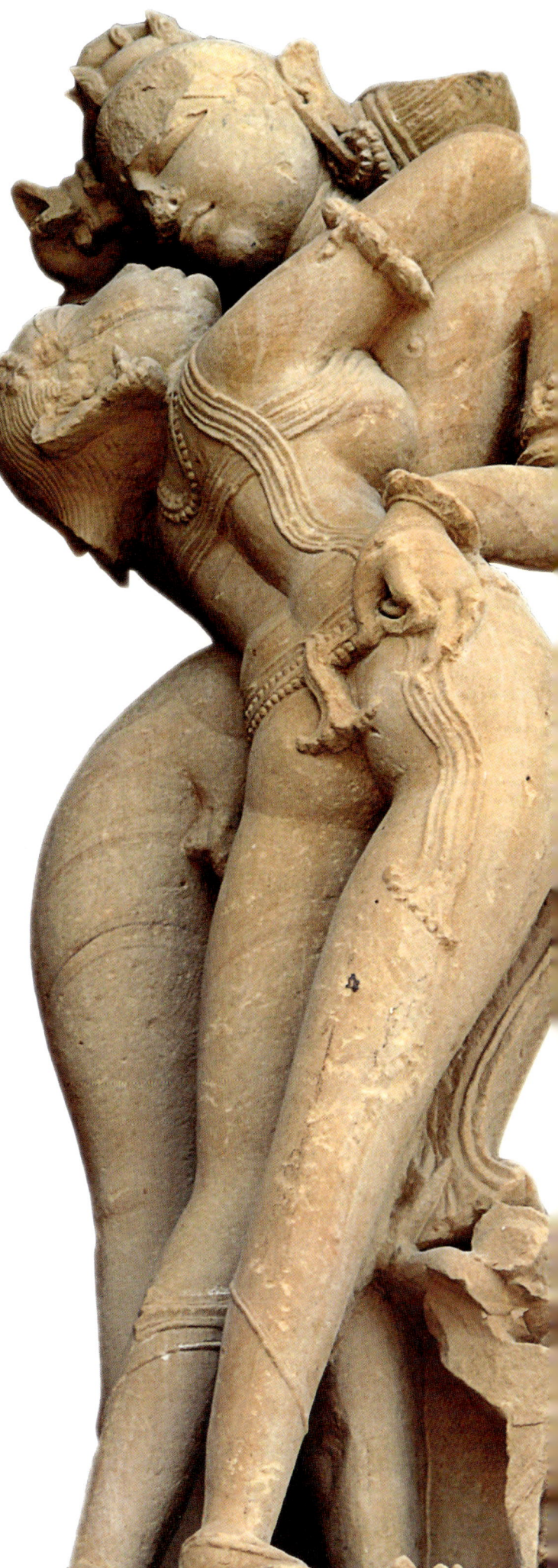

Acknowledgements	XI
Introduction	XIII
Natyashastra—the beginnings	3
Navarasa—the embodiment of flavour	19
Shringara—the *rasaraja*, king of *rasas*	29
Kama—the erotic	45
Kavya—beauty in verse	61
Chitra—lines of pleasure	83
Shilpa Shastra—adornment in stone	101
Sangeet—food for the soul	119
Nritya—joy in rhythm	135
Solah Shringara—adorning the body	149
Shringara—in living culture	163
Shringara—from the ancient to the modern	173
Glossary	182
Bibliography	183
Photo Credits	192
Index	193

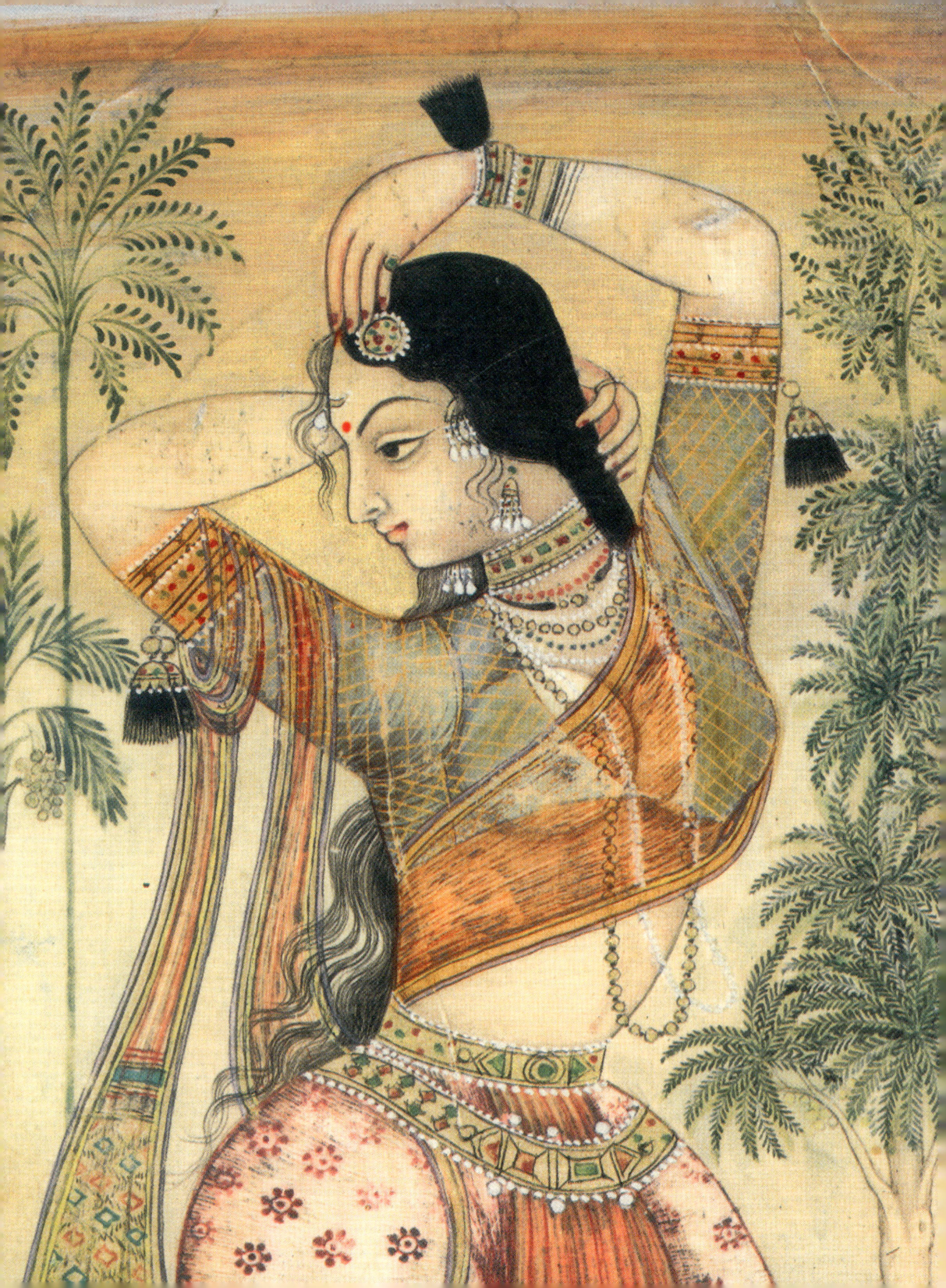

Acknowledgements

Shringara is about the aesthetics of beauty on the one hand and on the other, it is an ode to the beauty of my life and experiences with my friends and family. I may not be able to mention each one of them, but everyone I have met in the last six years—be they at the Habitat Centre where I work, or the Habitat gym where I work out with my set of many beautiful friends, my taichi group of friends, or colleagues I have met during my travels—I owe a debt of gratitude. Equally, to my publisher Shri R.K. Mehra, who started me on this journey by inviting me to do this book on beauty. It requires vision and love for aesthetics to commission a book of this nature in present times.

There have been a number of people who have walked the length of this journey of enriching the book with me in many ways. Peali Dutta Gupta, the designer, has worked on the book with utmost sensitivity and devotion. My sister Jyoti, who helped me through many difficult moments with her clear vision; my sisters Tripti and Dipti for simply being who they are.

Pramod K.G., Mita Kapur, and Sheema Mukherjee, who stepped in and gave me the wind beneath my sails.

To my friend Sanjoy Roy, who taught me the beauty of meeting the challenges at work; to Katherine Virgils and Melissa Apt, who sent me snippets of beauty through emails; to Rashmi Shanker, who I met after three decades and who helped me experience beauty at the Arboretum near Oxford.

This book has seen a lot of editorial help from Sonal Parmar in the initial stages, and later from Asha Spaak. However, the book has seen many changes since then.

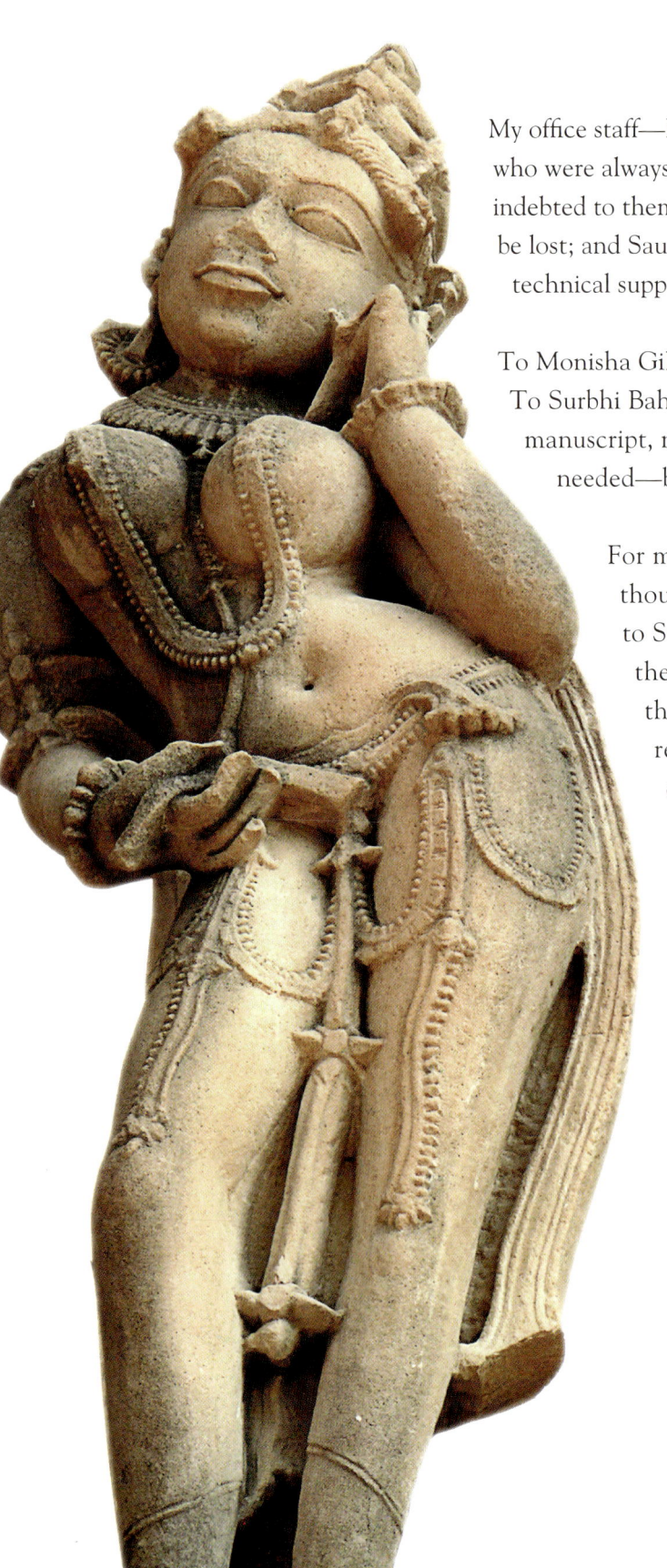

My office staff—Krishna Kapur, Suprabha Nayak and Shweta Sawant—who were always ready to help out in whatever way I wanted. I am deeply indebted to them for their help. Kushal Singh, without whom I would be lost; and Saurabh Rai, who stepped in and gave me huge amounts of technical support.

To Monisha Gill, who removed many a foggy thought during the period. To Surbhi Bahl, who worked quietly on the many changes I made in my manuscript, never complaining and always chipping in with the help I needed—both with research or verification of information.

For my friend Rukmini Sekhar, who with her wisdom and thoughtfulness provided many relaxed moments and cheer; to Sonal Mansingh and Rama Vaidyanathan, who shared their images so generously to be used in the book; to all the contemporary artists featured in the book, who so readily sent me the relevant photo support. The book could not have become such a visual delight without their generous support.

To the Rupa team led by Kapish Mehra, Stuti Sharma, Nandita Bhardwaj and Vijay Sharma. And of course, to the memory of Mulk Raj Anand, who too was looking at the beauty of Indian miniatures.

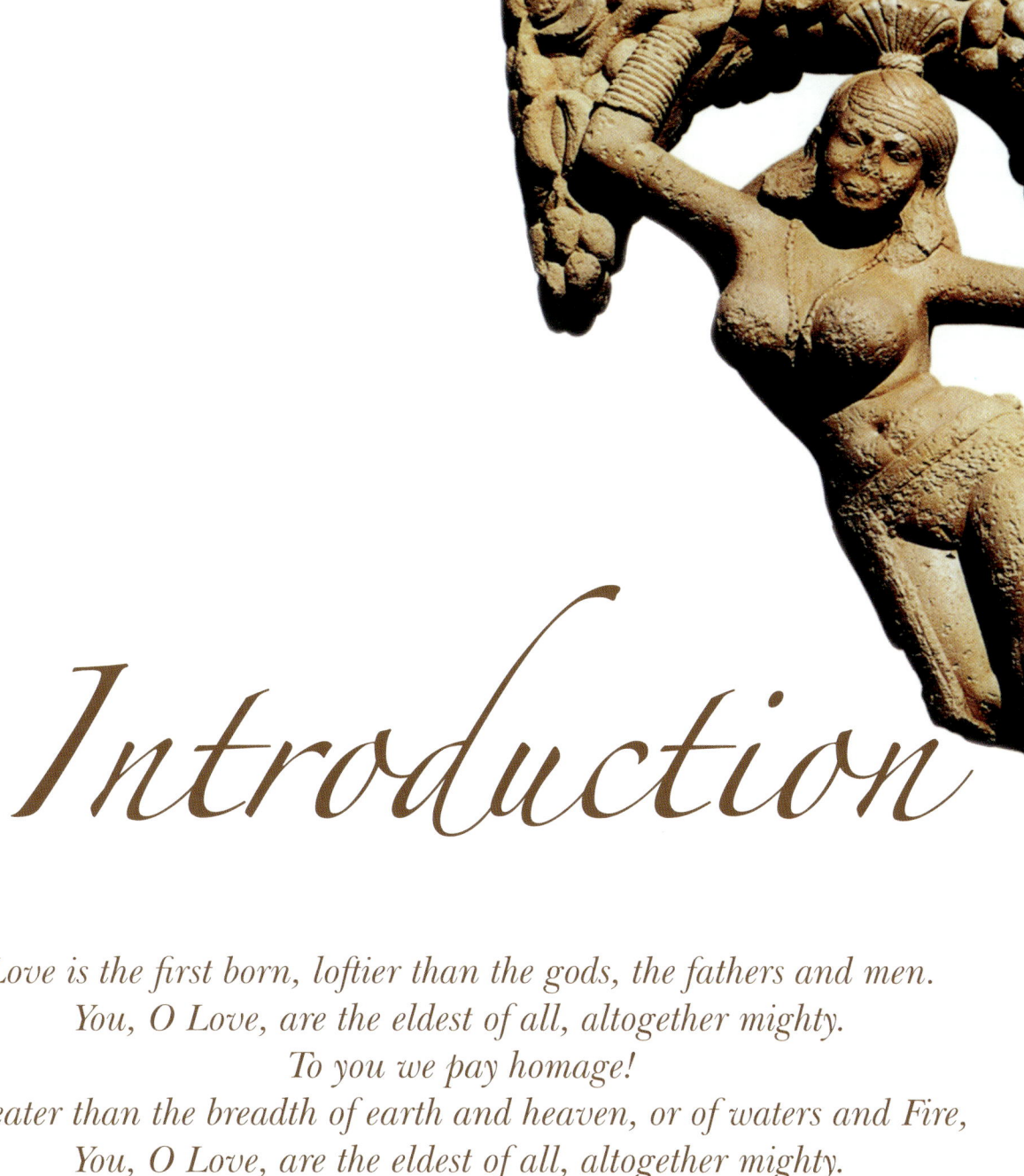

Introduction

Love is the first born, loftier than the gods, the fathers and men.
You, O Love, are the eldest of all, altogether mighty.
To you we pay homage!
Greater than the breadth of earth and heaven, or of waters and Fire,
You, O Love, are the eldest of all, altogether mighty.
To you we pay homage!
In many a form of goodness, O Love, you show your face.
Grant that these forms may penetrate within our hearts.
Send elsewhere all malice!

Atharva Veda

(Page X)
In Rajasthani miniature paintings, the costume and attire of the heroine is always given an added flourish. The wearing of 'sindhoor' is expressed in all its sensuality

(Page XII)
A female figure, Chitragupta Temple, Khajuraho

(Page XIII)
A sensuous yakshi, Great Stupa, Sanchi. Yakshis symbolize fertility and vegetation

(Page XV)
The contemporary painter Sidharth adorns and embellishes the two paintings from the Lotus Series with gilded gold

(Below)
Bronze statuette of The Dancing Girl, Mohenjodaro

As an art historian, I am often asked to define beauty in a word, phrase, or even as a concept. I see beauty essentially as a value connected to the perception of different affirmative aspects of human emotionality. When we perceive something that is in harmony with nature and generates feelings of joy, fulfilment and pleasure within us, we describe it as being beautiful.

The concept of beauty and aesthetics are both part of the European tradition. The closest parallels in the Indian lexicon are *shringara* and *saundarya*. Their ambit lies in the untranslatable—the slippage that occurs when shringara is translated into beauty. In fact this book belongs more to the domain of that slippage, the spaces between the concepts of beauty, shringara and its further dimension, saundarya.

Many-layered Meanings

Beauty, in its quintessential sense, is innate rather than created. It is to be discovered, rather than ornamented, and possessed rather than sculpted. Its appeal is different when seen through the eyes of the *samajika* (lay person) and the *rasikam* (trained aesthete). The lay person derives a visual delight, while the aesthete moves beyond the sensual beauty of the subject to an inner, subjective and private perception, rendering the concept more philosophical. Saundarya is this half-received and half-perceived phenomenon. Through the dual realms of shringara and saundarya, I discovered that the concepts and traditions of Indian aesthetics and beauty were like an onion: for every layer peeled, another notion waited to be unfolded, and yet another lay beneath.

The notions of Indian beauty have been drawn from *Saundarya Shastra*, a compendium of the ideas of philosophers, poets, aestheticians, dancers, musicians, religious texts, secular texts and the Puranas. At the base of the pyramid is *Natyashastra* in which is embodied the first written canvas of the performance and appreciation of beauty or the *shringara rasa*, also known as the *rasaraja* or the king of all *rasas*.

The notion of beauty defies any attempt at limited and compartmentalized generalization. All over the world, at different times in human history, the idea of beauty has meant different things to different people, whether it be in terms of aesthetic experience, concepts of divinity, perceptions of nature or physical form.

Beyond Definition

The concept of 'beauty' has never been an absolute and it will never be—for there are so many manifestations, so many ways of perceiving it, so many definitions, so many notions. The most immediate is physical beauty—the outer image that pleases in its very appearance and is easy to behold since it boasts perfect proportions. The human form provided the most universal inspiration for the depiction of perfect physical beauty. The Greek poets idolized it, painters painted it, sculptors sculpted it, philosophers pondered over it, and the bards sang of it. In the Indian context, physical beauty was always linked to nature. For instance, a maiden with beautiful eyes was referred to as *kamal nayan* (lotus-eyed) and flowing black hair was compared to dark monsoon clouds.

Experiencing beauty involves extending its landscape to include the performing arts, the senses, the fragrances, and the ambience that the viewer experiences and derives joy from.

Ways of Perceiving Beauty

There are myriad ways in which one can experience and appreciate beauty:

Beauty through participation is of the highest order, since this is beauty beyond utility. The creation and celebration of beauty through objects of beauty is an integral part of the Indian psyche. Whether it is adornment of the body or the dwelling, or making beautiful objects of daily use—there is a vibrant connection between the maker, the object itself and the users of these objects. From the Indian point of view, the very act of creating something new, integrating the beautiful in daily living, is an evocation of Vishvakarma, the Divine Architect.

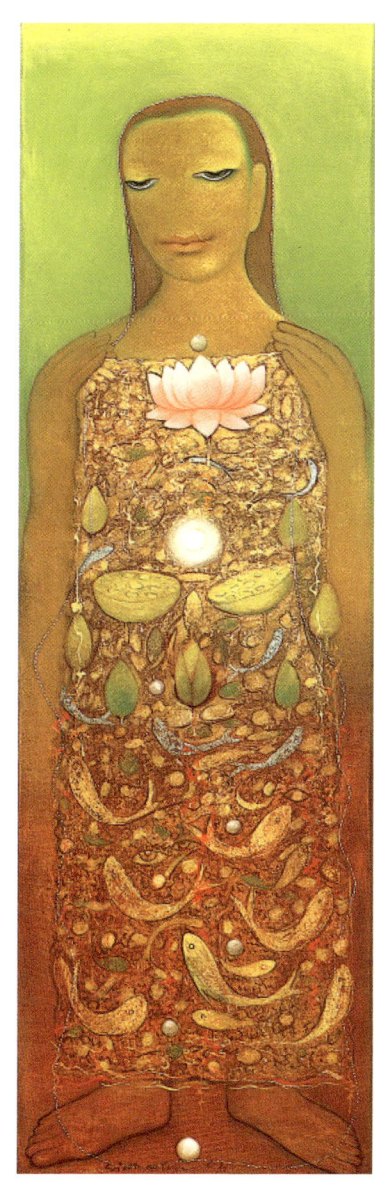

Beauty through ritual establishes a correspondence between the microcosm and the macrocosm, between the world of humans and that of the gods, between chaos and order.

Beauty through narrative is where the narrator and the listener are bound together within

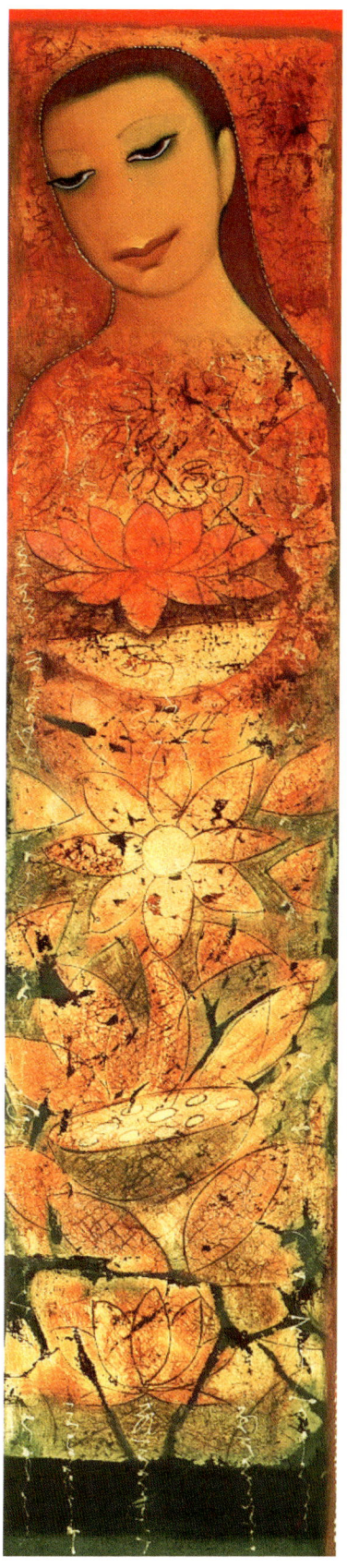

Introduction XV

the magic of the story that unfolds through the *geet* and the *patua* (the song and the scroll) till it becomes a living theatre. The beauty in this instance is intertwined with the story itself, whether it is from the epics or the Puranas, folk legends, or the deeds of local heroes—in what becomes the multi-sensory epistemology of a narrative communicated at many levels simultaneously.

Beauty through shringara, or adornment, operates at more than one level. In Indian literature the sixteen traditional adornments of a woman do not merely enhance her beauty—they are also an *arpana* (offering) for her beloved. This is an important part of shringara rasa.

The performing arts are an important vehicle of beauty. Classical and popular music and dance, folk, religious and festive songs, are all part of this experience. The human voice is the most ancient of musical instruments and the human body the most primal repository of beautiful forms. Together they convey an idea, narrate a story or communicate our deepest longings.

The non-verbal attributes of beauty are created through sensuality without language, form or structure. Music, dance, *ranga* (colour), *rachna* (texture), and arrangement can convey a whole gamut of emotions, create myriad sensations, and indicate harmony and order. While classical forms incorporate non-verbal features of beauty, it is in the folk arts, where the non-verbal element operates innately and intuitively.

An appreciation of beauty through the classical arts requires a strict adherence to the canons of art and aesthetics. These include rasa (emotive juice), *rupa* (form), *vastu* (architecture), *tala* (rhythm) and *nada* (sound). The true perception of the classical arts can only be obtained through *pratyaksha* (contemplative perception) and *anumana* (thoughtful inference). The trained aesthete not only avails himself of a variety of *sakshatartha* (surface meanings) that come from the first sensual contact with the art object, but more importantly, those that call upon his intellectual resources to find the *parokshartha* (suggested and hidden meanings) contained in the art object. In fact, *artha* (semantics) is the bedrock of the contemplative aspect of the classical arts and it is this that makes the aesthetic experience spiritual or idealistic.

Aesthetic beauty and philosophical beauty are not mutually exclusive as they represent two poles on a continuum. In the

Uma-Maheshwara, Pala sculpture, National Museum, New Delhi. The work depicts the slender body form of the Pala period sculpture

first sense, beauty is associated with lightness and balanced order; it has a decorative quality to it. In the second sense, it is the much darker form of beauty, one that is associated with profundity and truth. This is the sublime, occidental concept of beauty.

Western Theories on Beauty

In the West, beauty has, traditionally, been the defining parameter of an aesthetic experience, although voices such as those of Plato and John Ruskin argued for a social and/or moral purpose in the art experience. The early understanding of beauty in the West was linked to the various arts that conveyed it: in sacred music beauty was expressed by the harmony of the cosmos, in poetry by that enchantment that makes men rejoice, in sculpture by the appropriate measure and symmetry of the parts, and in rhetoric by the right rhythm.

Untitled, 16" x 16", medium acrylic on canvas, painting by Viren Tanwar

Plato, Immanuel Kant and Hegel spoke of beauty in terms of the sublime and the blissful. The beautiful object is an object that, by virtue of its form, delights the senses. But aspects that are perceivable by the senses are not the only features that express the beauty of that object. There are others, too, like the soul and the personality that are perceived by the mind's eye rather than the eye of the body.

The complex Greek value of beauty is best expressed in Plato's *Symposium*:

> *But what if man has eyes to see the true beauty – the divine beauty, I mean, pure and clear and unalloyed, not clogged with the pollutions of morality and all the colours and vanities of human life – thither looking, and holding converse with the true beauty simple and divine? Remember how in that communion, only beholding beauty with the eye of the mind, he will be enabled to bring forth, not images of beauty, but realities (for he has hold not of an image but of a reality), and bringing forth and nourishing true virtue to become the friend of God and be immortal, if mortal may. Would that be an ignoble life?*
>
> —***The Glance,** Plato*

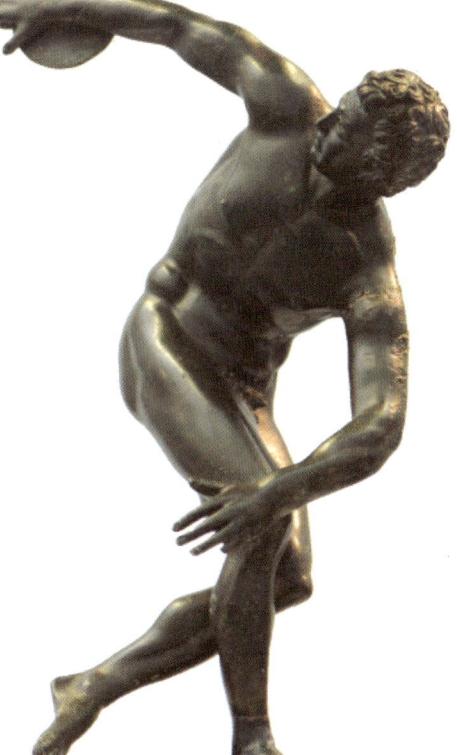

Roman bronze reduction of Myron's Discobolus, 2nd century AD. A beautiful depiction of rhythm, harmony and balance

The ancient Greeks had an early understanding of beauty, but it was closely connected to the arts. Beauty was defined as the 'appropriateness' of the object for its function. 'Appropriateness' was then paraphrased as the power to perform its function. However, function may not always have been productive of good; so was the power to produce evil also 'beauty'? No, beauty was always generative of good; beauty was goodness.

Socrates identified at least three aesthetic categories: Ideal beauty, Spiritual beauty, and Functional beauty. Plato's position was a more complex one. He identified beauty as harmony and proportion between the parts, and beauty as splendour. In Plato's viewpoint, beauty could exist independently from the physical medium that expressed it. It was not bound to any material object, it rather shined brightly on its own. Plato believed that the body was a 'dark cavern' within which the soul was trapped. And so, not everyone was able to grasp true beauty. Art was a fake impression of true beauty and could corrupt pure minds.

Aristotle had an influential school of aesthetic thought that strongly believed *mimesis* or imitation to be the greatest end for all art. There has, ever since, been extensive debate over what constitutes 'imitation' and, although no definite conclusion to the debate was ever reached, by the mid-eighteenth century the concept of *imitatio naturae* (imitating nature) had firmly ensconced itself as the dominant model of the aesthetic ideal.

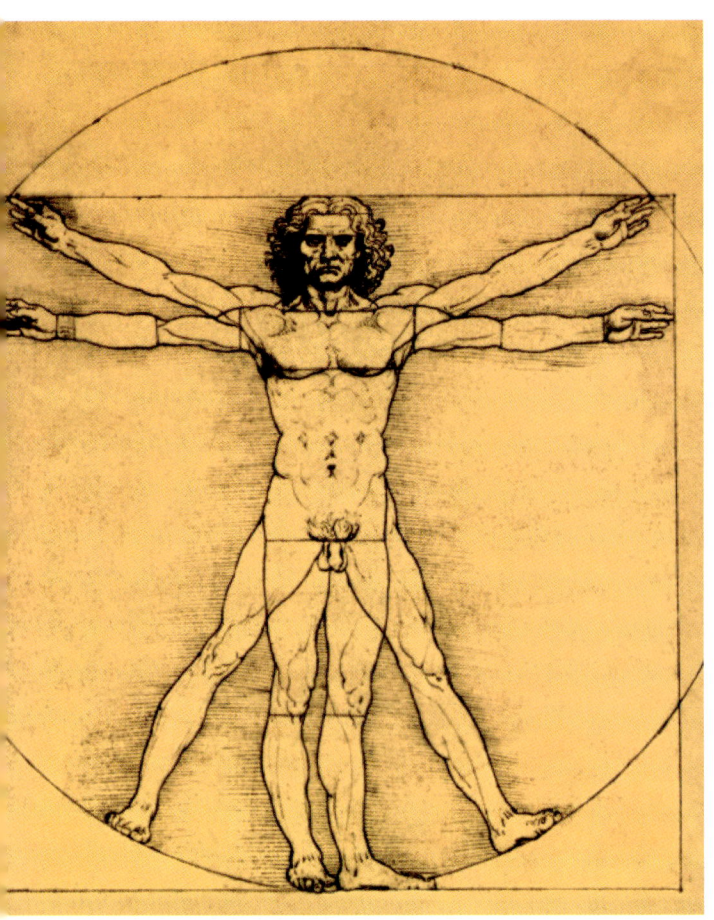

The Vitruvian Man by Leonardo da Vinci. Geometry and nature reconciled

French philosopher Rousseau believed that beauty was an expression or manifestation of nature. Most pre-Romantic aestheticians were agreed upon the fact that the highest form of beauty was natural beauty and the highest form of art its imitation.

I have always believed that good is none other than Beauty in Action, that the one is inextricably bound up with the other and that both have a common source in well ordered nature. From this idea, it follows that taste is perfected with the same means as wisdom and that a soul open to the seduction of the virtues must be sensible in like measure to all the other kinds of beauty.
—**Julie or the New Heloise, Jean Jacques Rousseau**

George Wilhelm Friedrich Hegel's approach to natural beauty was significant in its departure from the history of aesthetic theory. Hegel spoke of beauty as the 'ideal', the idea in its spirituality and universality given determinate form. He also believed that beauty is inseparable from truth and goodness. But the 'ideal' as beauty requires a sensual appearance, whereas the 'ideal' as truth is realized in thought.

According to David Hume, critics could only judge the standards of aesthetics if they could rid themselves of the external customs and prejudices that influenced their judgement. These should instead be based on internal qualities like good sense and freedom from bias as well as method, refinement and experience.

The influential German thinker, Immanuel Kant, interpreted beauty in terms of form, structure, balance and an incredibly detailed sense of proportion. He maintained that any work of art must approximate to some aspect or product of nature to fulfil the criteria of beauty. However, he saw sublimity in its unlimited magnificence and power that came within the realm of the beautiful rather than of the Divine. Kant believed that beauty cannot be judged by the unrefined or the uncultured; it can only be recognized and judged by the trained and educated eye of the critic or aesthetician.

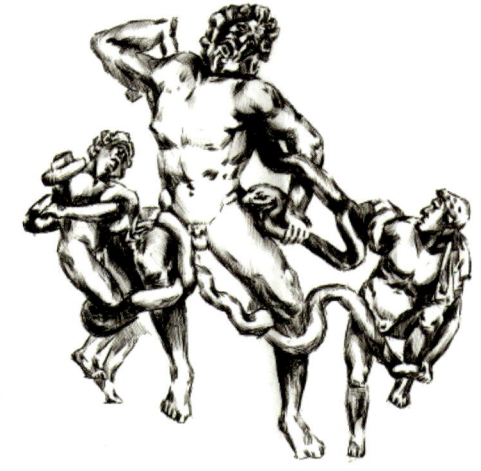

Ancient Roman sculpture of Laocoon and his sons

Saundarya—The Indian Approach

In the Indian tradition, there is no opposition between beauty and social responsibility, between aesthetics and ethics. Examination of any one form of art—say narrative art—shows the goals of all art spanning final liberation or *moksha* (personal ethics) to the establishment of *lokasangraha* (public ethics). Saundarya is not the overriding parameter of Indian art; nor is it its *atma* or defining property. Saundarya is, however, the property that enables art to fulfil its *prayojana* (goal). Further, its nature is to be understood not only from theoretical discussions but also from the practice of verbal art; not only by poets but also philosophers (like Adi Shankara's text *Saundaryalahari*).

Earlier Athenian painting on a pot depicting Dionysus

In literary theory, the formal discussion of art begins with Bharata who wrote *Natyashastra* in the 5th century BC. According to him beauty is both, the seen and experienced element of shringara rasa. It is significant to note that the words saundarya/*sundara* appear for the first time in the 8th-9th century AD in Vamana's *Kavyalamkarasutra*, where he states that *alamkara* (to adorn), is essentially saundarya (beauty).

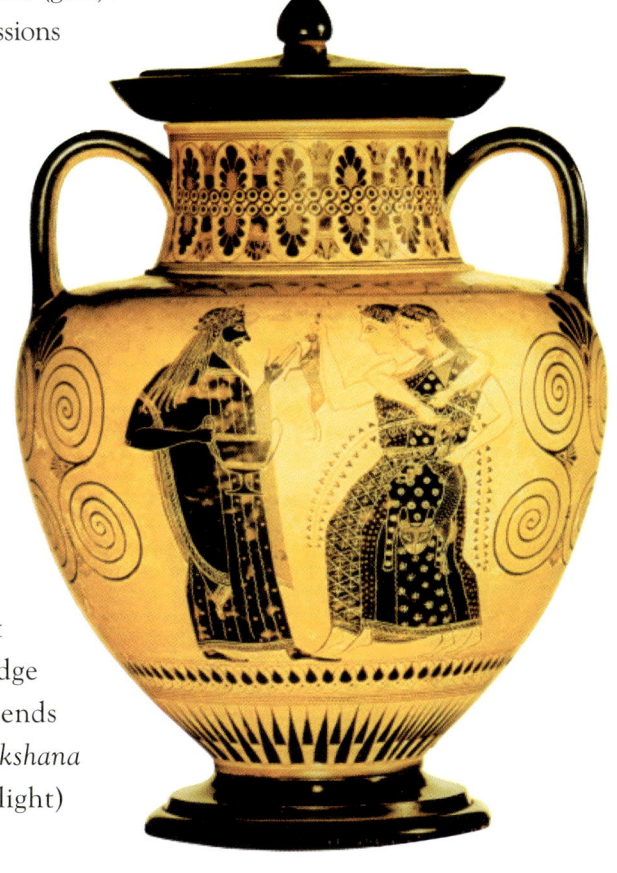

From Bharata to the highly-stylized Sanskrit verse of the Kashmiri poet Rudrata (9th century), it is clear that verbal art is closely related to the life of the people. As oral literature that is aural and visual in character, it is able to disseminate knowledge widely and this knowledge promotes the attainment of the four ends of life. Vamana addresses this question when he says that the *lakshana* (dominant characteristic) of verbal art is the *priti* or *ananda* (delight) that the audience experiences.

Almost four centuries later Abhinavagupta, the 12th century Kashmiri philosopher, says in his *Lochana* that of all the purposes served by *kavya* (literature) ananda is mainly for the spectator. If priti is not recognized as a characteristic of kavya, there is no difference between literature and other rational discourses.

Thus the primary purpose of kavya has to be *ananda sadhana*, a structuring of delight that, according to Abhinavagupta, is the ultimate end of all human effort. Abhinavagupta reserves the term saundarya for crafting the discourse—only when it is well crafted does it bring delight, generating new knowledge or awareness in the viewer. Beauty or saundarya is merely instrumental in the fulfilment of the primary goal of verbal art, it is not the end.

Satyam, Shivam, Sundaram

In kavya, sundar refers mainly to sensual or material beauty without any suggestion of the metaphysical, moral, ethical or spiritual. Morality and spirituality are subsumed in the concept of *dharma*. The concept of *Satyam, Shivam, Sundaram* (truth, god, beauty) was a much later addition in the Indian tradition. *Bhakti*, or devotional literature, does relate the concept of Sundaram to Shivam because, for the devout, beauty can only lie in Ishvara or God. The rasa doctrine, too, places rasa on the same level as *Brahmananda*, the Godhead, thus merging beauty with *sat* (truth). John Keat's union of Truth, Goodness and Beauty strangely coincides with this Sanskrit parlance.

Interestingly, in traditional Sanskrit usage, the word sundar is never used in a metaphorical sense. Essentially secular, the word is one of several that denote sensual beauty—*satchitananda*, truth is beautiful. In his essay titled 'The Hindu View of Art' from the book *Dance of Siva: Fourteen Indian Essays*, Ananda Coomaraswamy observes:

> *Delightful or disgusting, exalted or lowly, cruel or kindly, obscure or refined, actual or imaginary, there is no subject that cannot evoke rasa (sentiment) in man.*

Sahitya Darpana is a comprehensive text on all aspects of poetics including dramaturgy, ascribed to Kaviraj Vishwanath, the 14th century literary critic who apparently held a ministerial position in the Ganga dynasty in Orissa. Vishwanath observes:

> *Pure aesthetic experience is theirs in whom the knowledge of beauty is innate; it is known intuitively in intellectual ecstasy without accompaniment of ideation, at the*

Paintings by Dhara Mehrotra

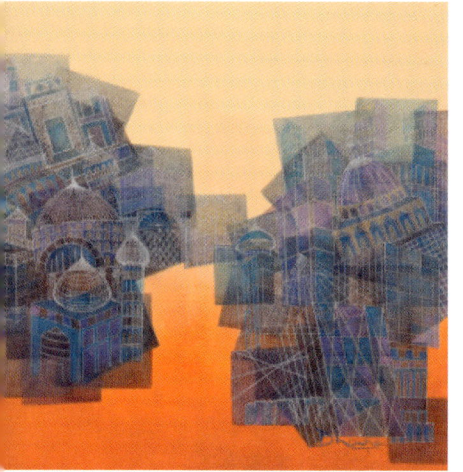

Untitled, acrylic and mixed medium on canvas

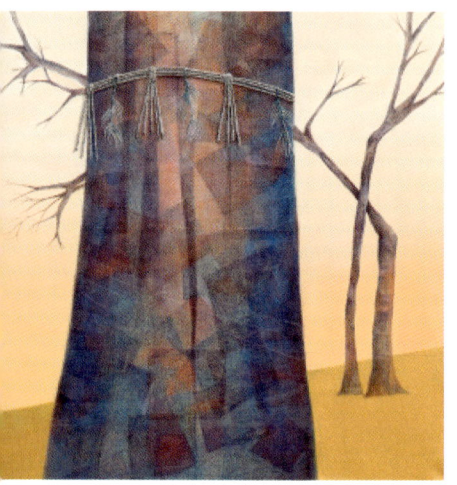

'Sanctified' acrylic and mixed medium on canvas

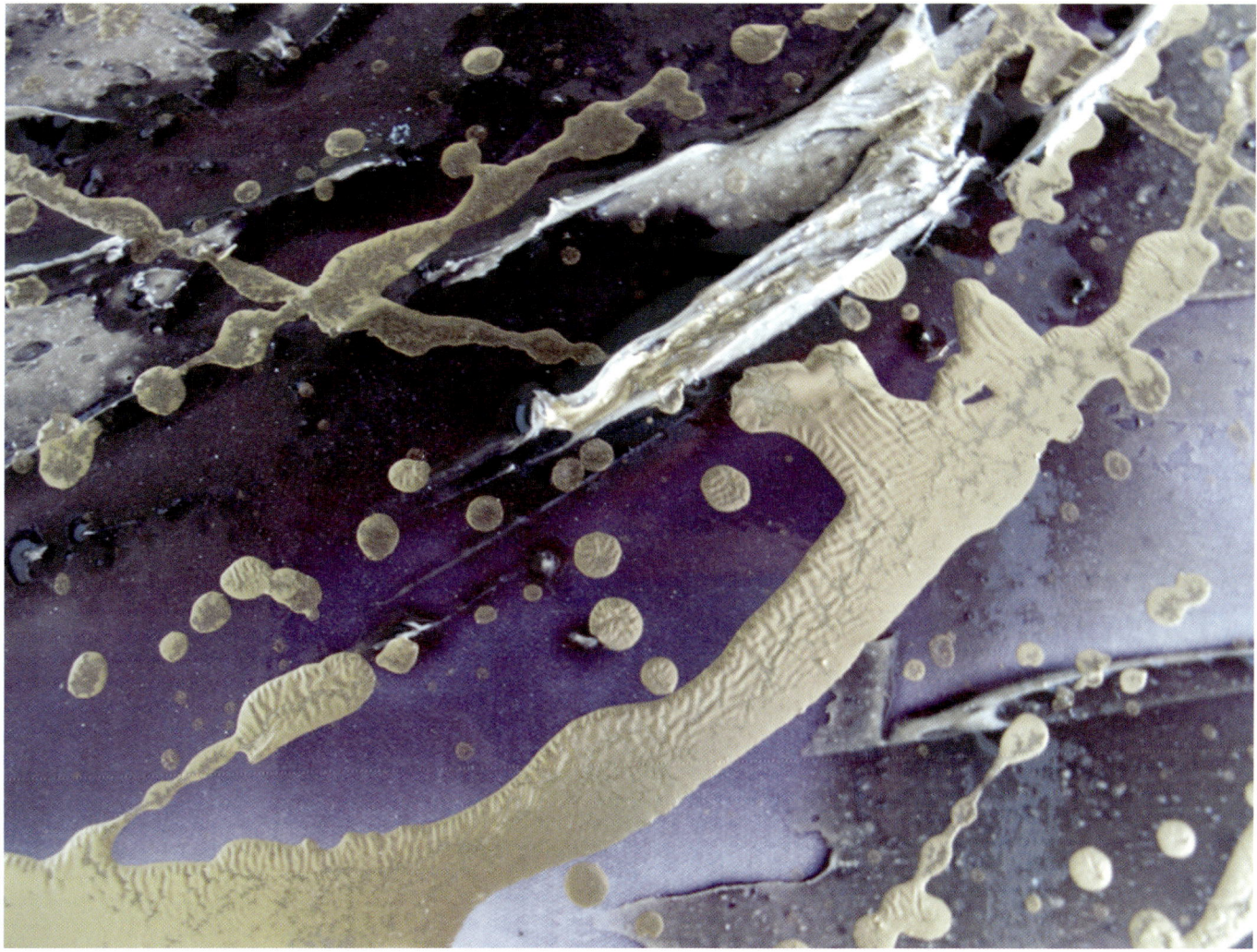

Acrylic on canvas by Shola Carletti

highest level of conscious being. Subjectively, beauty could be defined as that which gives satisfaction to the tushti, mind, *hence where the mind rests and finally merges in the bliss of that satisfaction.*

According to Kashmiri Shaivism, which has provided the most developed philosophy of aesthetics in Indian thought, beauty is inseparable from bliss, and bliss is not just a subjective feeling; it is the very *anandashakti*, or power of bliss of the Lord. If beauty is indeed an aspect of the anandashakti of Shiva, Abhinavagupta maintains that it belongs to the highest level of the *shaktis*. Indian scriptures define five shaktis: *chitta* (consciousness); ananda (bliss); *ichchha* (will or desire); *jnana* (knowledge); and *kriya* (activity). The first two are inseparable from Shiva—they do not belong in the realm of manifestation but of transcendence.

One must then conclude that beauty in the West has notions of the sublime, of bliss, harmony, geometry and balance. In the Indian tradition, however, notions

Sculpture of Uma-Maheshwara from Khajuraho, National Museum, New Delhi

of beauty are more complex because they have myriad manifestations: beauty as truth, desire, shringara/saundarya or beauty as the aesthetic. The erotic comes into play in the sphere of shringara and two distinct streams emerge out of it. The first is that of physical beauty; adornment, pleasure—where the sensual and the erotic become the principal ingredients of representational beauty. Here it is beauty of form, and the beauty of the ultimate union with atma and *parmatma* through bhakti, leading to ananda (supreme bliss).

The closest interpretation of saundarya is found in aesthetics where spirituality and philosophy become the handmaidens of beauty. Thus the sacred and the profane cross over, unite and finally lead to the purest essence: that of truth as ananda. In other words, while their paths are different, in the philosophies of both the East and the West—with beauty as ananda and beauty as sublime—the end result is the same: beauty is the path to godliness.

Side A   Side B

If one views this idea as a pyramid, the base of the pyramid consists of different notions of beauty – philosophical beauty, representational beauty, physical beauty, beauty that is experienced. The base also contains the sacred and the profane, the erotic and the sensual.

Side A

Side A then deals with the notions of Eastern beauty. In the east, an interpretation of the iconic trends from Bharata, Bhatta, Mamatta Lolatta, Abhinava et al. shows a constant re-interpretation of the treatises where complex notions of beauty range from the physical to the philosophical.

Side B

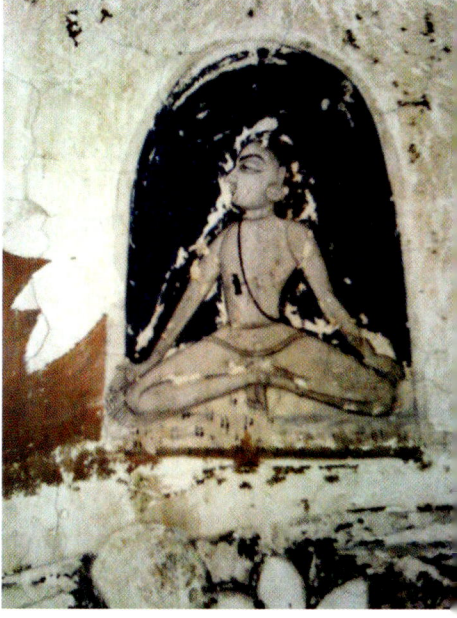

A royal painting from Jodhpur depicting a Nath yogi's greatness and also the 'Absolute'

Manjushri, Pala sculpture, 8th century, Nalanda, National Museum, New Delhi

Side B deals with the Western notions of beauty. The Western aesthetic model starts from the Greek philosophers like Plato, through to the Bible and on to contemporary writers, according to whom beauty becomes more subjective, less interpretative. The top of the pyramid finally leads to universal bliss, the Indian concept of ananda or moksha.

Beauty in Ugliness

Every culture has its own individualized concepts of beauty and ugliness. From antiquity to the Middle Ages, several theories on aesthetics looked at ugliness as the antithesis of beauty, a discordance that breaks the rules of that proportion on which both physical and moral beauty is based. Yet, one common view pervaded all these theories: although ugly creatures and things exist, art has the power to portray them in a beautiful way.

The beauty of the imitation makes ugliness acceptable. For example, medieval man set himself the problem of a beautiful representation of the Devil, a problem that was to resurface in all its intensity in the Romantic period.

According to Bonaventure of Bagnoregio in his 'Commentary on the Book of Sentences' in *The Beauty of the Devil* (1217-74):

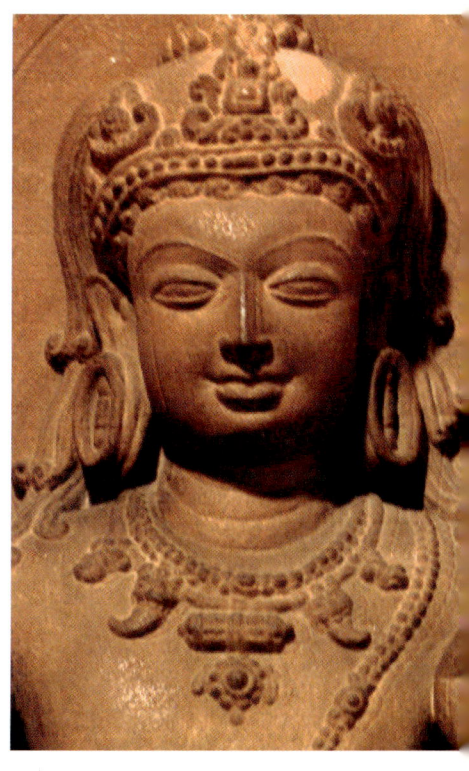

> *Two modes of Beauty may be found in the image, although it is obvious that there is only one subject of the image. For it is clear that the image is called beautiful when it is well painted and it is also called beautiful when it is a good representation of the person whose image it is. And that this is another cause of beauty emerges from the fact that one mode of beauty can be present in the absence of the other: which is precisely why we may say that the image of the Devil is beautiful when it well represents the turpitude of the Devil and as a consequence of this aspect it is also repugnant.*

In *The Aesthetics of Ugliness*, published in 1852, Karl Rosenkranz maintains that:

[it is impossible to appreciate beauty without] entering at the same time the inferno of evil, the real inferno, because the ugliest ugliness is not that which disgusts us in nature — swamps, distorted trees, salamanders, and toads, sea monsters that stare at us with goggling eyes, and massive pachyderms, rats and apes — it is the egoism that manifests its folly in perfidious and frivolous deeds in the wrinkled lines of passion, in grim looks and in crime … . It is not hard to understand that since ugliness is a relative concept, it may only be understood in relation to another concept.

This other concept is that of beauty which is its positive premise. If there were no beauty, there would be no ugliness, because the latter exists only as the negation of the former … There is an intimate connection between the beautiful and the ugly, in as much as the self destruction of the former is the basis of the possibility of the latter …

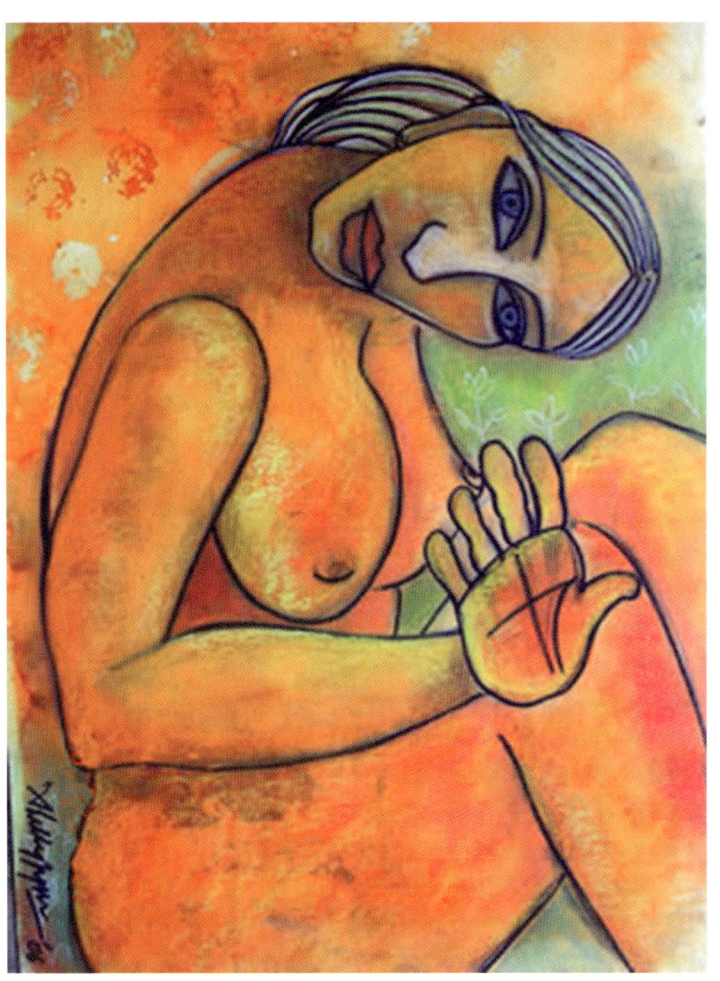

Evite, painting by Shelly Jyoti

(Page XXV) A Bundi painting of Krishna teasing the gopis. A distinct feature of Bundi painting is a lush landscape—well-laid gardens full of mango, peepal and plantain trees

What is the secret of Beauty? Wherein lies its power? The very concept of beauty itself is elusive, as all arguments and interpretations point out. This book attempts to probe the profusion of interpretations through the phenomenology of beauty, through the philosophical discourses on beauty, and finally, through the physical representations and experiences of beauty where even the anti-aesthetic becomes an integral part of beauty.

Within Indian aesthetics, I am convinced, beauty moves beyond the spheres of the more esoteric *Saundarya Shastra*. The defining moments in Indian poetry, painting and sculpture have derived their inspiration from the sensual and beautiful bordering on the aesthetics of the erotic. And erotic in this context is the stimulatory, the exciting soaked in the rasa or sentiment of shringara. This sentiment finds expression in music, poetry, flowers and gardens and all other things associated with love and lovemaking. I am concerned with the expression of the erotic or shringara that underlies much of ancient Indian art, be it music, dance, literature, sculpture, poetry or painting.

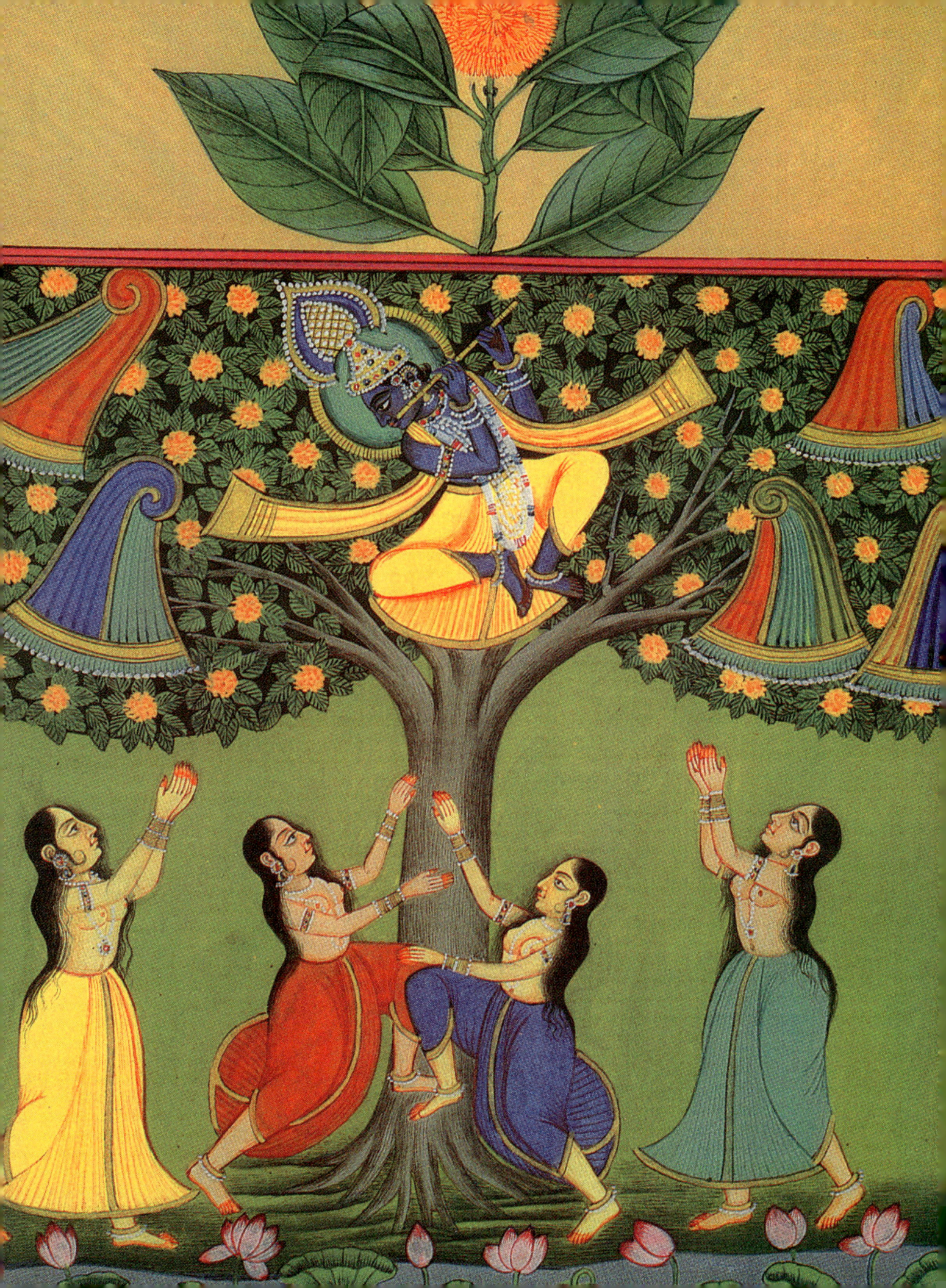

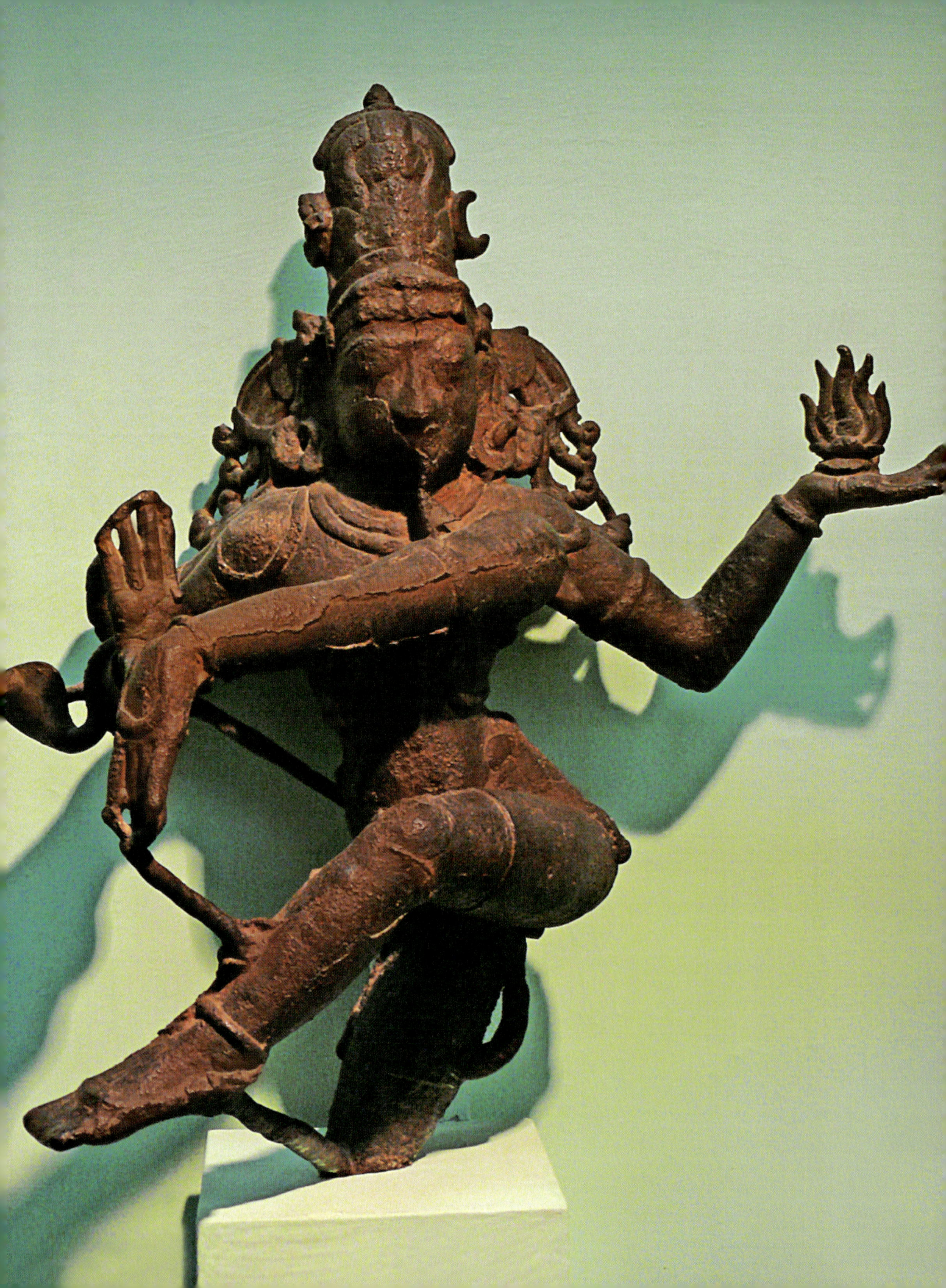

CHAPTER 1

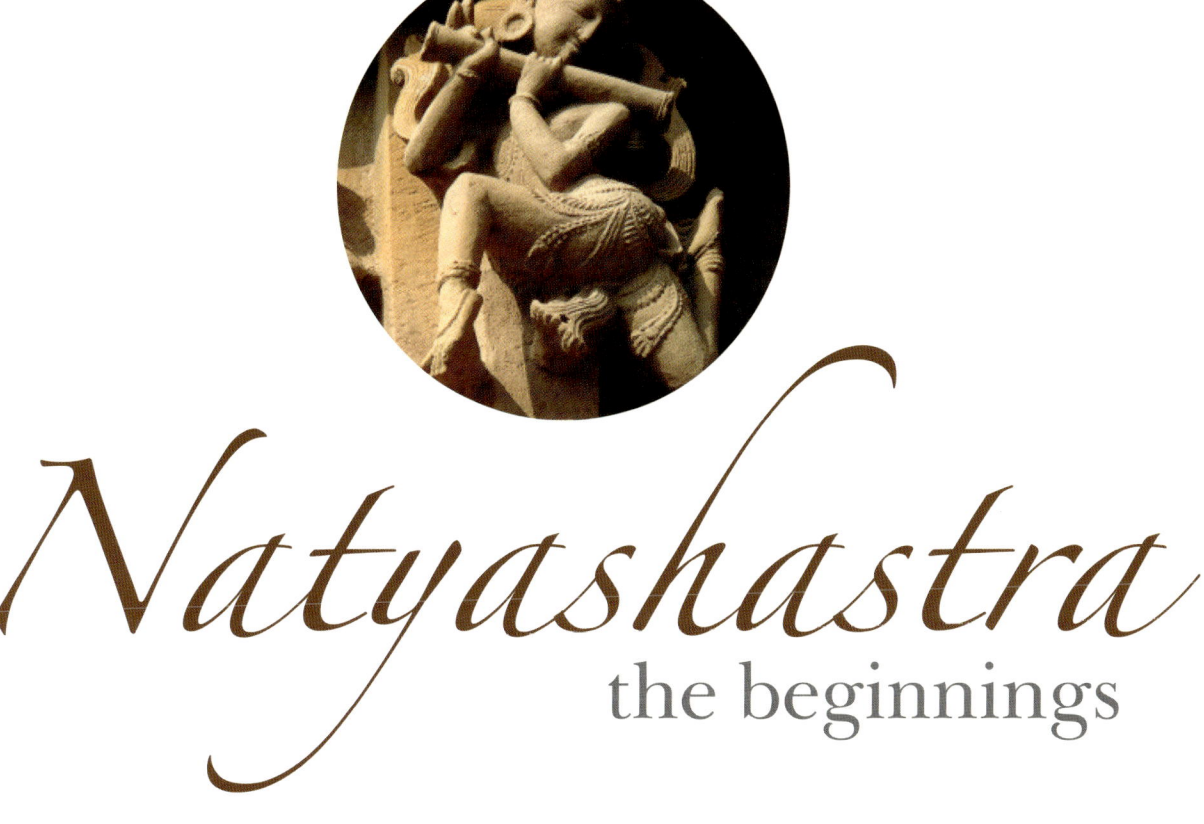

Natyashastra
the beginnings

Tatra Shringaronam rati-sthayeebhav prabhava.
Ujjwalveshatmaka. Yat kinchit loke
schuchimedhya-mujjwalam
darshaneeyam va tachrangarenomiyate-avamesh acharsidho
hridyojjwalveshatmakatatwachrangaro rasa.
Sacha stripunsahetuka uttamyuvaprakati.

NATYASHASTRA, BHARATA MUNI

Ancient and medieval India has witnessed prolific and lengthy discourse on the arts. The seeds being laid in Bharata Muni's *Natyashastra* in the 1st or 2nd century BC, a series of technical treatises on poetics, dance, drama, music, sculpture, painting, architecture, and other allied arts grew over the 4th and 5th centuries, continuing right through to the end of the 17th century. Among these Sanskrit treatises were *alamkara-shastras* (on poetics, rhetoric and prosody), *sangita-shastras* (on music), *natya-shastras* (on music, dance and drama), *shilpa-shastras* (on sculpture and painting), *vastu-shastras* (on architecture), and more. Strictly speaking, none of these can claim to be treatises on aesthetics; nevertheless they are deemed to be fully adequate compendiums on the respective arts.

Among these, *Natyashastra* is the most inventive and seminal work of all and is often referred to as the 'Fifth Veda'. Without doubt, it is the iconic text for aesthetic theory in ancient Indian arts. Its author, Bharata Muni, one of the most important thinkers of the time, laid the foundations of the rasa theory which became the theoretical base, not just for dance and drama or *natya*, but also for all art forms.

(Page 2)
Nataraja, the Lord of Dance, Unfinished Chola, 11th-12th century, National Museum, New Delhi

(Below)
Bhairav Raga depicting Radha-Krishna, Ragamala painting 1770, Rajasthan Miniature

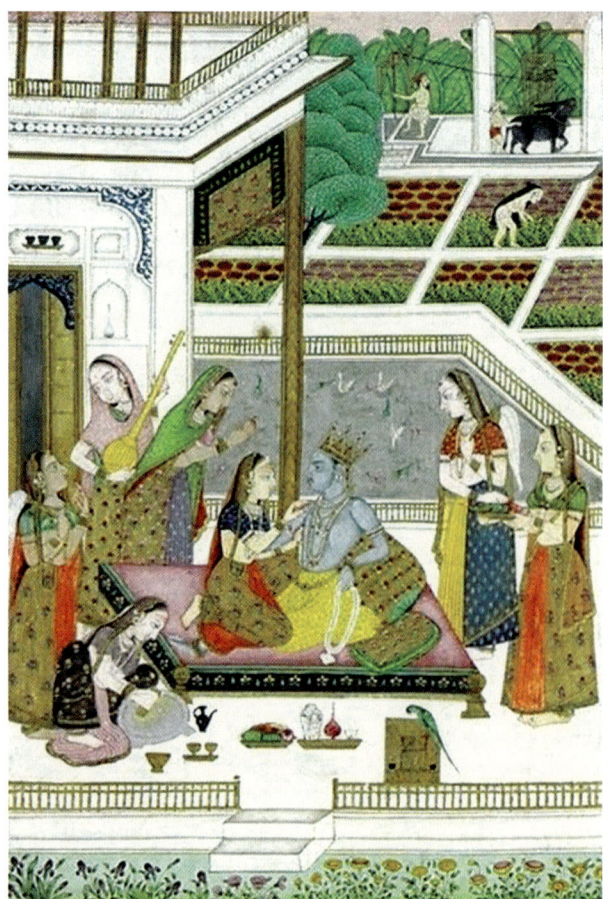

Beginning with *Natyashastra*, theoreticians took the philosophy of aesthetics forward by elaborating on every aspect of artistic practice. Among them were Bhamaha and Rudrata of the Prachina School (AD 650-850), Bhatta Lollata and Sri Sankuka (AD 800-840), Anandavardhana of the Navina School (AD 850), Pratiharenduraja (AD 900-950), Kuntaka (AD 950-1000), Bhatta Nayaka (AD 900-1000), Abhinavagupta (AD 980-1020), Mahimabhatta (AD 1020-1100), Mammata (AD 1050-1100) and Jagannatha (AD 1620-1660). One of the greatest philosophers, mystics and aestheticians of his time, Abhinavagupta exercised a strong influence on the study of arts. Born in Kashmir, he is best known for *Tantraloka*, an encyclopaedic treatise on the philosophical and practical aspects of Kashmiri Shaivism. He also wrote *Abhinavabharati*, perhaps the most canonical work on the philosophy of aesthetics.

The Indian Way of Aesthetics

In the *Natyashastra* Bharata describes the importance of poetics and the power of language, words and their meanings. The relationship of the rasa experience and

4   *Shringara*—the many faces of Indian beauty

poetic vision is exemplified in poetry, and rasa lies at its very soul. Poetics was studied in accordance with the rasa theory and aestheticians developed the idea that poetic experience was also a rasa experience. Emotion, in such a case, could be experienced not through any empirical knowledge but through aesthetic susceptibility alone.

Aesthetics can broadly be defined as that which aims to lay down and develop the principles of art, creativity and beauty. It can be further divided into the philosophy of art and the philosophy of beauty. The philosophy of beauty explores aesthetic experience beyond art, such as in the natural world, and in disciplines like ethics, science or mathematics; it is concerned with art only in-so-far as art creates beauty. This is essentially a view held by Western aestheticians.

In India, however, we have no text before us to show that there was any systematic intellectual discipline or autonomous speculative thought relating to aesthetics, as known in the West. Indeed, the question of beauty in nature and art was hardly ever a subject of serious investigation by our thinkers (*tattvajnanis* and *darsanikas*) except maybe incidentally. This could be because art was, for our ancestors, an activity directed towards the enrichment of the maker, viewer, reader or listener. It thus fell under the purview of ethics.

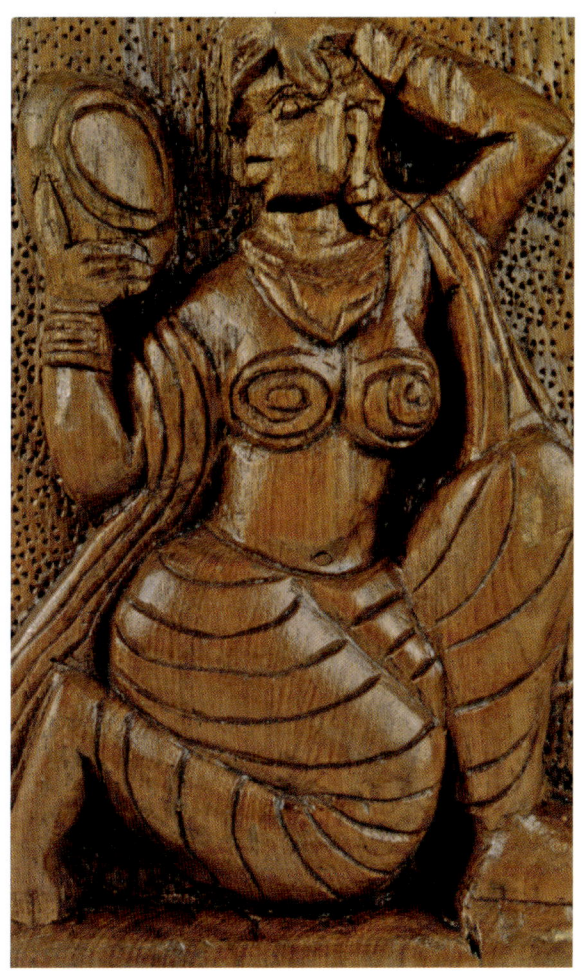

Wooden carving from Madhya Pradesh, Crafts Museum, New Delhi

In Indian speculative thought, the idea of the good belonged to the realm of epistemology and logic, while the idea of the beautiful was associated with psychology, the theory of rasa and *bhava*, which we shall discuss in detail in the pages to follow. Aesthetics was, thus, not regarded as an autonomous intellectual pursuit. The comprehension and conception of the good (*sivam, mangalam*) was coupled with the joy of bliss and beauty (*anandam, sundaram*). Ethics and aesthetics appear, therefore, to have been regarded as a single entity.

The definitions of art are legion and as unconvincing as they are multiple. Yet the minimum descriptive definition may be more faithful to the real nature of art than the more elaborate ones, for art is inescapably the organization of the sensuous particulars of a physical material. Like 'beauty', 'art' as a term is also a generalization that bases its meaning on no specific context; its terms of reference can therefore vary according to the context within which it is placed.

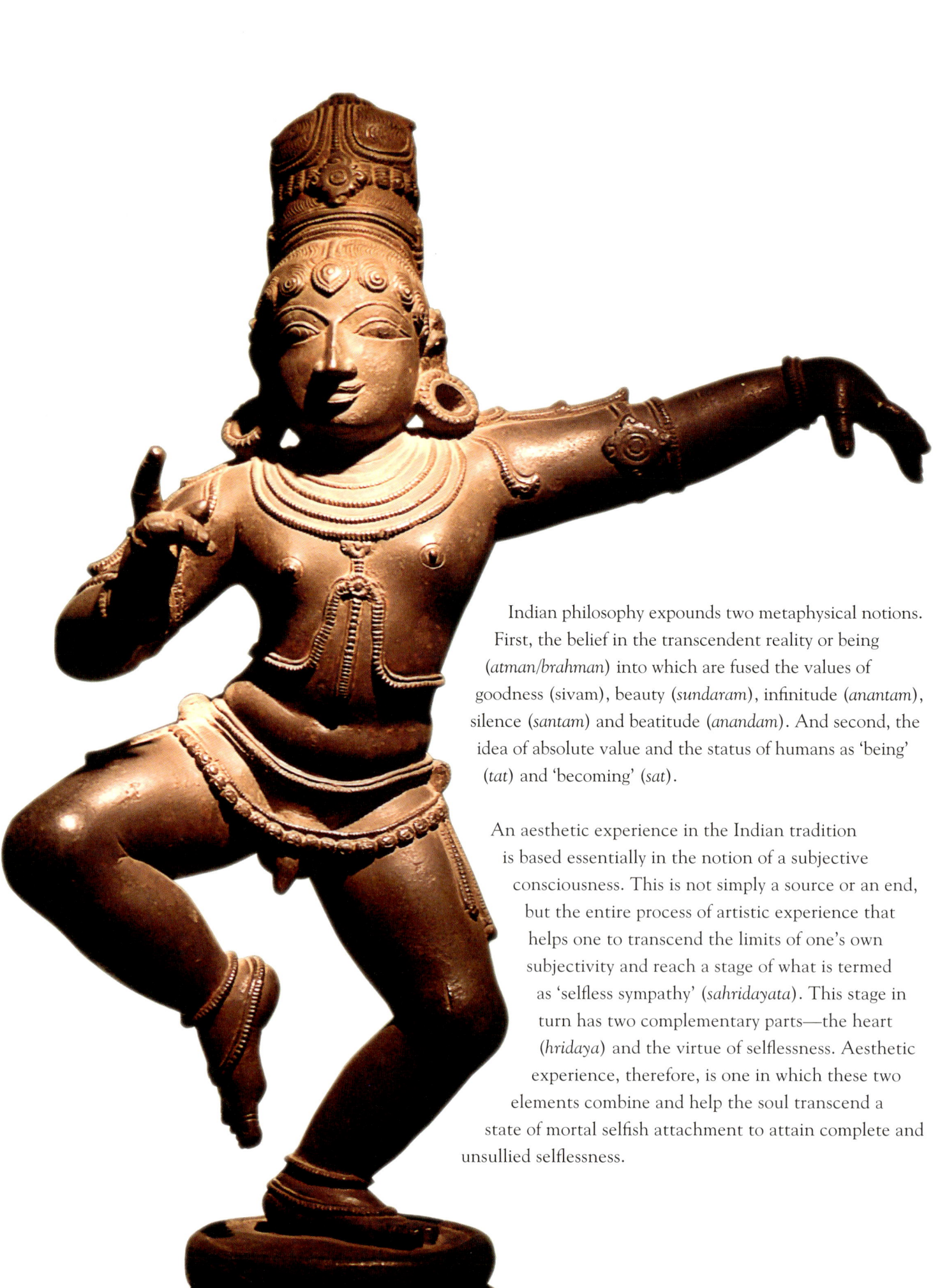

Indian philosophy expounds two metaphysical notions. First, the belief in the transcendent reality or being (*atman/brahman*) into which are fused the values of goodness (*sivam*), beauty (*sundaram*), infinitude (*anantam*), silence (*santam*) and beatitude (*anandam*). And second, the idea of absolute value and the status of humans as 'being' (*tat*) and 'becoming' (*sat*).

An aesthetic experience in the Indian tradition is based essentially in the notion of a subjective consciousness. This is not simply a source or an end, but the entire process of artistic experience that helps one to transcend the limits of one's own subjectivity and reach a stage of what is termed as 'selfless sympathy' (*sahridayata*). This stage in turn has two complementary parts—the heart (*hridaya*) and the virtue of selflessness. Aesthetic experience, therefore, is one in which these two elements combine and help the soul transcend a state of mortal selfish attachment to attain complete and unsullied selflessness.

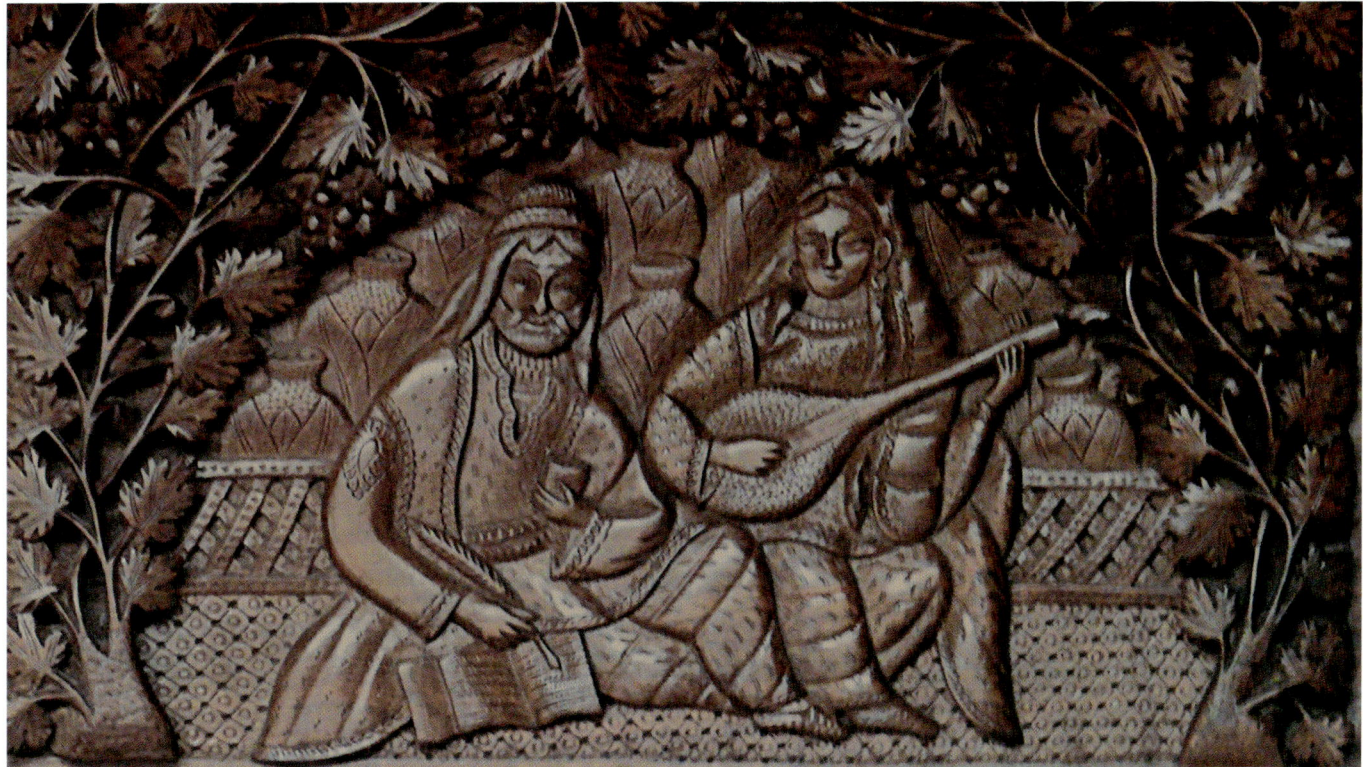

Wood panel, Kashmir, Crafts Museum, New Delhi

(Page 6) Balakrishna in a dancing posture, Vijayanagara, 15th century, National Museum, New Delhi

The central idea rooted in Indian classical art is that beauty is inherent in spirit, not in matter. The ancient treatise *Shukraniti* clearly states that while making images of the gods, the artist should trust only his spiritual vision, and not rely upon the appearance of objects perceived by the senses. All the same, naturalism and realism were not completely subordinated to the classical symbolism of iconographic values. Spiritual fervour was often coupled with deep reverence and love of nature. *Vishnudharmottara*, a 5th century treatise, enjoins the painter to study the picture and mood of nature and depict the seasons he sees around him through flowers and fruits, and the joy of men, animals and birds. Philosophical as it may be, Indian art theory is also realistic in its minute observations. Its aim is not just to evoke sensuous delight; reality, instead of being veiled, is simply idealized.

The Vedanta School expresses one of the earliest views on poetics. Brahman-centred, it posits the realization of the 'ultimate reality' through art, namely the attainment of moksha or final liberation from this existence. Other views exist in ancient and medieval philosophy, such as the popular belief that art affords personal pleasure to the viewer; the Samkhya view is that art is an end in itself.

Scholars, particularly the *navina* or later scholars, Bhatta Nayaka, Anandavardhana and Abhinavagupta, concerned themselves with the art of poetry supported by the entire classical heritage of Sanskrit verse and drama in its noblest manifestations. Through Kalidasa's plays like *Abhijnana Shakuntalam* and *Meghadutam*, they came to the inescapable conclusion that a mere analysis of technical skill and formal construction did not afford them a unique artistic experience. This had more to do with an emotional state or bhava created and induced by skill and formal construction.

Yashodhara came to much the same conclusion with respect to the plastic arts. Of the six canons or *shadanga*, meaning the six limbs of the art, *rupabheda* (differentiation of form), *pramanani* (proportion, balance, rhythm), *sadrishyam* (verisimilitude to natural forms), and *varnikabhangam* (literally, waves of colour, high and low, surface and depth, gradation and tonality) are purely formal qualities characterizing the body of the work. The other two, bhava (emotional state of being) and *lavanya* (grace) are qualities that constitute what has been called the atman or soul of art.

The Cradle of Rasa

According to the Upanishads, the ultimate source of all enjoyment is the concept of rasa, the embodiment of the entire gamut of human emotions. In its most identifiable, physical sense, rasa refers to the sap, or juice of plants. But rasa also signifies the essential, non-material, non-tangible core of something that can be experienced but not touched. At another level it bears reference to the fundamental flavour of something that needs to be savoured in order to experience pleasure. Hence, when it is applied to the realm of art and aesthetics, rasa merges all these different connotations and takes on the essence of something that elevates an experience from the ordinary and physical to one of spiritual bliss and joy (ananda).

The aesthetic experience is described as the 'tasting of flavour' or *rasavadana*. The viewer, or more specifically the scholar or connoisseur, is referred to as a *rasika*. A work of art bearing rasa is often described as being *rasavat* or *rasavant*. The artist strives for rasa in his work and the rasika or connoisseur intuitively detects it. Rasa, it must be kept in mind, is bestowed, not made. It was once believed that only those with a philosophic bent of mind could perceive the quality of beauty in a work of art, independent of the theme.

Nine rasas, or the *Navarasas* are generally listed in most texts on the subject. Bharata, however, speaks only of eight in *Natyashastra*: shringara (erotic), *hasya* (comic), *karuna* (pathetic), *raudra* (furious), *vira* (heroic), *bhayanaka* (terrible), *bibhatsa* (odious) and *adbhuta* (marvellous). Later writers added the ninth rasa:

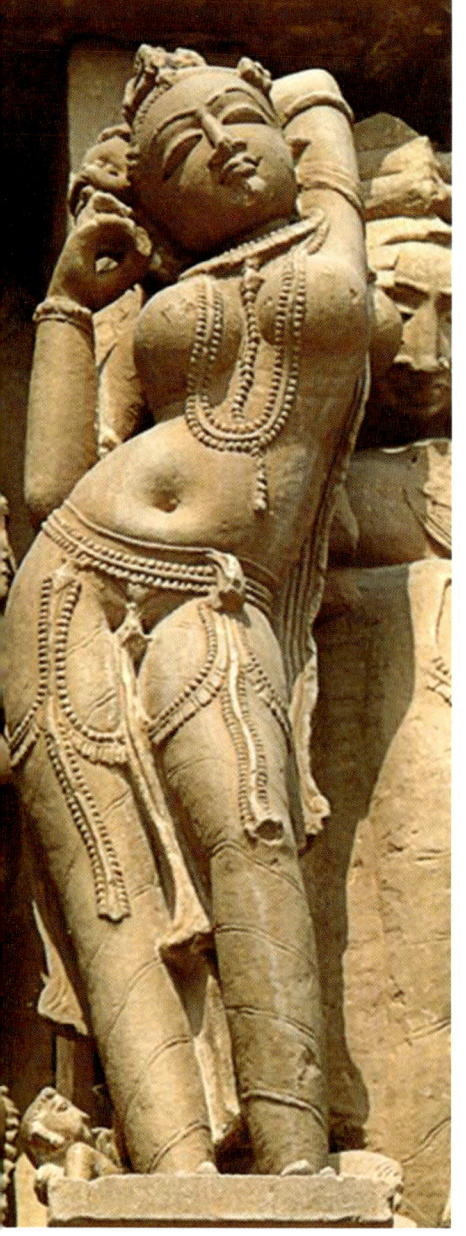

Personification of shringara, Vamana Temple, Khajuraho

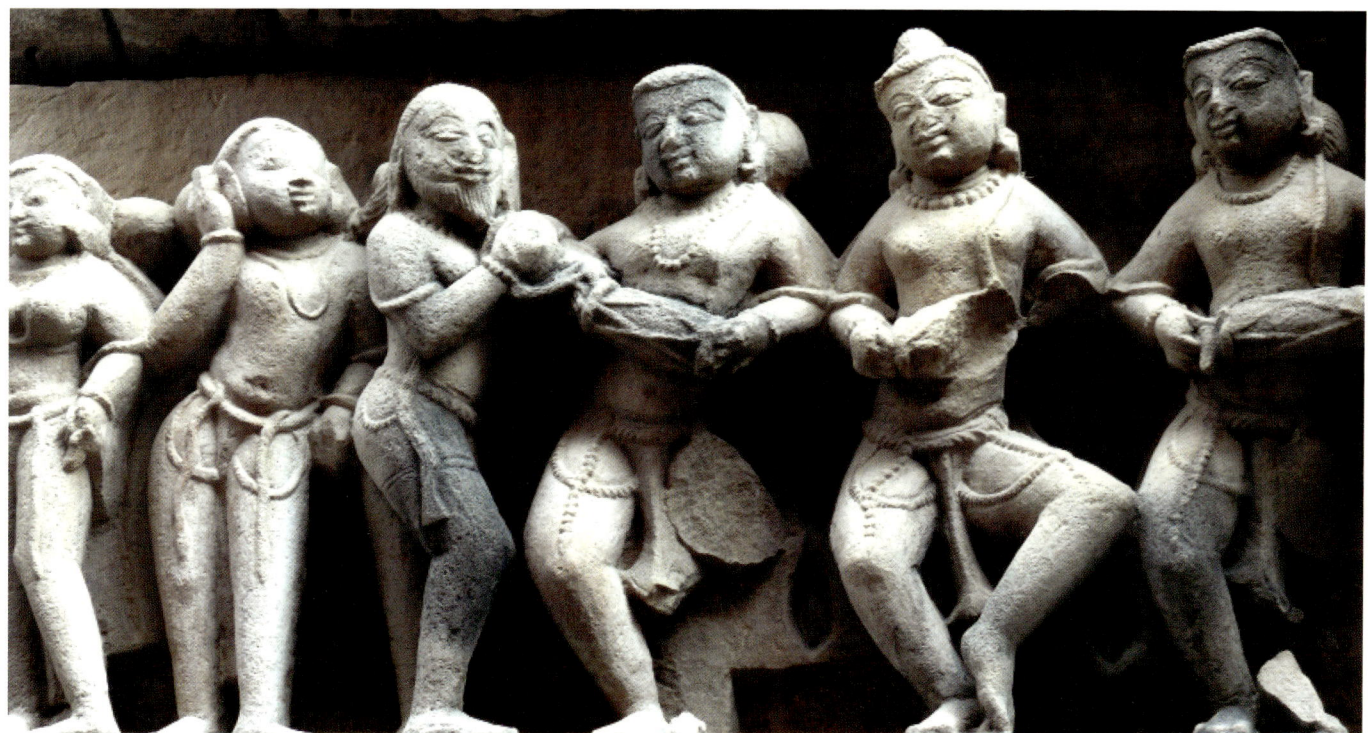

A group of musicians, Lakshmana Temple, Khajuraho

shanta, which is variously translated as the quiescent or peaceful. It is, in effect, a state of superconsciousness, which is the ultimate end of any yoga. Shanta was not recognized as a rasa in the early texts as it was considered to be devoid of emotion or *niras*. Images and sculptures of the Jain and Buddhist tradition are the most visible examples of this ninth rasa.

Although rasa is defined as one and undivided, one particular sentiment or flavour emerges as dominant, and through it the spectator experiences a specific emotion. Bharata goes on to say: *vibhavanubhava-vyabhichari-samyogad rasamspattih*. This means that rasa originates out of a combination of *vibhavas* (excitants), *anubhavas* (ensuants) and *vyabhicharibhavas* (accessory feelings), along with the *sthayibhava* (permanent feeling).

This emphasis on emotional states may appear paradoxical, in light of the views held by our writers on poetics. They believed that the aim of art was to induce in the mind of the beholder, listener or viewer, a state of detachment, impersonality, disinterest and non-involvement. These were the essential pre-conditions to attain pure bliss or ananda inspired by the aesthetic experience. According to the rasa theorists of the Navina School, this detachment was easier for the viewer whose feelings were already cultured and disciplined. Art, poetry, music and all the other arts, thus gradually came to be acknowledged and drawn on as a means of refining human feelings, emotions, sensibilities and perceptions.

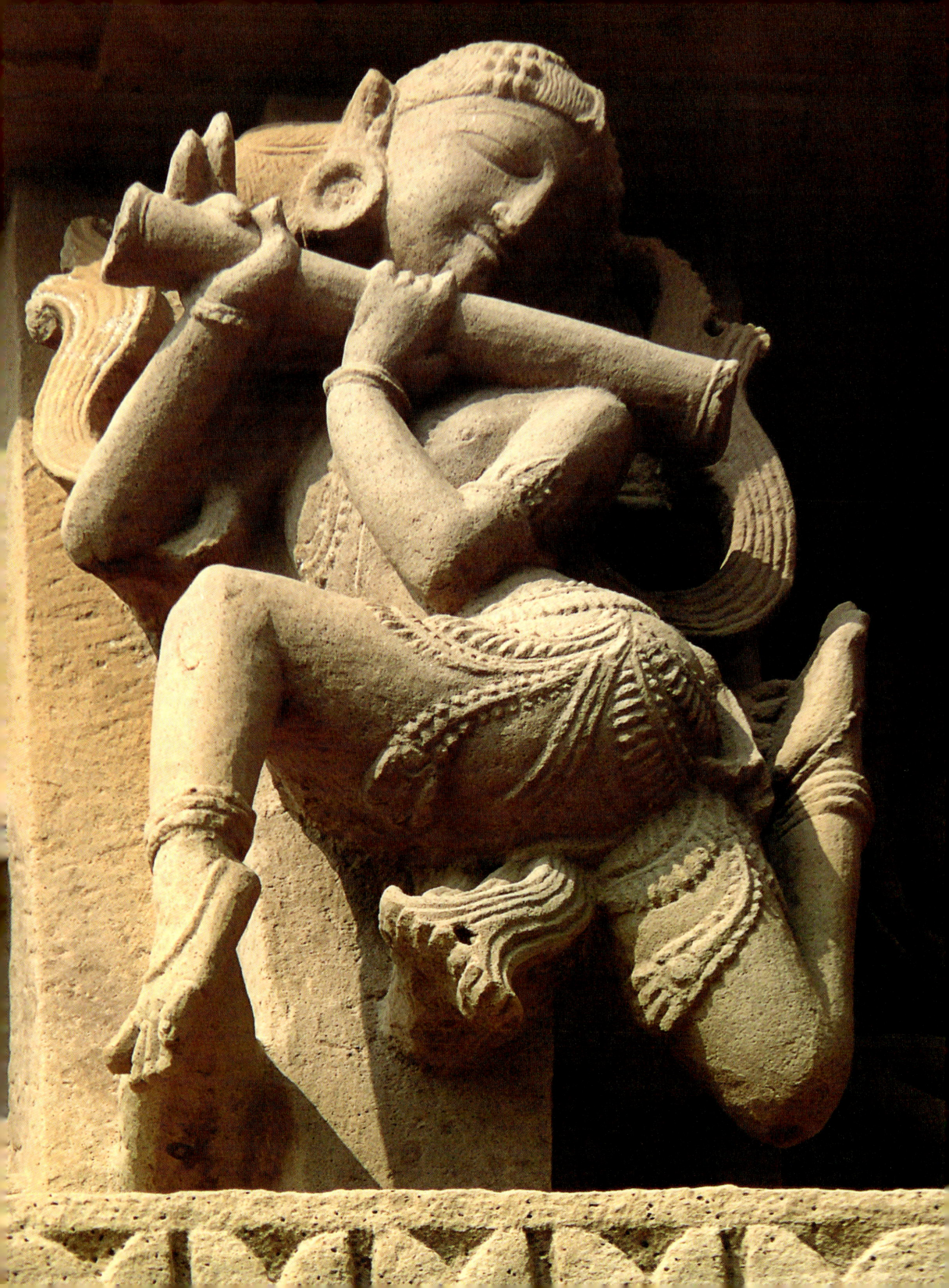

While most Indian philosophers believe that creativity is something one is born with, and is an essentially spontaneous occurrence, some like Rudrata contend that creativity (*pratibha*) may be acquired or developed by training and knowledge. The creator is considered a seer (*muni*) who has the skill (*kaushala*) to represent his insights in concrete form as the ultimate reality, Brahman. His skill lies in his ability to perceive the unity and harmony of the universe which, to the ancient Indians, signifies 'perfect beauty', and then to convey this unique insight of the Brahman to the viewer.

The creator does this in three stages. First, through the perception of cosmic beauty by 'self-forgetful' activity: this is made possible by the use of his imagination (pratibha), when contemplating a common experience or observing facts. Second, by using pratibha to transform these observed facts and experiences into a general idea symbolizing the 'ultimate reality' or perfection in perceived beauty. And finally, by converting this general symbol into concrete material form.

Many scholars assert that the rasa experience belongs not to the poet or to the actor but exclusively to the viewer who, to fully appreciate the work of art, should ideally be similar in temperament to the artist or creator, that is, *sahridaya* or of similar heart. Many authorities, including Vishwanatha of the Kashmir school, also maintain that the artist 'may obtain aesthetic experiences from the spectacle of his own performance'. The actor is moved by the passions he depicts just as the musician, dancer and image-maker is deeply involved in the emotions that he or she brings to the performance or work. However, the emotion during the act of creating or performing is different from the rasa experience. The rasa experience has an illuminating element—'a lightning flash of delight' that can be experienced by the artist only when in the position of a spectator. The process of appreciation is the reverse of the process of creation. The work of art stands midway between the two, effecting a transition from the one to the other. This transition is made possible by the fact that the viewer is of the same nature as the artist. 'But the viewer differs from the artist in the degree of that nature, and this is the reason why appreciation waits upon creation.' (Ramachandran, 1979)

The Keystones of Aesthetics
Indian aesthetic theory revolves on an axis of key concepts such as rasa (taste, flavour), *dhvani* (poetic resonance), alamkara

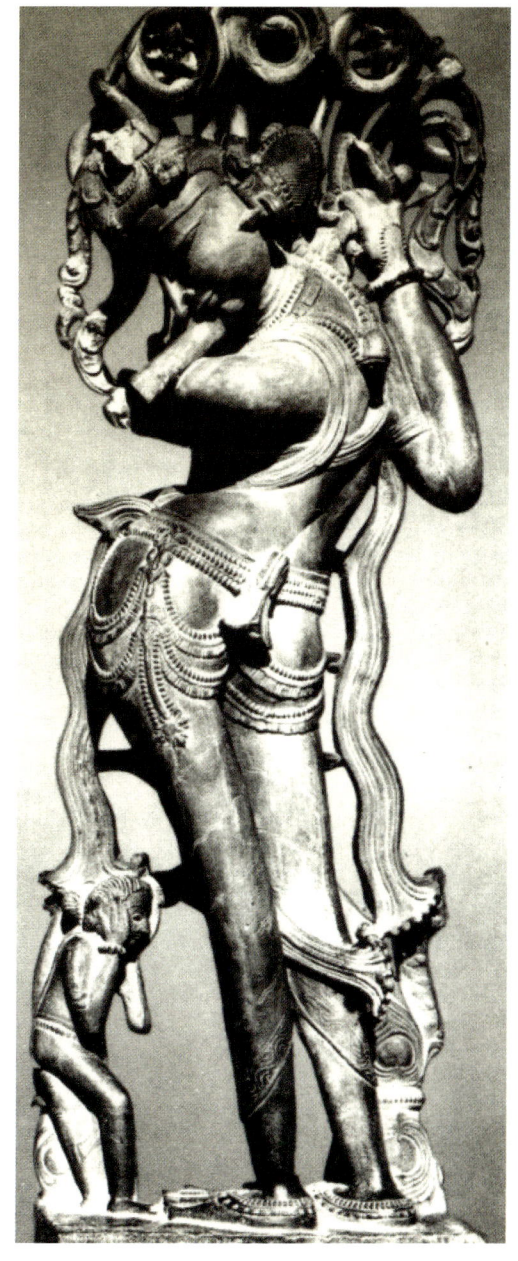

(Page 10)
A celestial damsel playing a flute, in typical pose of languor and ecstasy

(Below)
Flute player, Visvanath Temple, Khajuraho

and lakshana (poetic ornaments and marks), *sphota* (blossoming, sprouting utterance), or *shabda* (sound), all of which act as a bridge between the physical and the metaphysical. The emphasis is on the subjective dimensions of aesthetic experience, which translates itself into an overwhelming feeling of *advaita* (oneness or non-duality).

The true function of art is the quest for the beautiful. Art expresses beauty that is not just limited to visual appreciation. It encompasses both the intellectual and spiritual sensitivities. Beauty defies definition, explanation, and prescription. Every culture, at any given time, has its own ideals of beauty. So does beauty lie in the eye of the beholder, or is it a quality inherent in the art object? Is beauty based on a canon or principle, or is it a quality entirely projected by the observer? The meaning of beauty could be approached in many ways; it could be subjective or objective, and therefore not defined by any one single absolute.

According to the sages, the pursuit of art was not left to the mercy of occasional sparks of inspiration, nor to individual taste and tendency found in people of high birth. *Chatuhshashthi-kala,* or sixty-four arts recognized by the ancients, were an integral part of the syllabus for aristocratic schooling. Every prince and princess, every son and daughter of an aristocrat, had to be proficient in most, if not all these arts, failing which he or she would be denied a place of privilege in society.

In his romantic work *Kadambari*, Banabhatta, the court poet of Emperor Harshavardhan (606-647), has given a list of subjects in which Chandrapida, his hero, gained mastery of the various disciplines. Among the arts he mentions

Frieze of dancers and musicians, Lakshmana Temple, Khajuraho

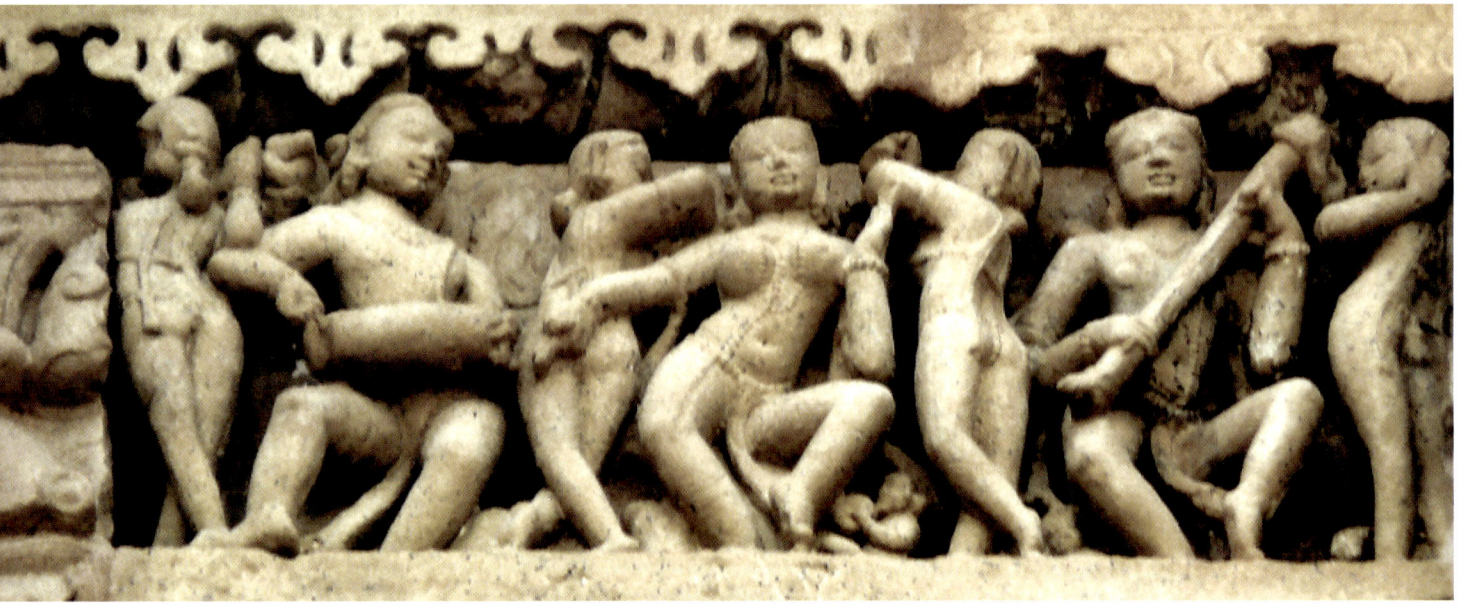

vyayamavidya (physical culture), *ayudha* (use of weapons), *rathacharya* (chariot riding), *gajaprastha* (elephant riding), *vadya* (instrumental music), *nritta* (dance), *gandharvaveda* (dance and music), *hasti-shiksha* (training of elephants), *turangavayojnana* (ascertaining the age of a horse), *purushalakshana* (determining the nature of a person), *chitrakarman* (painting), *patracchedya* (decoration), *lekhyakarman* (engraving), *sarva dyutakala* (the gambling arts), *sakunirutajnana* (interpretation of the sounds of birds, a part of *nimittajnana*), *grahaganita* (astronomy), *ratnapariksha* (appraising of jewels), *darukarman* (wood-craft), *dantavyapara* (ivory-carving), *vastuvidya* (engineering), *tarana-lan-ghana-pluti* (swimming-rowing-jumping), *indrajala* (magic), *sarvalipi* (all the scripts), and *sarvadesabhasa* (different dialects and languages). And despite all that, the list is incomplete, for the poet concludes with an etcetera!

Besides the *shilpa-shastras*, references have been made to the arts in the Puranas (*Vishnu Purana* and *Bhagavata Purana*), holy scriptures of the Buddhists and Jains, and in *Harivamsha*. The latter, also known as the *Harivamsha Purana*, consists of 16,374 verses. Vatsyayana's *Kamasutra* is also replete with references to both the performing and decorative arts. Art, therefore, has a well-defined function to fulfil in the graduated scheme of life, the definitive goal of which is anandam, moksha or *bodhi*, terms used to symbolize a state of joyous, blissful existence achieved through an experience of absolute freedom and perfect bliss. In one of his devotional lyrics, Rabindranath Tagore says: 'I dive into the sea of forms (*rupsagar*), hoping that I may come upon the gem of the formless (*arupa*, or absolute Brahman)'.

Tagore echoed the thoughts of the ancient seers and medieval *santas* or poet saints: If the experience of bliss, absolute freedom and wisdom is the final aspiration of life, then art should be a step towards the achievement of that final destination. In truth, art experience is intended to arouse interest in the final goal by giving the viewer a preview of this goal.

Shringara—The Supreme Rasa
From the earliest times, Indian art, philosophy and literature have not only been preoccupied with, but in many ways, obsessed with shringara rasa, or the erotic flavour. Bharata, for example, recognizes shringara as a primary emotion and then sets out a detailed classification of the various stages and types of romantic love and lovers, and their depiction on the stage through natya.

According to the rasa theory, all genuine aesthetic experience is essentially transcendental in nature. For the artist it lies in the act of creation, and for

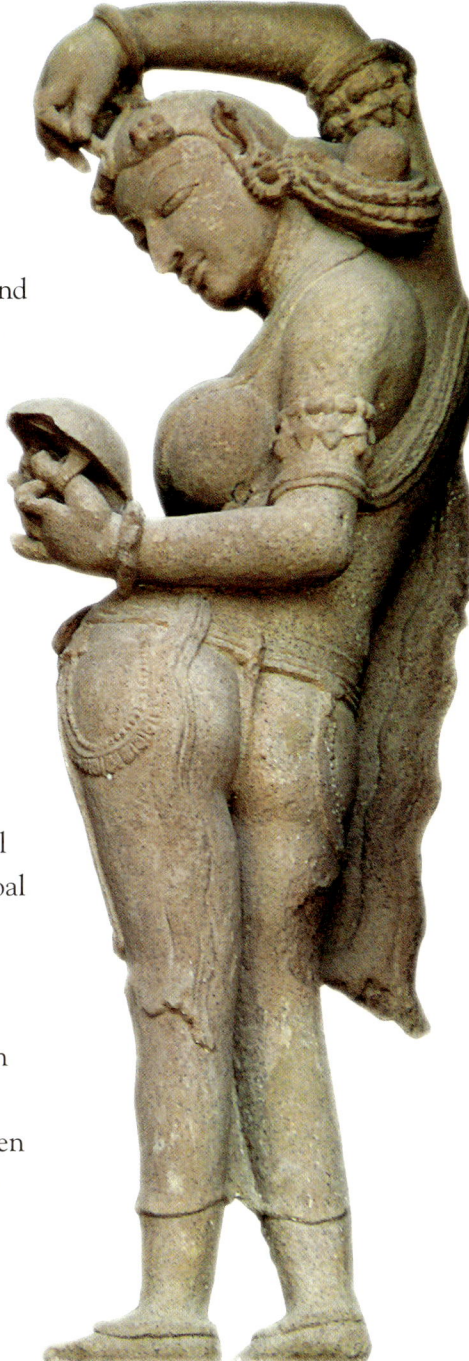

A lady adorning herself, Lakshmana Temple, Khajuraho

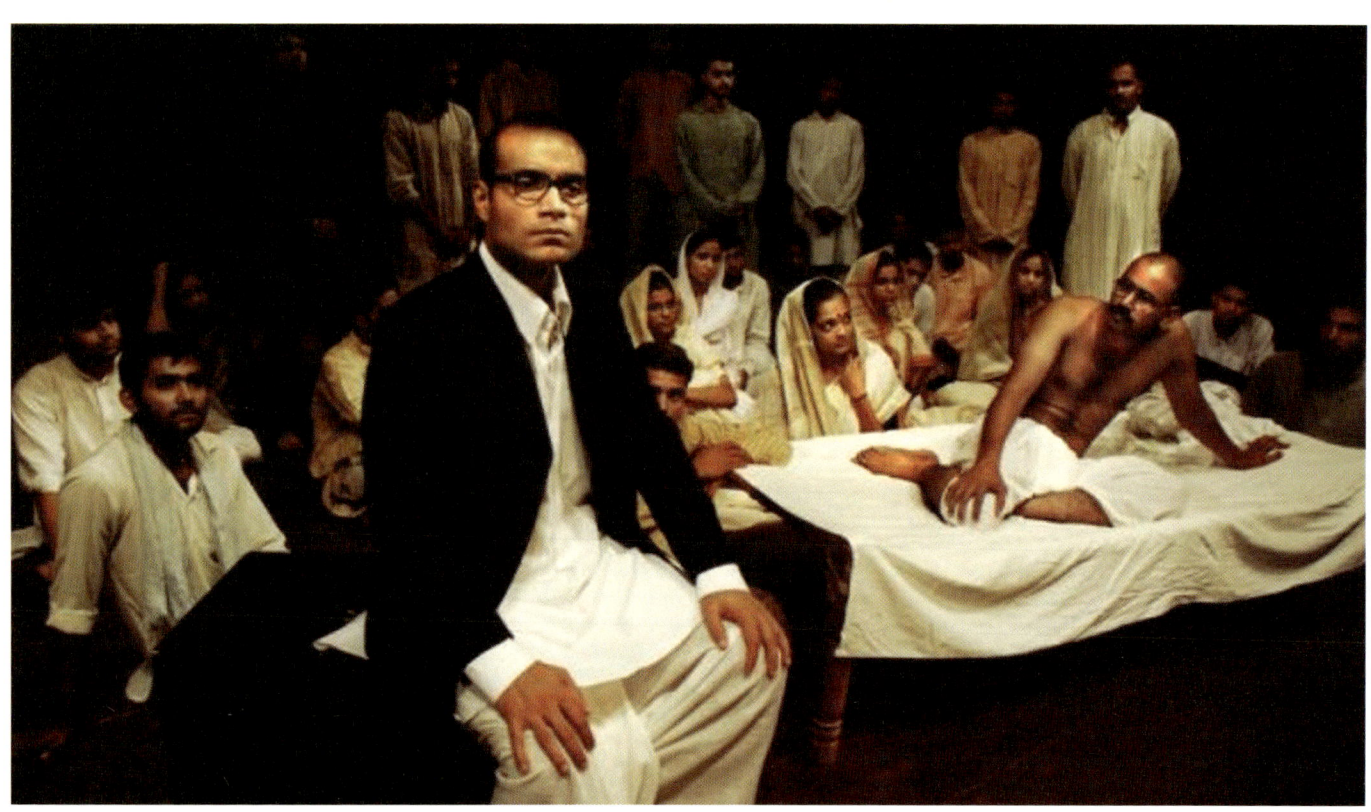

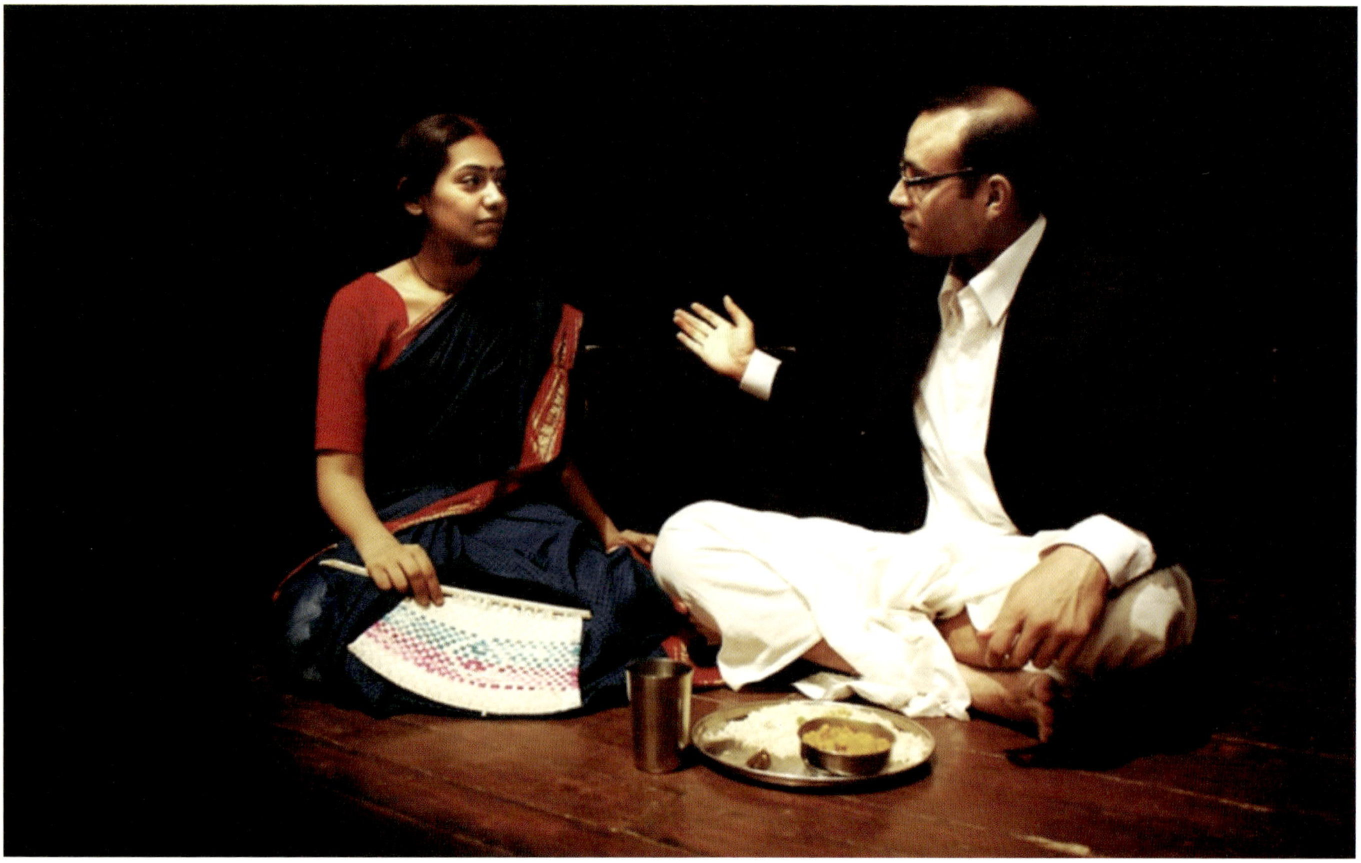

14   *Shringara*—the many faces of Indian beauty

the spectator, it is inherent in the act of observation; they are both therefore inextricably connected. The aesthetic experience results, eventually, in a state of transcendental bliss. This, in turn, stems from the one and only source of all ananda—the divine. Divinity, in fact, manifests itself through every art form, each reflecting one or more of its myriad shades of beauty, sublimity, magnificence and joy.

But the rasas do not stand alone. Each aesthetic experience is based on one dominant rasa, the sensitive portrayal of which will evoke a corresponding bhava in the rasika, the connoisseur or viewer. Bhava comes from the Sanskrit and Pali word 'bhu', or 'being' in the sense of ongoing worldly existence. Where rasa is the art of communication, bhava is the emotion contained in that rasa. The generation of this bhava is a fundamental prerequisite to the successful portrayal of any particular rasa. And if the rasika remains unmoved and untouched, the artist has failed to communicate the depth and sublimity of the aesthetic experience in a worthy manner.

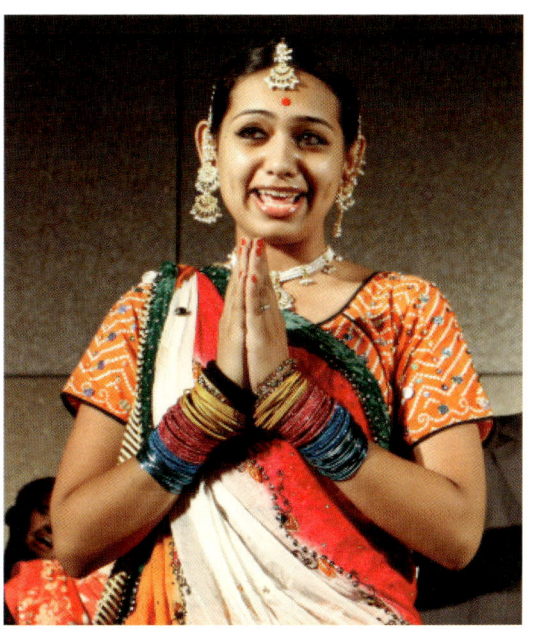

(Pg 15)
A scene from the play Moteram ka Satyagarh *based on a story by Munshi Premchand and directed by Arvind Gaur, a Asmita Theatre Group presentation*

(Pg 14)
Scenes from Rajesh Kumar's Ambedkar Aur Gandhi *directed by Arvind Gaur, a Asmita Theatre Group presentation*

Natyashastra holds that acting (*abhinaya*) comprises four features: body movements (*angika*), voice (*vachika*), spectacle (*aharya*), and sentiment or emotion (*sattvika*). Sentiment is emphasized in the context of the religious foundations of theatre. The integrity of emotion is vital, for theatre is perceived as a visual offering to the gods. The actors are required to be of a high calibre, as individuals and as performers, and their skills on stage are supposed to evoke responses that cover the entire gamut of human emotions.

The gods are perceived as the ultimate witnesses of theatre, for *Natyashastra* accepts that spectators can never embody all the qualities demanded of them by the text. These qualities are character and birth of high order; honesty and all-round virtue; and a mind that is quiet, perceptive, discriminating, alert, and knowledgeable. The treatise further states that while the plays are to be written in Sanskrit, the language of the priests and kings, the songs should be composed in the Prakrit language. These songs are meant to mark an important mood or action, introduce a character, or fill a gap (as when the actor has to leave the stage for a change of costume). Unfortunately, none of these early songs have survived.

The final chapter of *Natyashastra* tells us that Bharata Muni and his sons incurred the wrath of the sages since they were angered by the dramatization of themselves. However, royal patronage came into play and kings replaced the gods in protecting the actors.

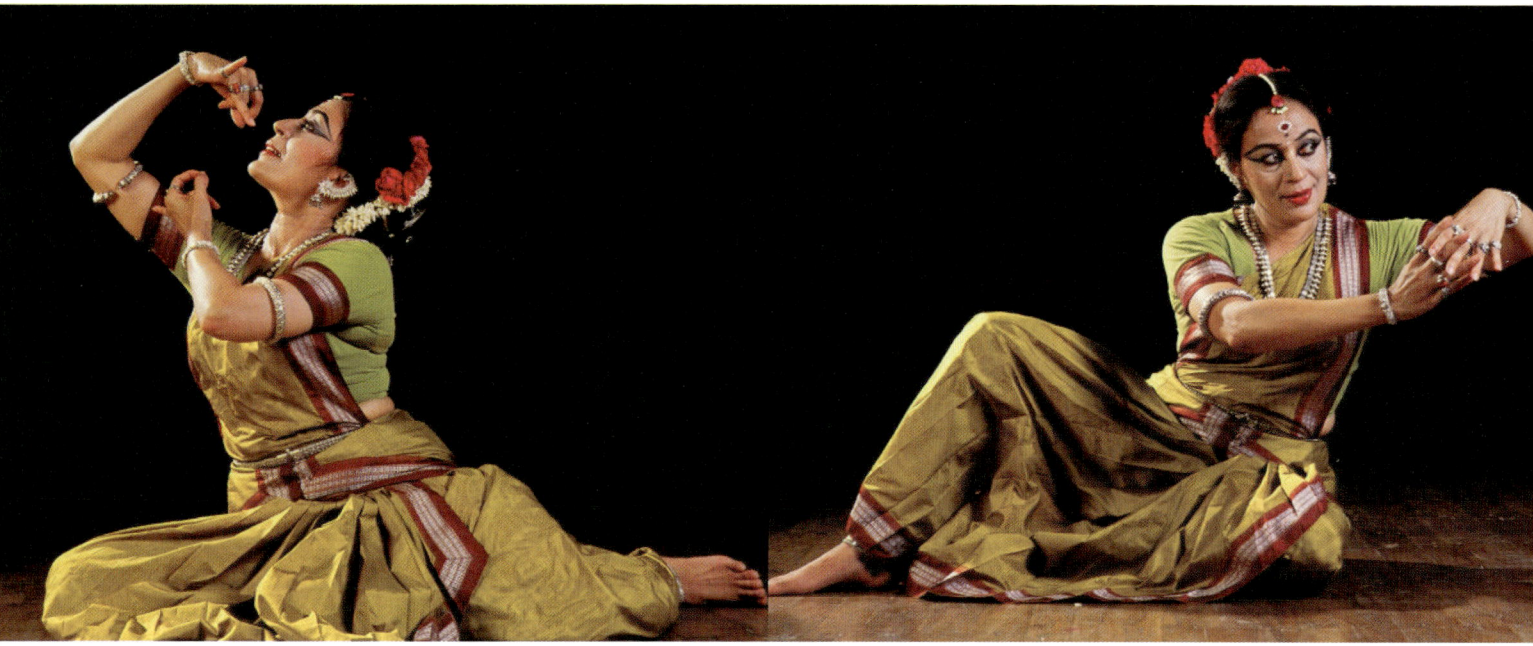

Dancer Sonal Mansingh expressing the detailed nuances of emotions

By the Middle Ages, there already existed a complex and hierarchal structure of human emotion with an extremely detailed and carefully described set of traits in Indian aesthetic thought and theory. Apart from *Natyashastra*, several other texts added to the wealth of ancient Indian aesthetic practice such as the *Shilpa Shastras, Shilpa Ratna, Samaranganasutradhara* and *Vishnudharmottara Purana*.

Ancient aesthetics emphasize the artist's role as the subjective beholder expressing himself in a highly detached and objective fashion. He meditates upon his experience and is able to give form to the formless. Art, therefore, plays a multiple role—it is a means of self-expression, a record of the artist's experiences, a form of communication satisfying man's need to be part of a group, and a way of searching for and understanding the virtues of life.

Like all other worldly as well as spiritual pursuits, literature is also measured by its social and individual value. Bharata, at the very beginning, asserts unequivocally that literature is a discourse of knowledge, *pancham veda*, as it mediates between philosophy and the layperson who actually needs the ideas of philosophy but cannot access them. It ensures, he says, righteousness, good reputation, long life, well-being and an increase in mental ability. Literature also provides the layperson guidance in the conduct of his life.

Bhamaha, a significant thinker of the 6th century AD, says that kavya produces ability in dharma, artha, kama, moksha (*Kavyalamkara*). He is emphatic about literature being a rational discourse, and according to him, a non-philosopher

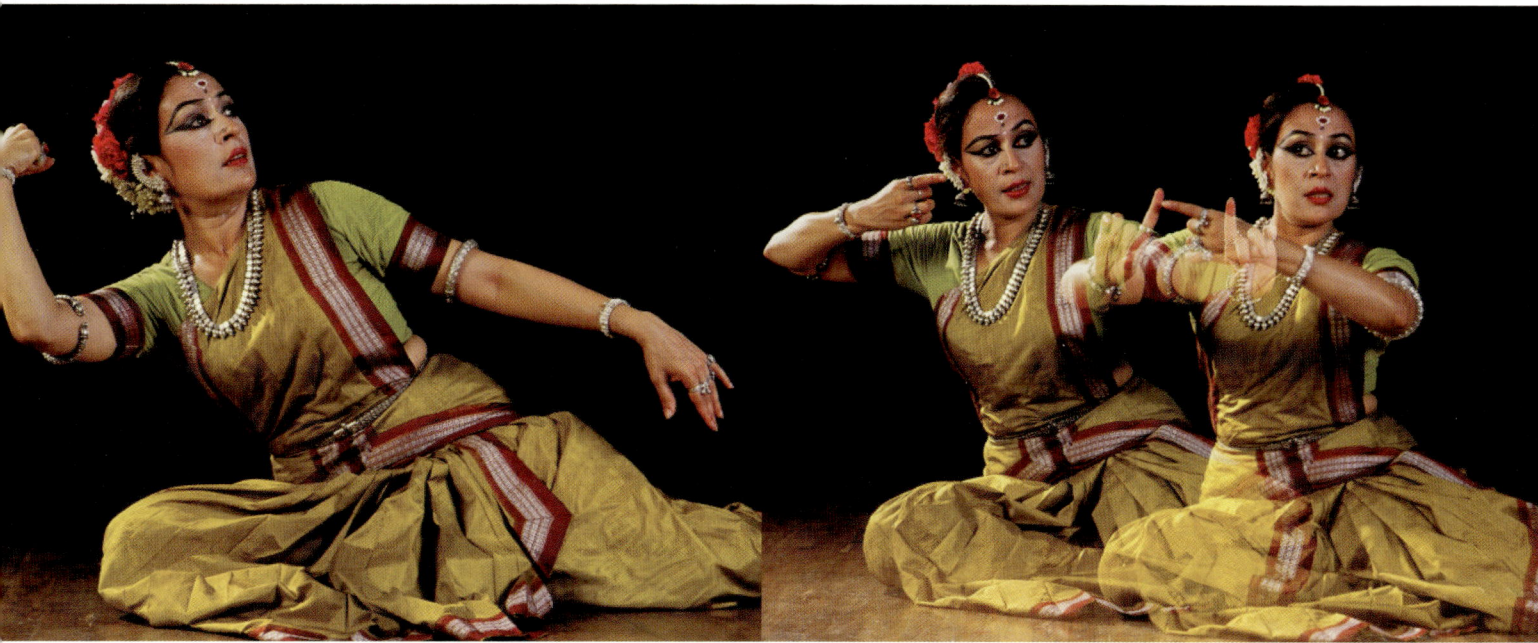

cannot be a poet and a non-poet cannot be a philosopher. Dandin, in the first half of the same century, also says that apart from a natural talent and practice, knowledge of the *shastras* is an important component of a poet's skill (*kavyadarsa*). Vamana (late 8th century AD) introduces the idea that kavya, from which stems ananda or bliss, is productive of a visible, concrete worldly fulfilment. Rudrata, also of the same period, talks of the fulfilment of knowledge and maturity of speech through grammar and logic, which makes kavya beautiful.

Abhinavagupta reserves saundarya for the purpose of crafting the discourse, for only when so crafted does it delight and generate new knowledge or awareness in the audience. Thus beauty or saundarya is merely instrumental in the fulfilment of the primary goal of verbal art. People recognize the beauty of public morality (*lokachara*) only from superior compositions—this is the 'beauty of novel experience laced with propriety' (*vakroktijivita*). Kuntaka goes on to say that the fulfilment of the four ends of life lies in the future, but the rasa of a literary composition produces *chamatkara*, an extraordinary feeling of delight experienced immediately on listening to or reading the composition. It repeatedly gives the experience of ananda.

Aesthetics becomes specially relevant when the sensory world takes over and when the otherwise latent ethical imperatives are developed around an emotional core; when creative energies are kindled and brought in contact with other models worthy of emulation; and when the perceived chasm between the sacred and profane, the sexual and spiritual, the sensuous and intellectual is bridged.

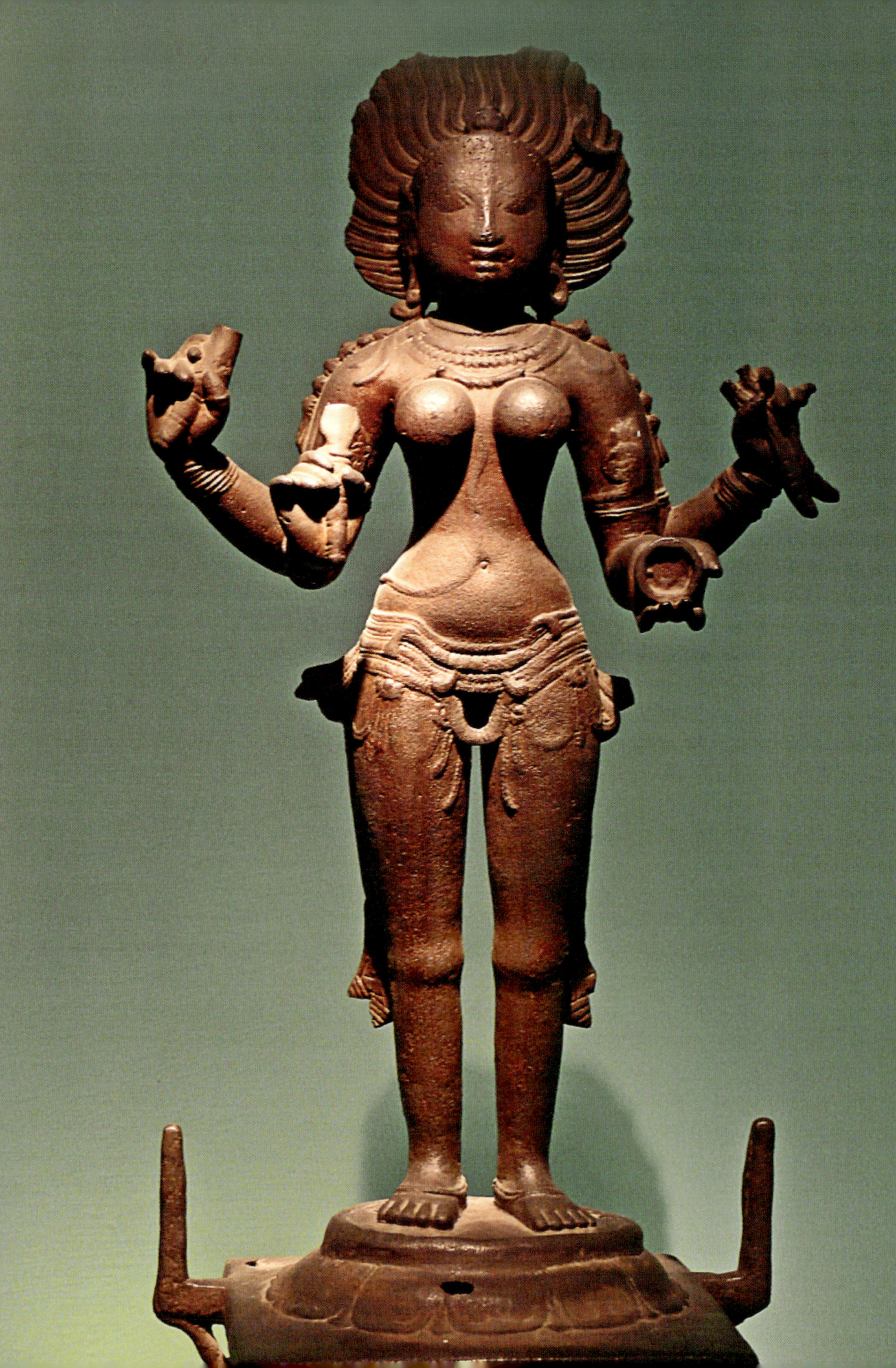

CHAPTER 2

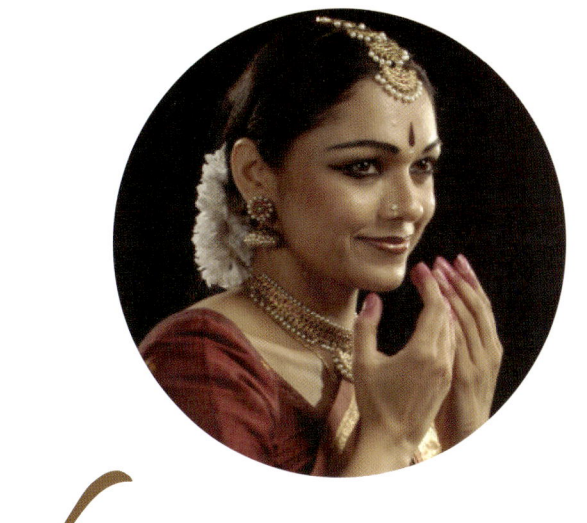

Navarasas
the embodiment of flavour

*Delightful or disgusting, exalted or lowly,
cruel or kind, obscure or refined,
actual or imaginary,
there is no subject that cannot evoke rasa in man.*

DASHARUPA, A TREATISE ON HINDU DRAMATURGY
DHANANJAYA

(Page 18)
Kali, Chola bronze, 11th century, National Museum, New Delhi

(Below)
'Kalia daman', a depiction of Krishna overpowering Kalia, an allegory of triumph over evil

Rasa is god-given and evanescent like perfume, says Bharata in his *Natyashastra*. It comes from matter but is not easy to describe or comprehend. Rasa does not take a physical form and the emotions it arouses are intangible. In its most refined form, rasa gives rise to a climactic bliss that can be experienced only by the spirit. It is a work of art that can make a human being experience ultimate happiness or ananda. This kind of enjoyment is described in Hindu scriptures as the 'taste of the mind'. It is the delight of the intellect. It comes as a burst of inspiration that overcomes the viewer when he or she comprehends the essence of artistic endeavour in a flash. Rasa, as has been said in the earlier chapters, is an essential part of the theory of art in India.

Rasa is the connecting link between the emotion, mood, and creative process of art, and the appreciation and perception of these in the viewer's mind. Rasa is indeed unique, but it is not one, for the aesthetic experience perceives varied flavours for several emotions. *Natyashastra* speaks of eight primary rasas: shringara (erotic), hasya (comic), karuna (pathetic), raudra (the furious), vira (heroic), bhayanaka (terrible), bibhatsa (odious), and adbhuta (marvellous). The poet Abhinavagupta added a ninth rasa—the shanta rasa, or tranquil sentiment—associated with mystical experience.

Degrees of Tasting

This essence, or literally 'juice', is to be 'tasted', and can be understood only by virtue of 'tasting'. Indian art appreciation believes that for a true aesthetic experience to be grasped, emotion and intellect have to come together, giving rise to a distilled knowledge that leads to ecstasy. This sense of ecstasy is inscrutable and illuminating and, therefore, cannot be described or judged.

Rasa creates a unique bond with a work of art. Vedas describe rasa as a 'gustative image' that can only be experienced as a flash of supernatural illumination. Everyone cannot experience this. It is only a few who have that intuitive knowledge of ideal beauty, and a heightened imagination and intellectual power. A rasa will only express itself to the degree that it has been tasted.

Transcending the Divide

In the field of Indian classical music, dhvani (resonance) plays an important role in enhancing a rasa, and thus suggesting the meaning of a work of art. The refined improvisations in classical music are meant to heighten the experience of a rasa. It is believed that the essence of a musical composition is appreciated through conscious listening. Thus the experience of Indian classical music is similar to that of meditation, or being centred around the divine. The listener, musician and the music being created are united on a single plane. This aesthetic experience can later be recalled by reawakening the flavour or rasa it has left in our consciousness.

In Indian art theory there is no divide between art and life, performer and audience, taste and truth, emotion and intellect. To experience the true creative process, one transcends this gap and creates a full circle. Emotions and thoughts play a dual role in colouring our perception of art. If we compare human emotions as clear and transparent water, when our thoughts flow through this medium, they add colour and vibrancy. If we are able to bridge the gap between thoughts and emotions, we experience emptiness of consciousness (*shunyata*). This is the feeling of liberation that both Hindu and Buddhist philosophies strives towards.

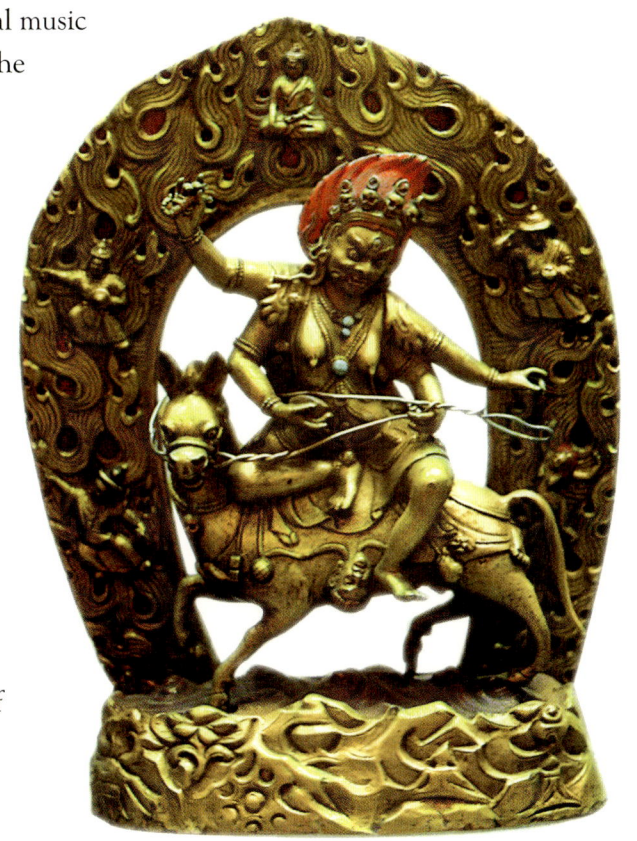

Devi, the female manifestation of the supreme lord. A folk image, National Museum, New Delhi

Emotions have a fundamental quality that makes them transmutable as a form of energy. Emotions can then be expressed both in the physical form and psychological form. In simple terms, they could take the physical form of a cloud and then condense into rain or assume the psychological form. When we allow the release of our emotions, we free ourselves from mental burdens. There is no need to control the way we feel, since this would imprison our emotions within the confines of the mental realm. Rasa is essentially indivisible. However, its academic division into spheres of emotion allows us the opportunity for further exploration. The variations, characterized as the nine sentiments, are like beams of different colours that we perceive when light passes through a prism, in this case 'enchanting the mind'.

The Spectrum of Rasas

It is believed that art evokes the shringara rasa, most frequently. It is related to passion among lovers, sensuality, and even the 'pain' of being in love. The emotion of love has a great range of modulations and complementary expressions. The associated colour is dark blue and is linked to God Vishnu.

Hasya or the comic sentiment suggests laughter and the experience of playful joy, celebration and fun. In philosophic terms, it reflects on the fact that life is illusory

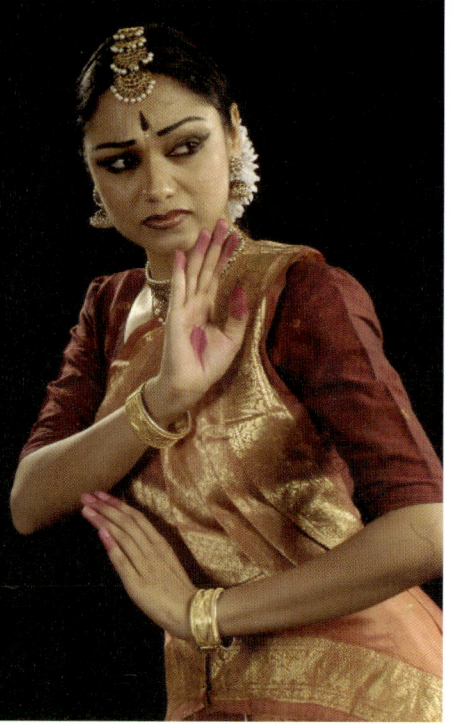 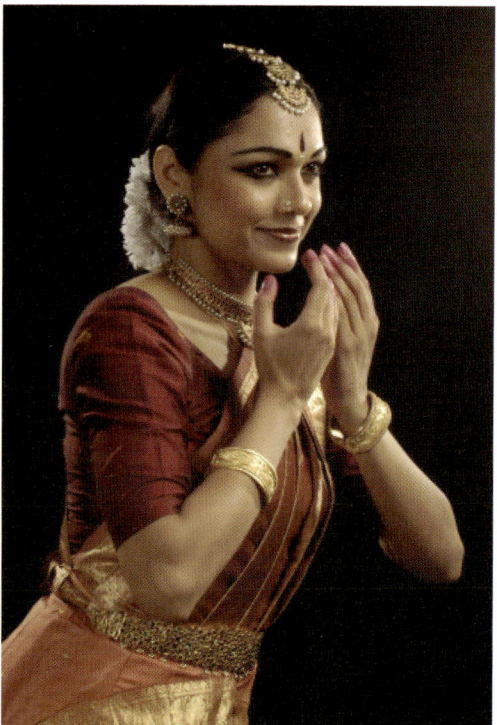 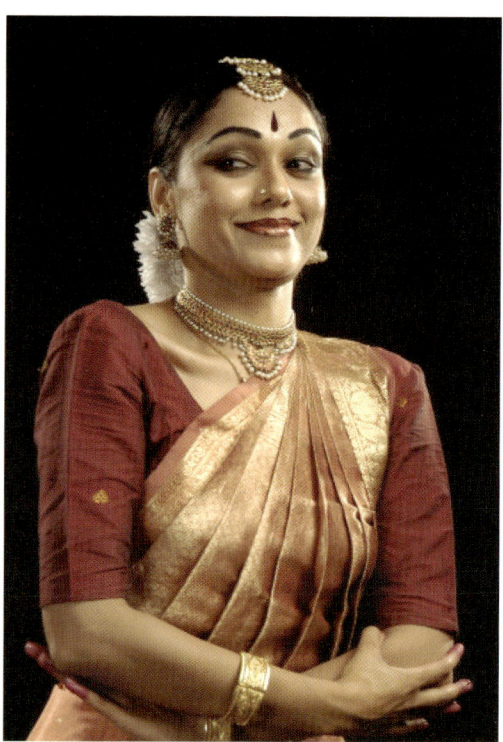

Bibhatsa, Shringara and Hasya rasas—Rama Vaidyanathan

(Page 23) Bhaya rasa—Rama Vaidyanathan

or *maya*. When combined with the intellect, humour can become satire. The colour associated with hasya is white and its god is Shiva.

Karuna or pathos suggests sadness, psychic pain, depression and desire of what we have lost. It is comparable to Sigmund Freud's majestic metaphor describing melancholy and grief: 'the shadow of the lost object falls upon the self'. Music evokes this particular rasa, expressing it through many shades and subtleties. In physical terms it is felt in the form of tears, a dryness of the mouth and loss of memory. The emotions associated with karuna are sorrow, anxiety, illness, weakness, insecurity, indolence, paralysis, tearfulness and regret. The intensity of these feelings, their almost devastating quality, has inspired many a masterpiece in our musical legacy. We can also see this rasa in the earthly lament of separation, or in a more mystical form of devotion suggesting compassion and unconditional love. In Sanskrit, the mystical dimension of karuna is referred to as an 'experience of spiritual service'. Associated with Yama, the god of death, this rasa is grey. Minor scales on the octave are generally known to induce karuna, and the music most descriptive of this rasa is found in the important Indian ragas and Meera's *bhajans* or other devotional songs.

Raudra (furious) is a sentiment displaying violent rage expressed by a character in art, music, or literature. The form of expression is aggressive and

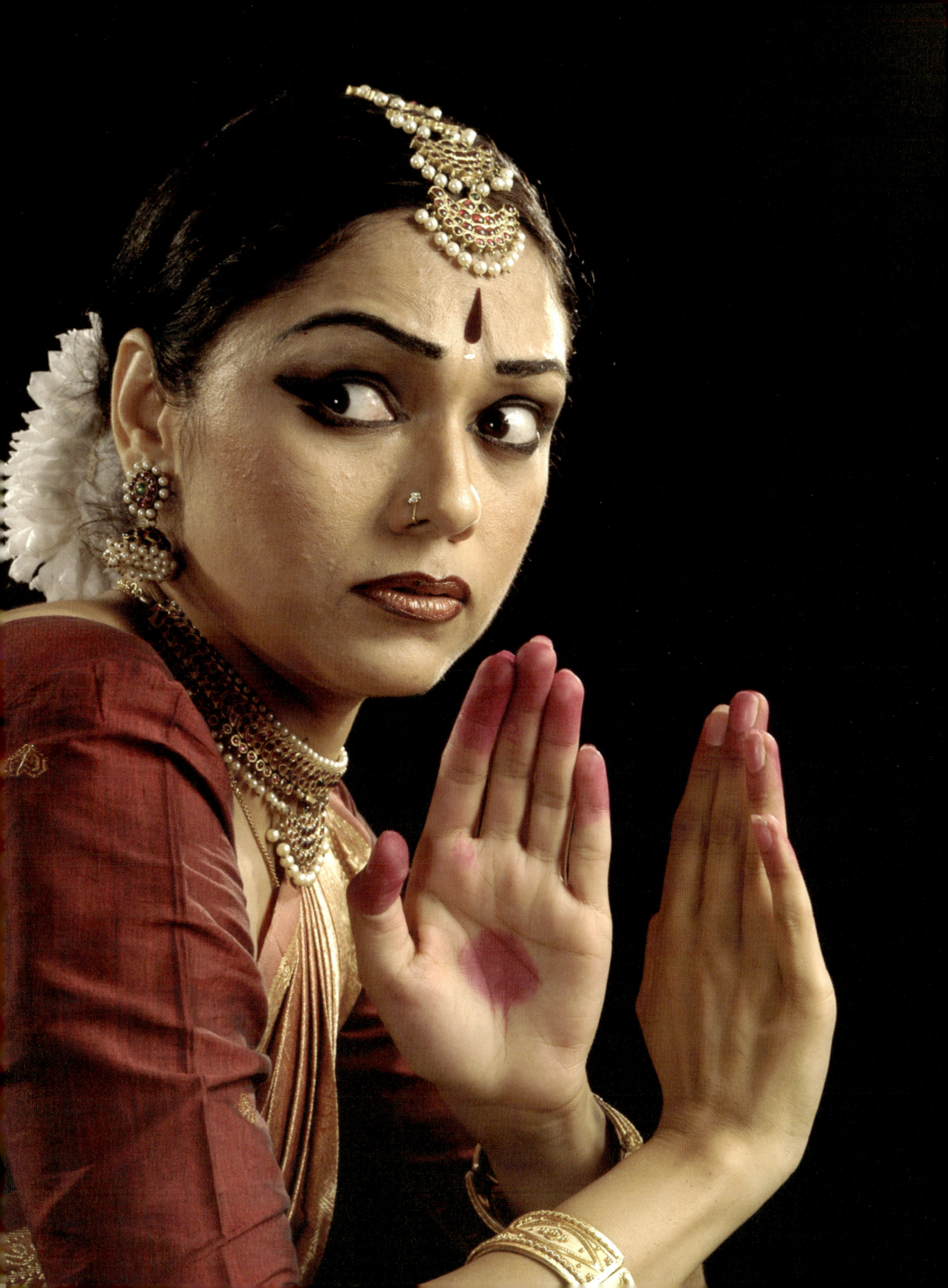

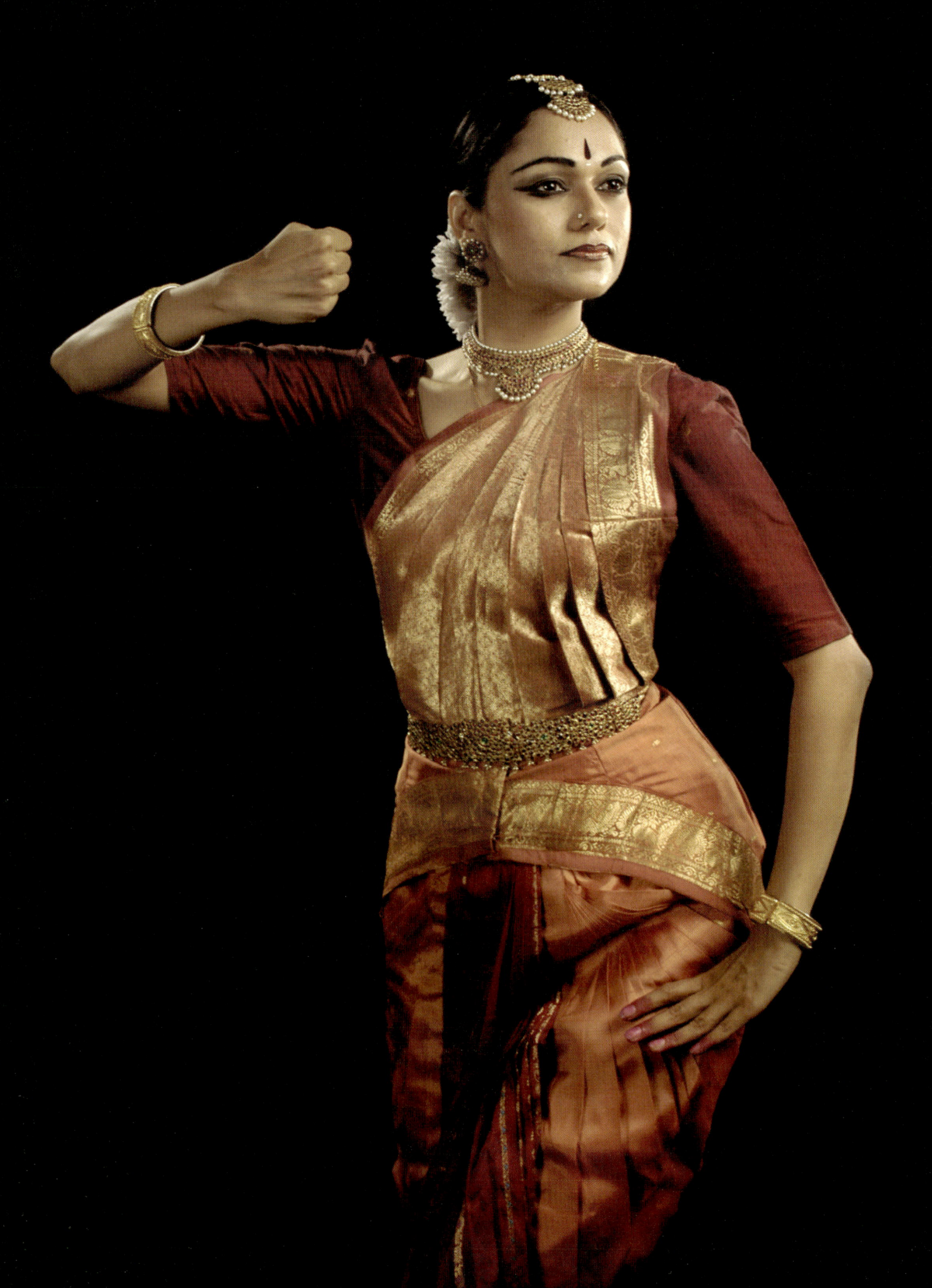

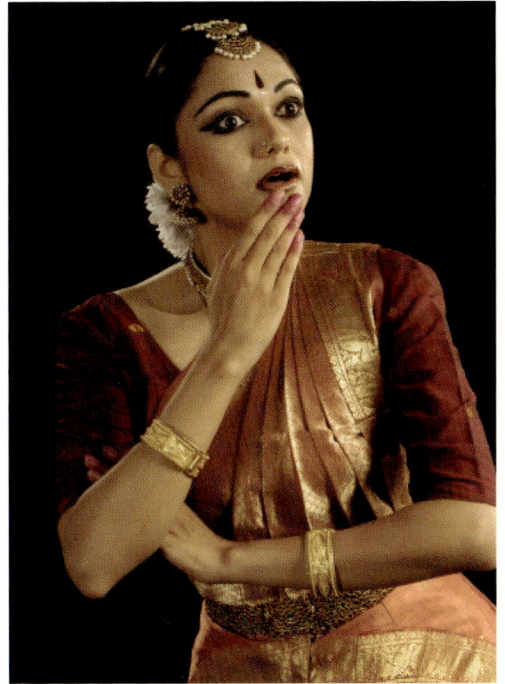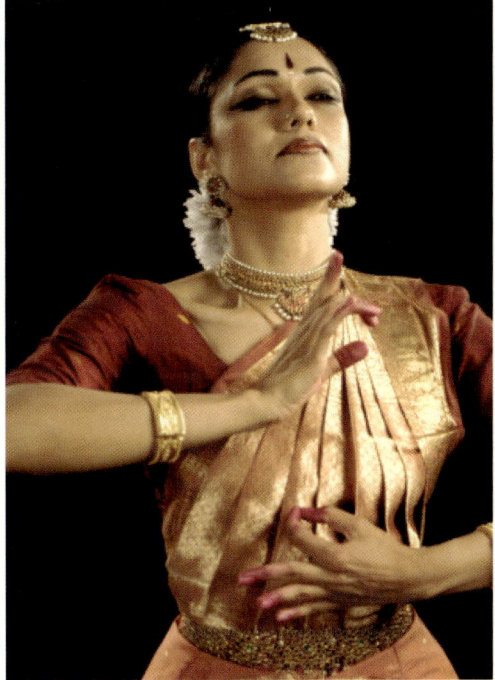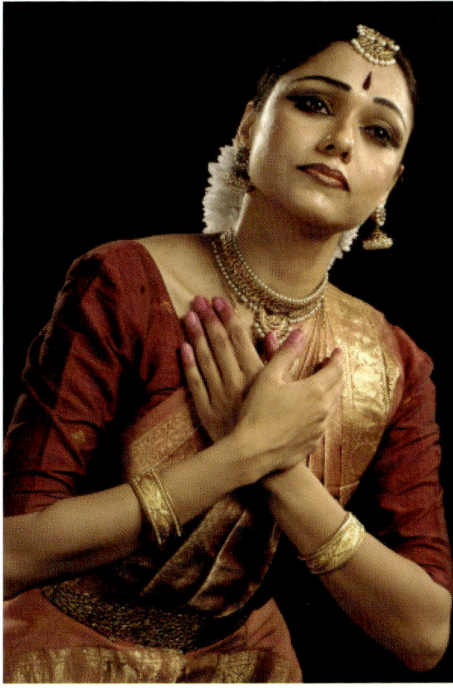

Adbhuta, Shanta and Karuna rasas—Rama Vaidyanathan

(Page 24) Vira rasa—Rama Vaidyanathan

the resultant feelings are of injustice, humiliation, revenge or envy. It may be experienced by good or evil characters, people from all walks of life, and by human and immortal beings. Raudra gives rise to the desire to avenge or defeat the enemy. An offshoot of this emotion is impatience. It is signified by the colour red and the god associated with this rasa is Rudra, the fierce god of storms in the Vedic hymns, who is also a manifestation of Shiva. Although musical texts do not mention this rasa in the evolution of ragas, it is reflected as a mood in drama and musical performances, and can be found in significant episodes of Ramayana and Mahabharata.

Vira or the heroic sentiment is characterized by valour, power combined with patience, and heroism with steadiness, tact and energy. Arising from this rasa are complementary feelings of confidence, pride and determination. Vira is the energy associated with those who are in a high position of authority and of virtuous character. Its colour is yellow and its guiding divinity is Indra, god of the heavens, who rules the celestial kingdom. In musical ragas the sentiment of vira is suggested through the challenging counterpoints between melody and rhythm that galvanize energy and strength.

Bhayanaka or the sentiment of fear suggests panic and aversion. It is physiologically characterized by a trembling in the feet and hands, a change in skin colour and a loss of voice. This rasa is the inspiration for many theatrical and film performances. It is also the favourite of film music, especially in the

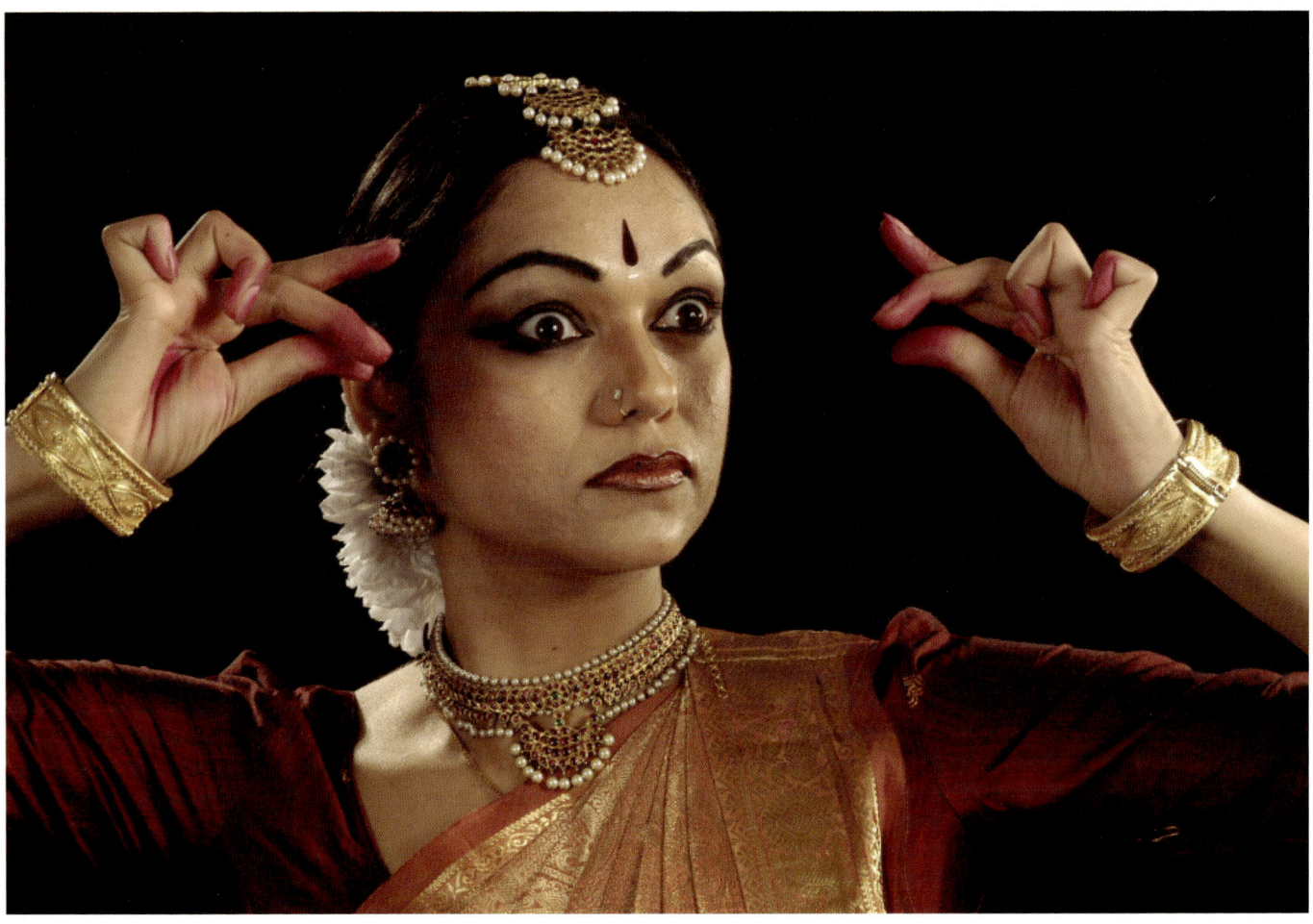

*Raudra rasa—
Rama Vaidyanathan*

*(Page 27)
Devi, Vijayanagara,
15th century, National
Museum, New Delhi*

melodramatic background scores. A favourite instrument used to create this suspenseful music is the theremin, an early electronic invention from Russia, which has a higher tone than a violin. Bhayanaka induces the suggestion of ghosts, devils and death; something that is more easily represented in painting and sculpture than in music. The associated colour of this rasa is black and the divinity is Kala, god of death and time.

Bibhatsa evokes disgust, hatred and odium. It repels the subject, and often arises out of feeling offended, or an argument that causes one to be disturbed or hurt. The body can be immobile or agitated. Feelings of nausea and repugnance arise, leading to unconsciousness, disillusionment, illness and death. It is like seeing or feeling annoyance, sensing the odours of a slaughterhouse or being compelled to close one's eyes during scenes of blood and gore in a film. Sometimes, however, feelings of repugnance can become delightful because of their power to excite the imagination. The safety of distance, or a psychic distance, often results in a pleasurable aesthetic experience. Bibhatsa is blue and the deity associated with it is Mahakala, an angry manifestation

26 *Shringara*—the many faces of Indian beauty

of Avalokiteshvara, the Bodhisattva who is known as an embodiment of compassion and wisdom, who is the protector of Buddhist law. Pictorial examples are found in the Tibetan tantric *tankhas*, that represent the wrathful manifestations of the protective divinities of the dharma (teachings) and the *sangha* (spiritual community). This rasa does not appear in the classical music of India, but can be found in other visual and performance arts.

Adbhuta, or the sentiment of wonder and the marvellous, is inspired by a feeling of incredible surprise. It is associated with the fantastic, supernatural and the unknown. It is manifested by feelings of astonishment and excitement at an extraordinary event, sound or sight. This rasa is gold in colour and the deity is Gandharva, a male celestial being. Adbhuta is featured in images and sculptures of the gods, and finds a parallel in the surrealistic art of the early 20th century, Dadaism in particular. In the context of music it can be associated with the intellectual and abstract fascination produced by the avant-garde, modern music composed from the 1940s onwards. It is creative music that inspires detachment from the beauty of harmony, and at the same time nourishes the creative unconscious of archetypes, fantasies and novelties.

Shanta, the ninth rasa, is peace or inner serenity, an emotion experienced by one who has realized the emptiness, the vanity of all things, and achieved freedom from all desires and the material world. Shanta brings to mind holy hermitages, sacred places and shaded groves. It gives rise to happiness, mindfulness and kindness towards all beings. It is the sentiment associated with the ascetic or one who is on the spititual path.

Shanta rasa induces healing and calmness and is invoked by slow, meditative music. This rasa is linked to chanting and prayer. Unlike karuna, shanta does not imply devotion to humans, but rather a spiritual devotion. The colour that goes with it is white, that of the fragrant jasmine and the moon. The god of shanta is Narayana, the personification of Lord Vishnu's creative energy. The feelings conducive to this rasa are expressed in the pure melodic development of ragas (*alap*) that comes before the accompanying rhythm cycle (*tala*). Shanta is also suggested in some slow, evocative religious songs (bhajans). It is echoed in many forms of spiritual expression—the harmonic chanting of Tibetan monks, traditional mantras, syllables that are repeatedly sung to induce adoration and meditative states, and also the recitation of Vedas.

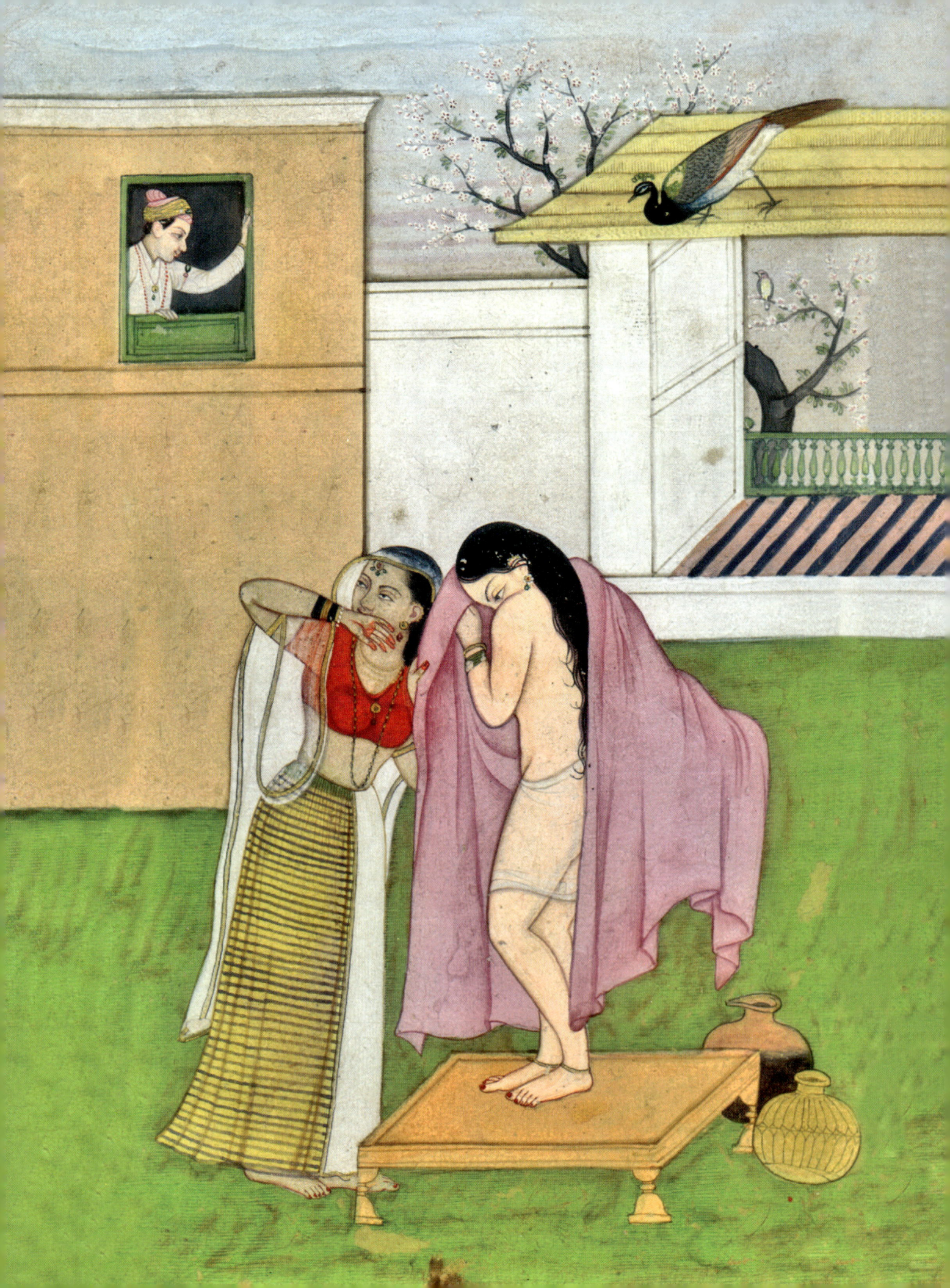

CHAPTER 3

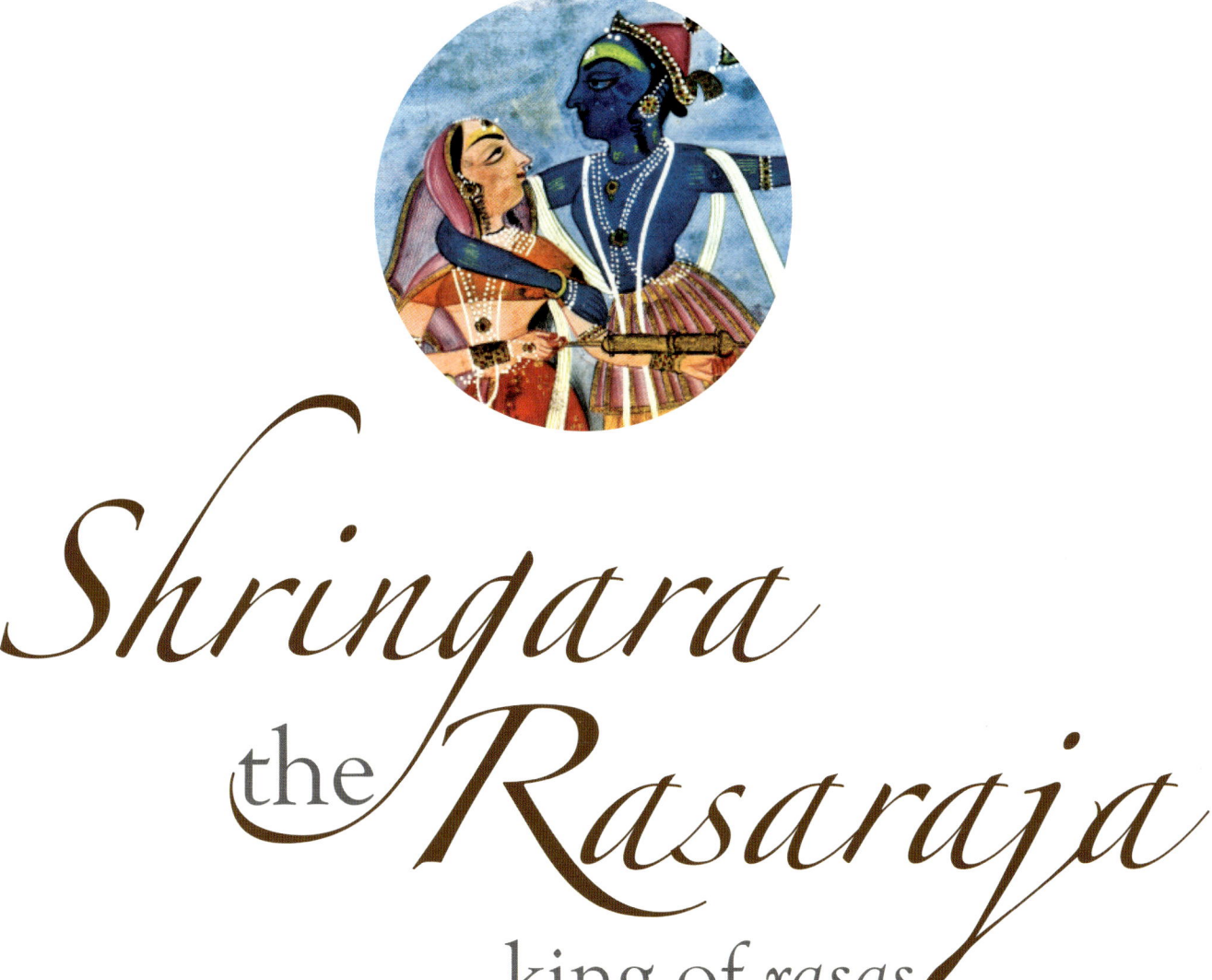

Shringara the Rasaraja
king of rasas

In India the union of the male and female has become the symbol, from the earliest times, for the union of all cosmic forces and the pleasure of the body in mating became, under accepted religious doctrines and social norms, linked with the sanctity of procreation and an end in itself. The concept of the original sin and sexual secretiveness never formed any part of the intense phrases of Indian culture.

MULK RAJ ANAND

(Page 28)
*'Lady Bathing in Courtyard',
Guler Kalam, Pahari, 1790,
N.C. Mehta Collection,
Ahmedabad*

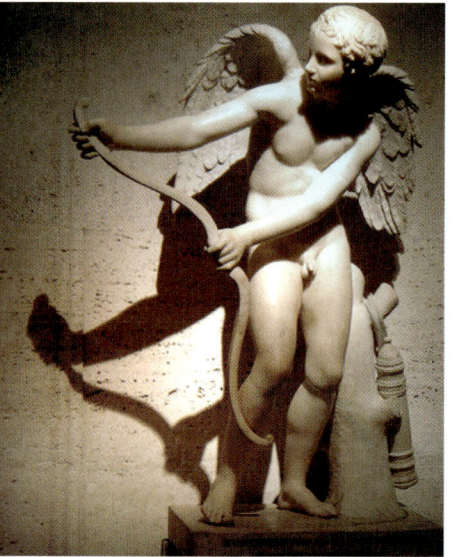

*Cupid, the Roman god of
erotic love. In contemporary
culture he is the personification
of love and courtship*

*(Below)
An 18th-19th century
painting depicting Kamadeva,
the Indian god of love. His
bow is made of sugarcane and
the arrows of fragrant flowers*

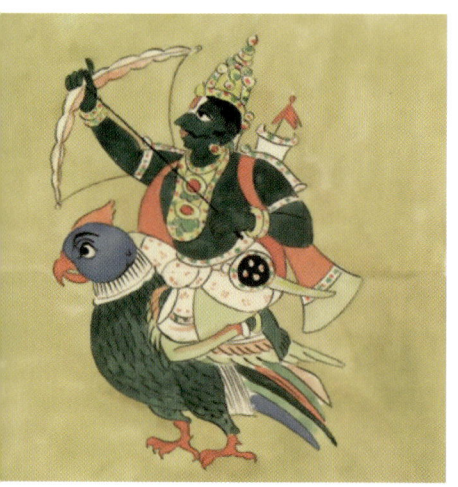

That which is amatory, stimulating, sexual; that which is between the romantic and the lascivious; that which evokes the shringar rasa and leads to the *vilasam* bhava (pleasure), which in turn leads to *maithuna* (sexual act) and ultimately to the state of ananda (bliss) is erotic.

Erotica is the name given to any artwork – written, pictorial or performed – that portrays sex explicitly yet possesses enough value to escape condemnation as pornography. The name derives from Eros, the Greek God of physical desire, whom the Romans called Cupid and the Hindus call Kama.
—**Academic American Encyclopaedia, University of Michigan**

The word erotica has its root in the Greek word 'eros', which means passionate and sensual love, and is also the name for the Greek god of love. The Hindus in North India call him Kama or Kamadeva and his foibles have, over the centuries, provided inspiration for artists and poets alike. In South India, he is known as Manmatha, whose arrows of love are a perfect parallel to those of Cupid. The shared metaphors of Indo-Greek literature and mythology are evidence of the close relationship between the two diverse ancient cultures.

In India, erotic symbolism is to be found in every facet of the social and cultural fabric from ancient to contemporary times. The openness of society can be seen in the explicitly erotic sculptures of the Khajuraho temples, and in articles of daily use like shringara combs and ornamented mirror frames. Most importantly, there are the detailed, almost clinical, treatises on physical love in its various forms, the best known of which is *Kamasutra*. Among others are *Koka Shastra, Anangaranga, Nimmat Nama*, the Aham poetry of the Tamil Kingdom, the Sanskrit poetry of Kalidasa, as well as the bold mention of physical desire in many musical and dance compositions, and in poetry. There is also an overt, as well as subtle, mention of the erotic in the love poetry of the Bhakti era.

A Way of Life
In a broad study of the world's religious traditions, it becomes evident that the erotic was an integral part of every society's culture. Sexuality and spirituality are inextricably linked to the mythology and texts of ancient India. The inevitable expression of the erotic finds its way in the various mythical tales and treatises on love and sex. Kalidasa's *Ritusamhara* established a sensual contact between the erotic and nature. Indian artists accepted the sensual and erotic as an integral part of life and dealt with it accordingly in their carvings, paintings and writing, manifesting the shringara rasa in several ways. To Western eyes schooled by Victorian standards, such imagery may appear offensive. Unless one is familiar with the ideals that governed the Indian mind, one cannot fully

appreciate erotic art and its representations. Indian art, born in a land 'teeming with gods and legends', is deeply rooted in philosophy and religion and more often than not, in its varied expressions. There is a sublime urge to search beyond.

Myths are the collective experiences of a society conveyed through the words of philosophers and saints. The tales, metaphors and symbols act as mirrors and interact with man on the archetypal level, reminding him that all life's processes are nothing more than *leela* or 'the divine play of the gods'. These ancient tales hold the key to the unconscious desires of people. Desire and delight are stages of initiation and kama, the consciousness of pleasure, arises from contact. Man must realise himself through kama, artha and dharma to reach moksha.

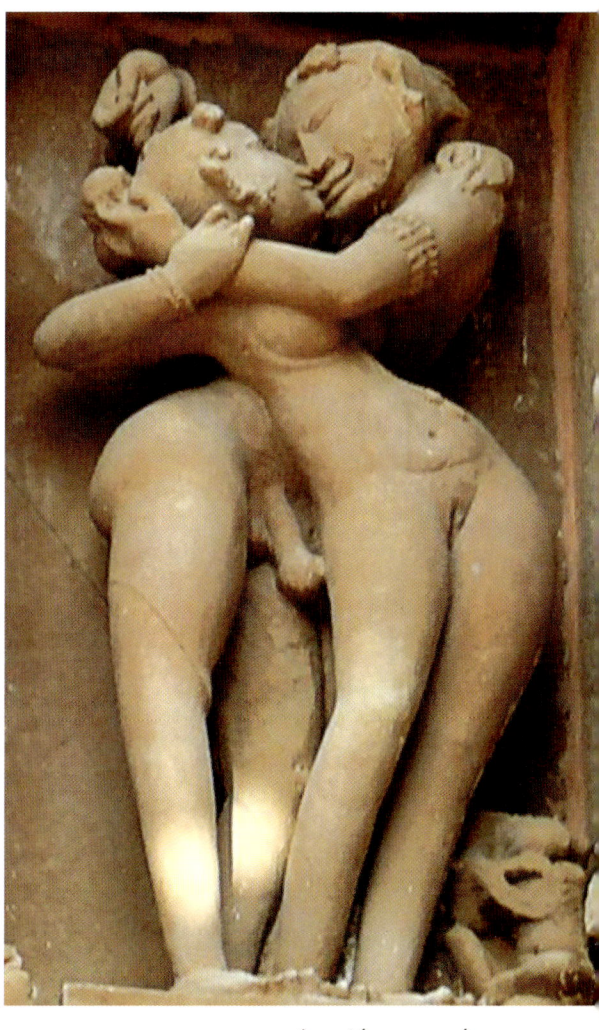

A maithuna couple, Lakshmana Temple, Khajuraho

> *Man, the period of whose life is one hundred years, should practise Dharma, Artha and Kama at different times and in such a manner that they may harmonize together and not clash in any way. He should acquire learning in his childhood, in his youth and middle age he should attend to Artha and Kama, and in his old age he should perform Dharma, and thus seek to gain Moksha, i.e. release from further transmigration.*
>
> *Dharma is the stability of society, the maintenance of social order, and the general welfare of mankind, and whatever leads to the fulfilment of this purpose. It is the obedience to the command of the Shastras, holy writ to the Hindus, to do certain things, such as the performance of sacrifices, which are not generally done because they do not belong to this world and produce no visible effect; and not to do other things such as eating meat, which is often done because it belongs to this world, and has a visible effect. Dharma should be learnt from the shruti, Vedas and from those conversant with it.*
>
> *Artha is the foundation upon which the whole structure of life is built and it is only in its fulfilment that the other purusharthas can be achieved. It is the acquisition of arts, land, gold, cattle, wealth, and friends. It is, further, the protection of what is acquired, and the increase of what is protected. Artha should be learnt from the kings, officers and from merchants who may be versed in the ways of commerce. Artha should always be first practised by the king for the livelihood of men is to be obtained from it only.*
>
> —***Kamasutra of Vatsyayana*, Sir Richard Burton**

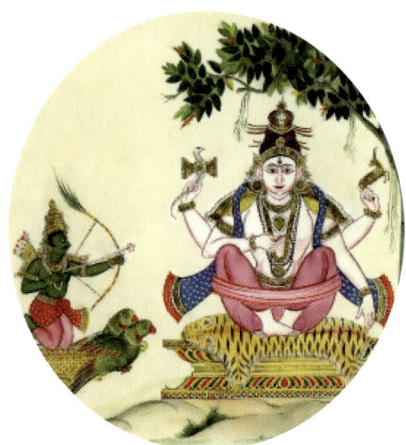

Kamadeva aiming his arrow at Shiva, Tanjore painting, c. 1820

A couple at Parsvanath Temple, Khajuraho

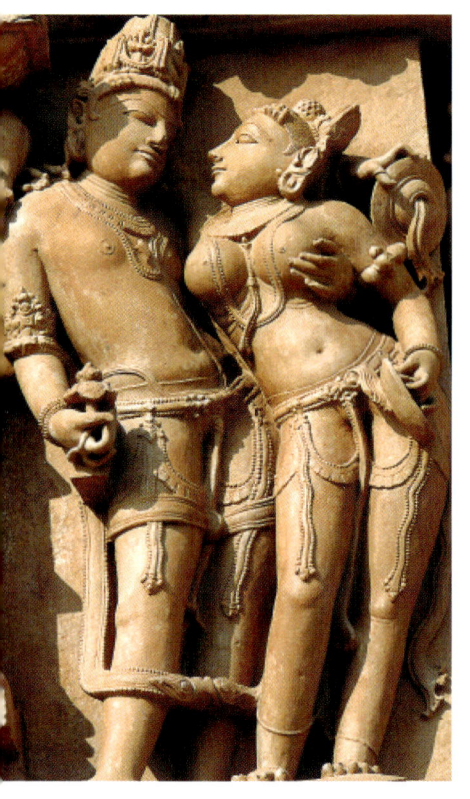

Kama is love, pleasure and sensual gratification. Kama is all desire that stirs the mind. It is the enjoyment of appropriate objects by the five senses of hearing, feeling, sight, taste and smell, assisted by the mind together with the soul. The principal ingredient in kama is a peculiar contact between the organ of sense and its object, and the consciousness of pleasure which arises from that contact.

Kama in the Scriptures

In *Atharva Veda*, kama is exalted as the supreme god and creator. In *Taittriya Upanishad* of *Yajur Veda*, *kama* is the first animator from whom space was created out of the stillness. *Bhagvad Gita* explains that kama is located in three places: the mind, senses and intellect. Desire begins by an enticement of the senses. Desire breeds a sense of incompleteness. Kama means desire of varying degrees.

According to *Kamasutra*, when dharma, artha and kama come together, it is dharma which is better than artha, followed finally by kama. Artha and kama result from the ultimate dharma. Artha and kama satisfy a human's psychological cravings and make up the dual core of the aspirations of every individual.

Central to Indian philosophy is the concept of moksha, which literally means the soul's deliverance from bondage. Our great philosophers argue that so long as the soul is imprisoned in the body and trapped in its material form, it will not be free from pain and sorrow. Such suffering is of three kinds: *adhi-bhautika* (originating from the body), *adhi-atmika* (originating from the mind) and *adhi-daivika* (that which is god-made). Moksha results from the extinction of false knowledge, which causes the extinction of lust and hate. Moksha extinguishes all sorrow, all karmas, and results in the cessation of rebirth.

Kamasutra aims to provide its readers, both men and women, with a 'guidebook', encyclopaedic in its scope, replete with detailed advice, that sets the framework in which erotic experiences are to be viewed. Side-by-side it also elucidates the social and moral underpinnings of the subject.

Ancient scriptures stand witness to the importance of the erotic in the Hindu way of life. The *rishis* (ancient Hindu seers) held the belief that within the womb is the red seed known as *rajas* (the counterpart of the white male seed known as *shukra*). The rajas wraps the soul in flesh and blood, while the shukra, besides being the medium for the soul, is also the source for the bones. Pleasure is one of the four aims of life in the Hindu cosmology, and it must be realized as fully as possible to attain the highest summits of sensual experience. It must also be realized in order to reach transcendental consciousness, the final aim of life, for which life itself is

32 *Shringara*—the many faces of Indian beauty

necessary. The body is thus the instrument, and the basis of all realization. The body's activities stem from desire that needs to be fulfilled, whether this need emanates from thirst, hunger, tiredness or sexual desire. The fulfilment of needs is intertwined with pleasure; and manifests itself as a form of pleasure. Mahabharata says, 'Without a taste for pleasure, even a rich Brahman would not eat fine food; without a taste for pleasure, he will ignore the joys of the body. This is why pleasure is the basis of all the other aims of life. And to attain a state of joy and permanent happiness, man must not forget the body that helps in the fulfilment of his destiny.'

Ananda—the Ultimate Pleasure

The extreme sensation of pleasure was, therefore, considered a reflection of the infinite ecstasy of the individual united with the universal or divine being. The female sex played a crucial part in this equation:

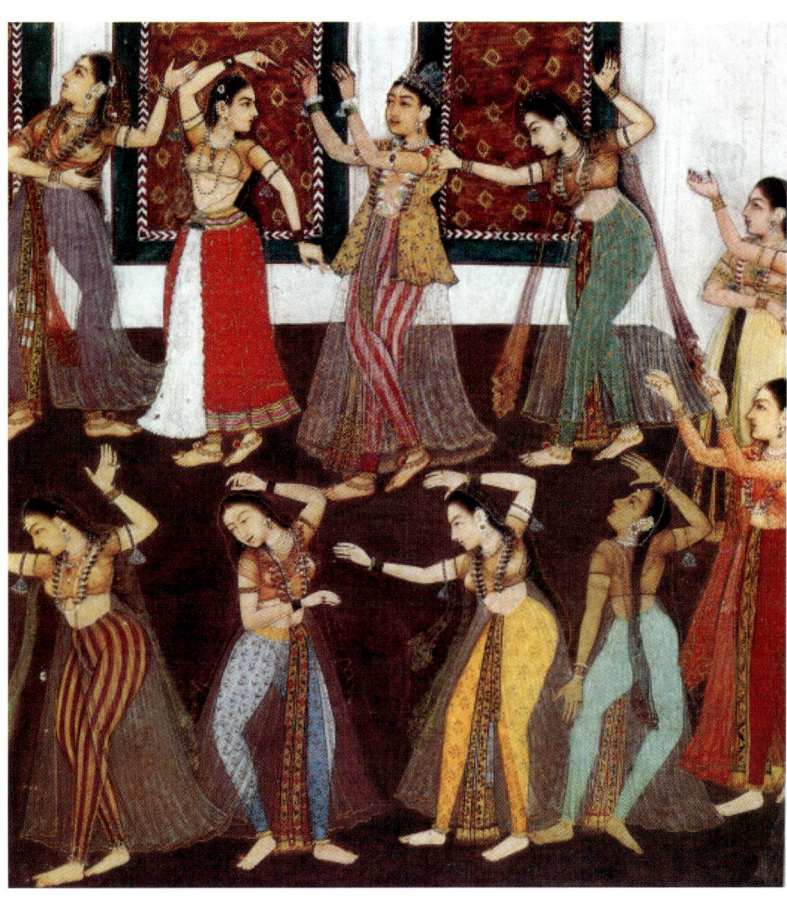

Celebration of New Year at the court of Shah Jahan, Mughal 1645. Paintings acquired a romantic flavour during Shah Jahan's time

in the Hindu pantheon, the various gods enjoy their existence and the ability to manifest themselves only when united with their corresponding feminine counterpart, their *shakti* or power. Talking of the *Shaiva Siddhanta* tradition, Alain Danielou in his book *Gods of Love and Ecstasy* says that 'Woman is the image of nature (Prakriti), and man the image of being (Purusha). When they unite, they dissolve into divine unity.' The uniting of the phallus (*lingam*) and the *yoni* (the female sex organ) is the very symbol of the divine being's creative potential, as well as the cosmic and physical reality of creation. This union was the beginning and end of existence and the cause of its continuation. Because of its symbolic and creative value, the sexual act was a most important ritual and was performed as a rite. All other rites were but its image and symbolically reproduced the original union—Agni, the God of fire and the male principle, burned in the *kunda*, the altar-hearth and image of the female principle. Upanishads interpreted all aspects of the sacrificial ritual as stages in the act of love.

The erotic search in this context translates into a basic and primal human expression. Sex is not considered outside the domain of religion. On the contrary, all religious conceptions emphasize the importance of the sexual force.

Shaivites, similar to the proponents of Dionysian orgy, consider erotic ecstasy not just a means of reproduction but also an inherent search for pleasure. In his aforementioned book, Danielou quotes from *Shiva Purana*, *Vidyeshvara Samhita*: 'The phallus is the source of pleasure. It is the sole means of obtaining earthly pleasure and salvation. By looking at it, touching it, and meditating on it, living beings are capable of freeing themselves from the cycle of future lives.' The yoni completes the picture of the creative element. It has been variously revered in the scriptures. 'The yoni represents the womb of the visible and the subtle world.' *(Yajur Veda)*. 'Because it is the origin of all life, nature is comparable to a womb.' *(Shiva Purana.)*

In Hindu ideology, the conflict between the ascetic and the erotic, passion and indifference, and birth and death is best expressed by the myth of the burning of Kama, the god of desire, by the ascetic god Shiva. Kama was called upon to distract Shiva, because the latter's resolve to remain an ascetic was considered inimical to the continuity of life. A close parallel is found in Buddhism where Buddha's ascetic powers posed a similar threat as he sat meditating beneath the Bodhi tree. Mara (Kama), the god of both desire and death, along with his bevy of beautiful *apsaras*, was sent by the gods to tempt the Buddha away from his meditation. The conflict was overcome by sublimating sensual pleasure into a higher state of transcendental pleasure, rather than by denying its importance or existence totally.

Early Gita Govinda *(Song of Govinda) illustration, Gujarat, N.C. Mehta Collection, Ahmedabad. The* Gita Govinda *was a work composed by the poet Jayadeva. It describes the relationship between Krishna and the gopis of Vrindavan, and, in particular, with Radha*

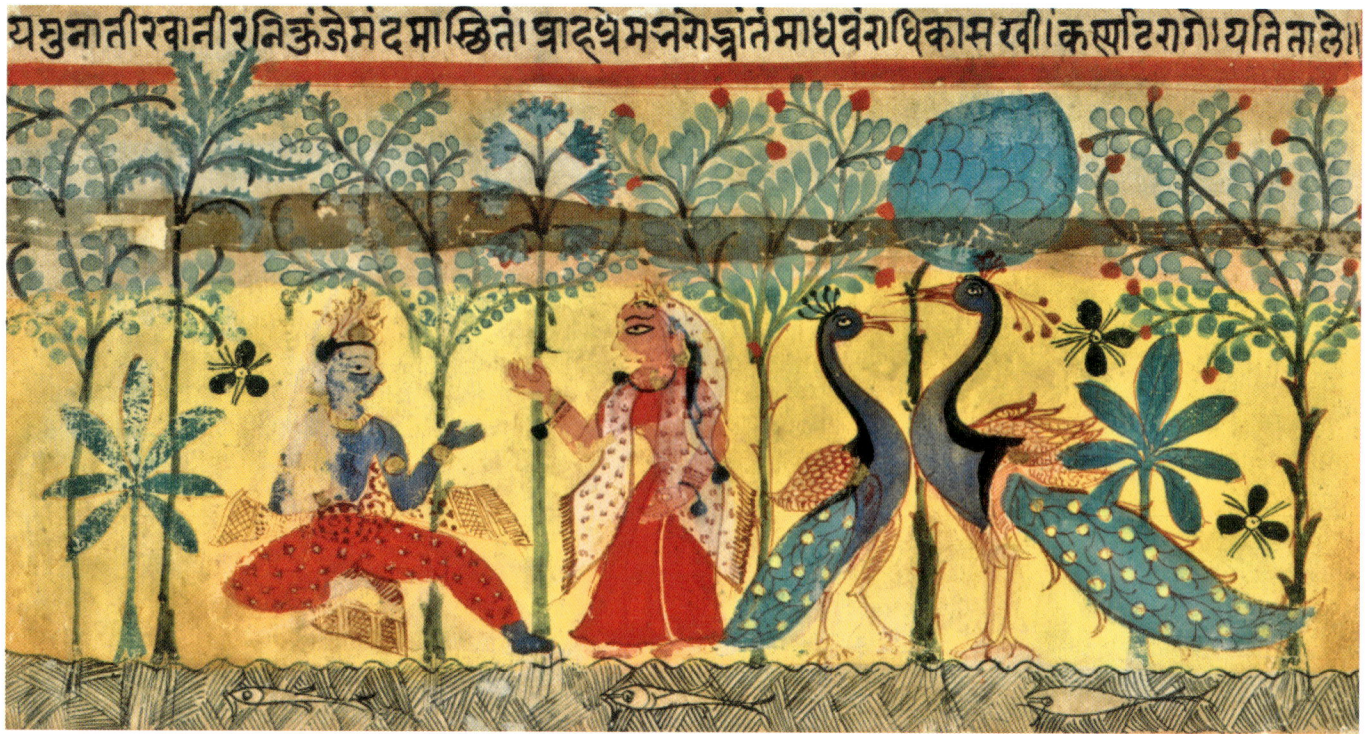

34 *Shringara*—the many faces of Indian beauty

While humans seek *sukha* (happiness) as the short-term and immediate goal, the penultimate aim is to achieve *mahasukha* (literally 'greatest happiness' or bliss). Buddhist philosophy has popularized the term mahasukha, while in texts this state is described as ananda, also synonymous with Parabrahma, or the Supreme Being. The blissful state of ananda (*anandaghana*) can be arrived at through a dual path of mystical and aesthetic experience.

Indian mythology is replete with stories of the gods enjoying intense amorous dalliances. However shringara, the greatest of all rasas, is best depicted by the legend of Radha and Krishna. Their relationship embodies the highest and purest love, passion and devotion that unite both the sacred and the profane. The *nayika* or heroine, dressing herself in anticipation of her lover, has been a recurrent image in the illustrated texts elaborating on shringara rasa. The image symbolizes the erotic, and the metaphor of divine love, through the human sexual act. Shringara bhava lends itself beautifully to the final goal of artistic expression, as well as of amorous love, that of union. And God becomes the Supreme lover and every devotee a nayika seeking union with Him.

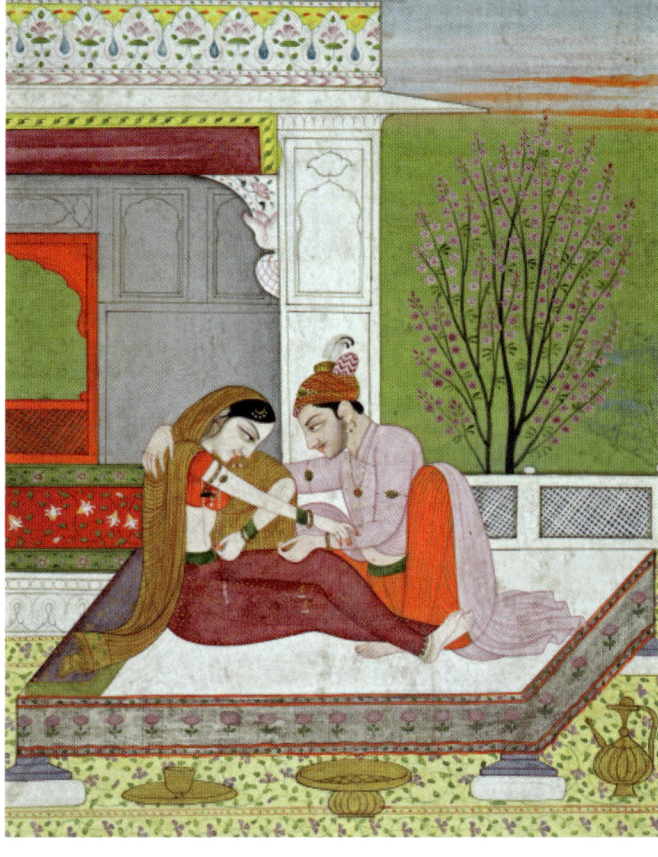

Love scene, Pahari-Guler, Chandigarh Museum

The Flowering of the Nayika

In his *Rasikapriya*, Keshavadas (c.1590) vividly describes the Vasaksajja nayika: 'O Sakhi, the Nayika, resembling the flame of a lamp, ran to hide herself in the grove of sandal trees entwined by lovely clove creepers of undimmed leaves where she conceals the lustre of her limbs in her blue garment. Startled on hearing the sound of wind, water, birds and animals, she looks around with eagerness for union with her beloved. Waiting for Krishna in the bower she looks like a caged bird.'

A Bundi painting illustrates this quite beautifully. We see the nayika seated on a bed of flowers amidst sandal trees entwined in flowering creepers. In the foreground are pairs of water birds. A peacock spreads its dazzling tail feathers before his mate, and on the side are deer in pairs. The animated scene reflects the nayika's desperate desire to meet her lover. Another Bundi painting, *Kamoda Ragini*, shows a beautiful lady seated on a bed of white jasmine. Clumps of bananas in the background and their swaying phallic-shaped leaves are suggestive of the nayika's unfulfilled desire.

Painters of the Kangra School of miniature painting symbolize the erotic very subtly and often used the *ashtanayika* listed by Keshavadas as symbols of the several stages of love. They are *abhisarika* who represents the aroused nayika; *kalahantarika*, the repentant one; *khandita* who symbolizes annoyance; *proshitapathika* who represents longing; *swadheenapathika*, the desired one; *vasakasajika*, the expectant lover; *virahotkantita*, who is separated from her lover and *vipralabda*, the disappointed one. The nayika who appears most frequently in Kangra art is abhisarika. The woman is dressed in blue in a jungle full of snakes creeping on the ground. The cobra emerging from a hole in a tree symbolizes the nayika's yearning to unite with her lover. The artists of Kangra also poignantly portray the *virahini nayikas*, the lovelorn women, represented with their pets, such as blackbucks, parrots, moon-pheasants and pigeons. The male animals and birds are symbolic of the absent lover or husband. The sight of a pair of sporting pigeons makes the nayika pine for her lover. The *madhavi* creeper entwined around the trunk of a mango tree is a subtle reference to the union of lovers.

Folk songs also express the pathos of the lonely wife separated from her husband. Nature sympathizes with her and as she weeps, mountains and rivers share her grief, and the trees shed their leaves. The mango blossoms and the love calls of the *koels* make her all the more miserable. The mango tree has been a significant erotic symbol in paintings as well as in poetry. Ripe mangoes are used as an analogy for a woman's full breasts. A colourful painting shows a lovesick lady standing on the balcony of her palace watching a flight of white cranes. A joyous peacock hails the dark monsoon clouds, while in the foreground are mango trees laden with fruit. *Raginis*, or the wives of ragas, are frequently portrayed as lovelorn heroines in the *Ragamala* paintings.

(Page 37)
Krishna and Radha playing Holi with sakhis, Bikaner, N.C. Mehta Collection, Ahmedabad

(Below)
Radha and Krishna in the Nayak-Nayika set, a Rajasthani miniature

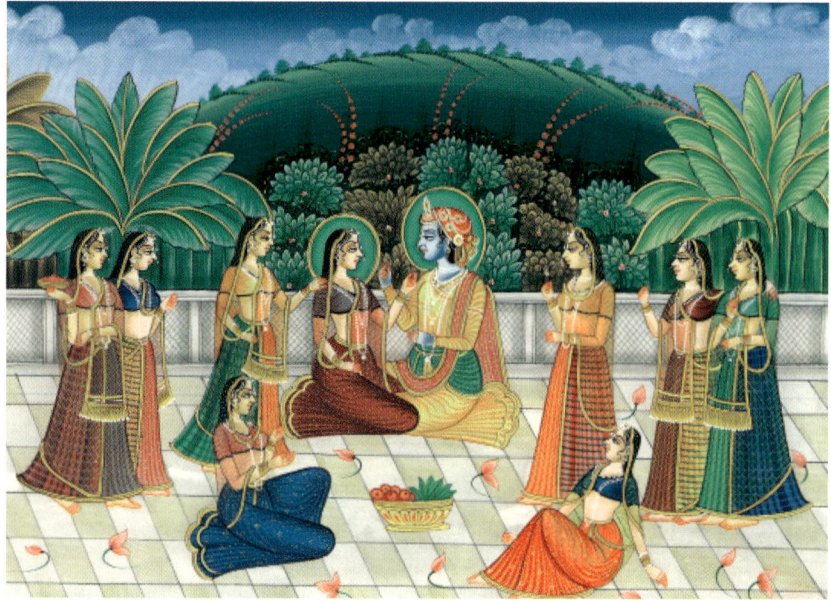

In the erotic paintings of Guler the elements most conducive to lovemaking are portrayed. A young prince and his beautiful wife are lying on a bed facing one another. They press their thighs and arms against each other. In front of the pavilion is a pool with lotus flowers, while on the roof is a peacock, symbol of the lover. In the crowns of the trees in the foreground are pairs of lovebirds. After a long summer, the rainy season (*sawan*) comes as a welcome relief, enhancing the physical desire of lovers. As Keshavadas says:

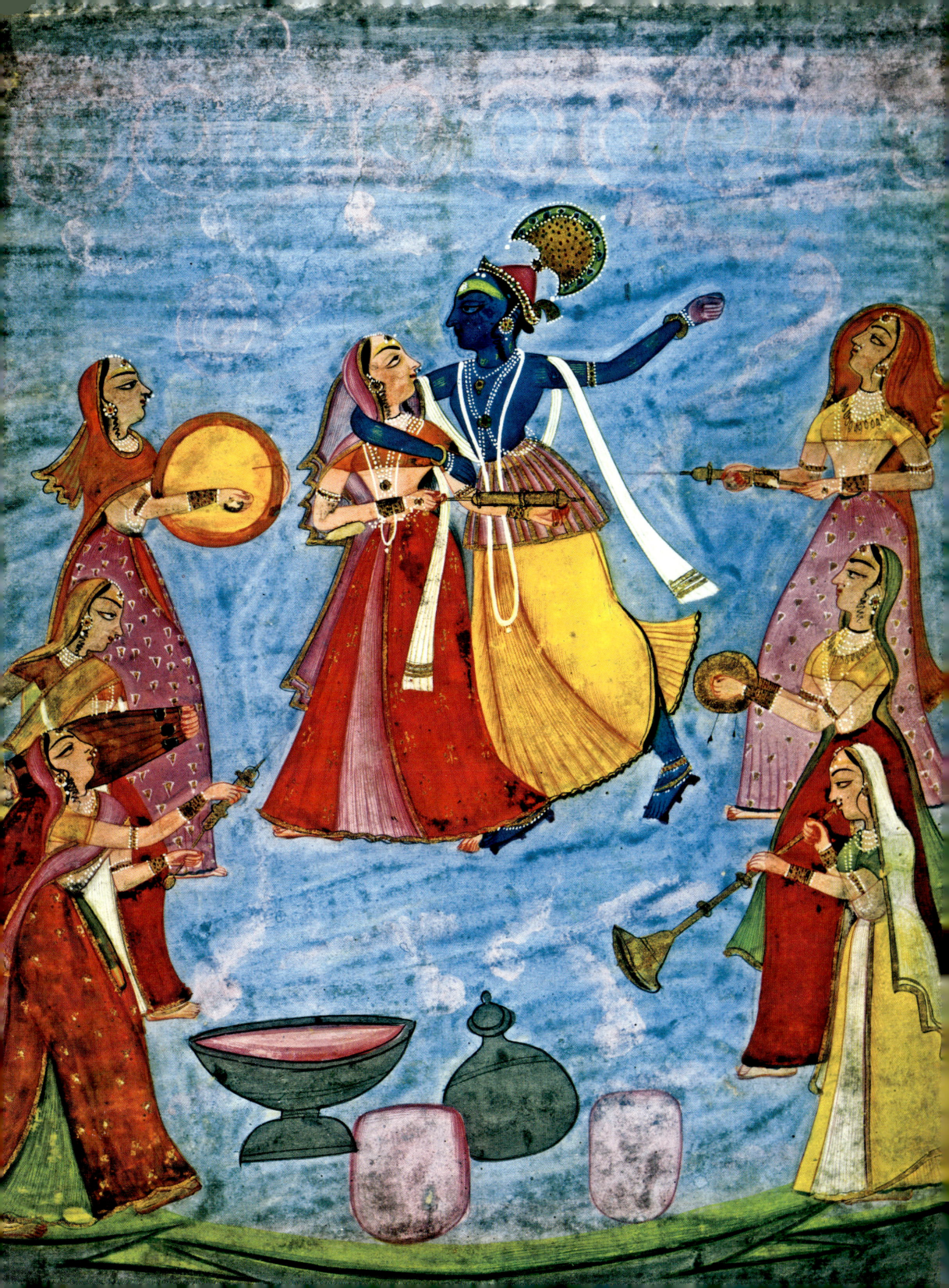

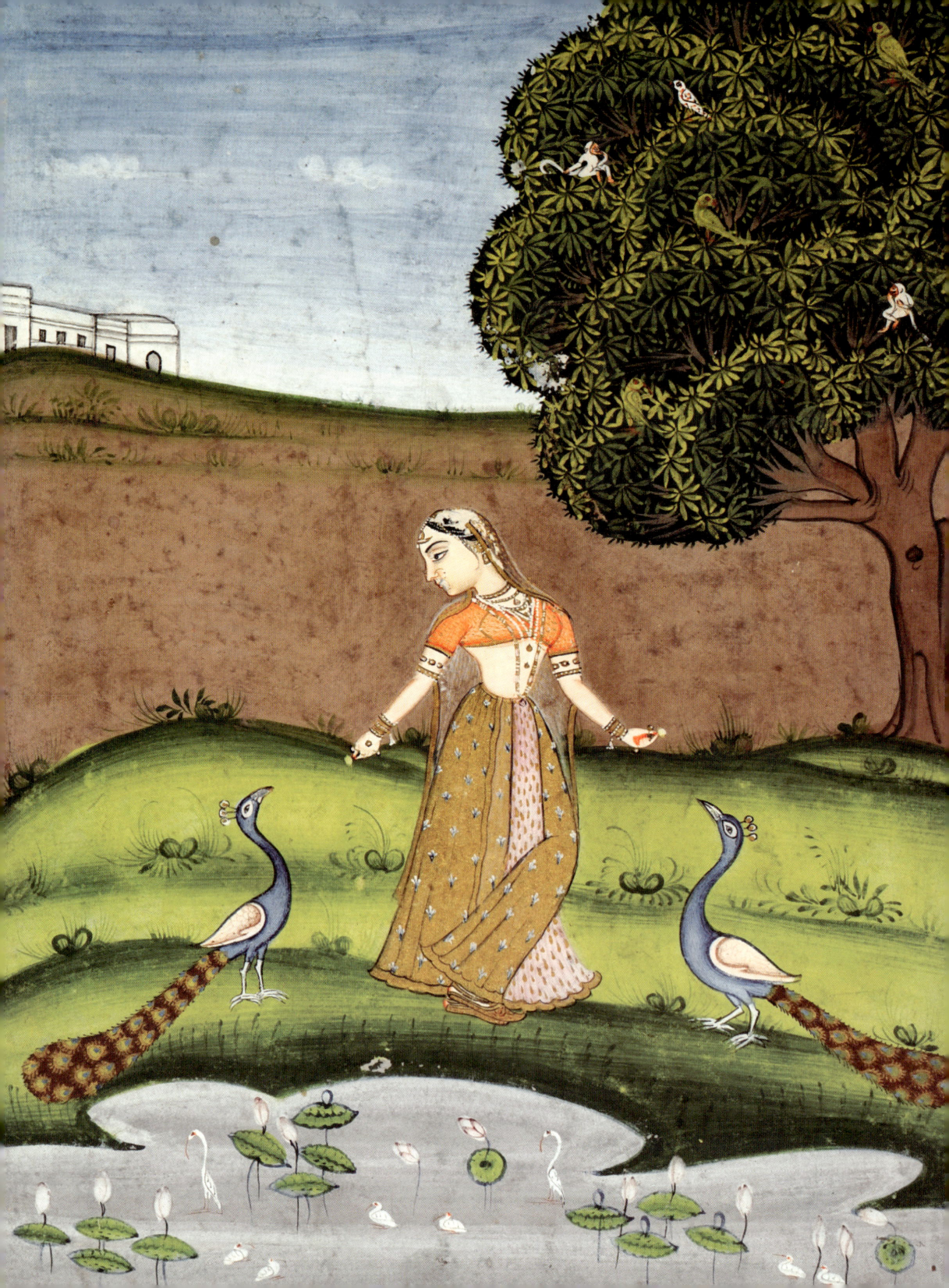

The creepers enchant the eye, embracing young trees lovingly.
The lightning flashes restlessly as she sports with rolling clouds.
The peacocks with their shrill cries announce the mating of the earth and sky.
All lovers meet in this month of sawan.

The creeper is the symbol of a woman, frail and tender, winding around the trunk of a tree, the symbol of man. The metaphors of beauty and the erotic in poetry, music, painting, sculpture and dance are derived from the artist's surroundings. And nature itself provides, in poetically symbolic terms, a description of a woman's orgasm:

Clouds are floating in the sky and the moon is, as if, coursing haltingly. The pigeon is cooing; the cluster of stars is drooping down and the lustre of the heavenly Ganges is tremulous.

Divine Ecstasy

With the spread of the Bhakti movement, erotic feelings were expressed as an outpouring of love towards a personal and intimate god. *Bhagavata Purana* and *Harivamsha* established the romantic tradition of *shringara-bhakti*, or ecstatic devotion. Krishna, the grandest god of the Hindu pantheon, is extolled as the beloved of Radha, and with the development of Krishna Bhakti, the poets portrayed him as a romantic hero. Erotic expression was depersonalized and universalized, bringing about a harmonious relationship between spirituality and sensuality. Sri Chaitanya, absorbed in the consciousness of Lord Krishna, and singing bhajans to the deity, was filled with divine ecstasy. Mirabai was a devotee of her beloved Krishna and composed many songs expressing her heartfelt longing for union with Govinda, or Krishna. She sang:

O my mind,
Worship the lotus feet of the Indestructible One!
Whatever thou seest twixt earth and sky
Will perish.

Bhaktikaal, or the period in which the Bhakti movement was the strongest, is known as the golden age of medieval Hindi literature because of the shringara rasa and the beauty of the concepts that were portrayed, and the words chosen to present them. Kabir writes about the Bhakti path:

The bhakti path winds in a delicate way.
On this path there is no asking and no not asking.
The ego simply disappears
the moment you touch him.
The joy of looking for him is so immense that you just dive in,

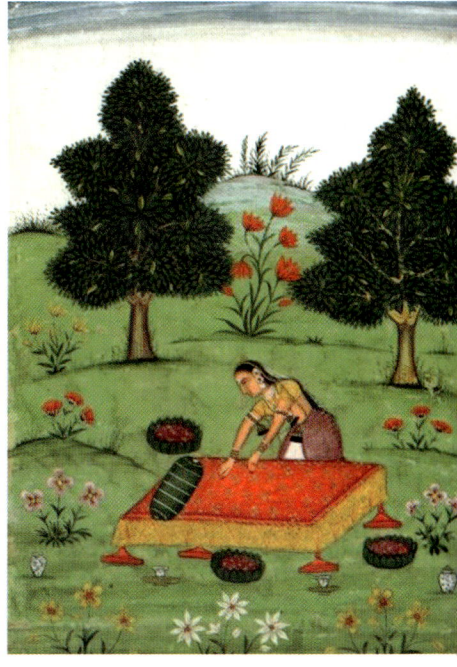

Malasri Ragini,
Ragamala painting,
1620, Rajasthan

(Page 38)
Kukambh Ragini,
Ragamala painting,
Jaipur, Chandigarh Museum

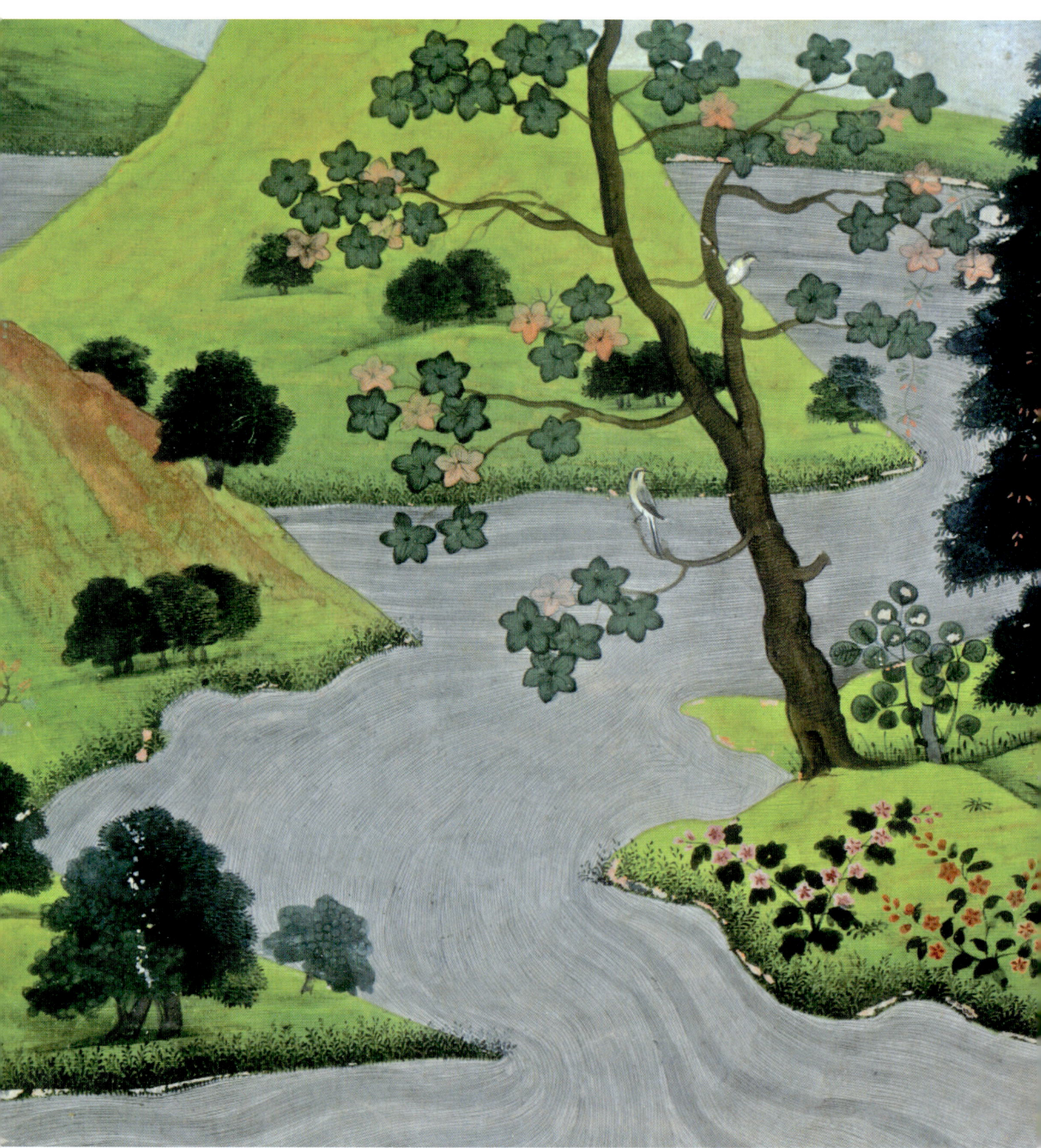

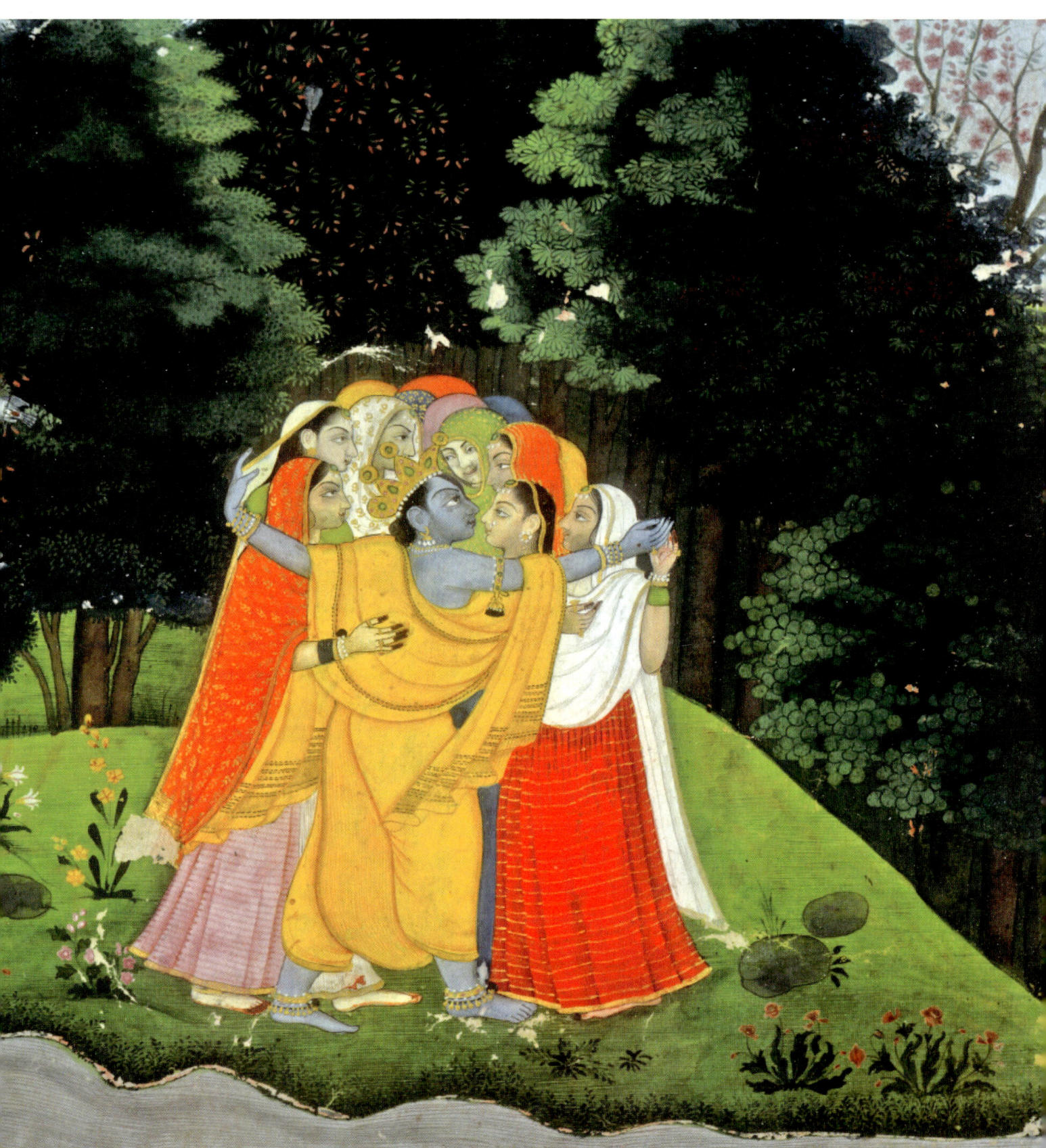

Shringara—the *Rasaraja*, king of *rasas*   41

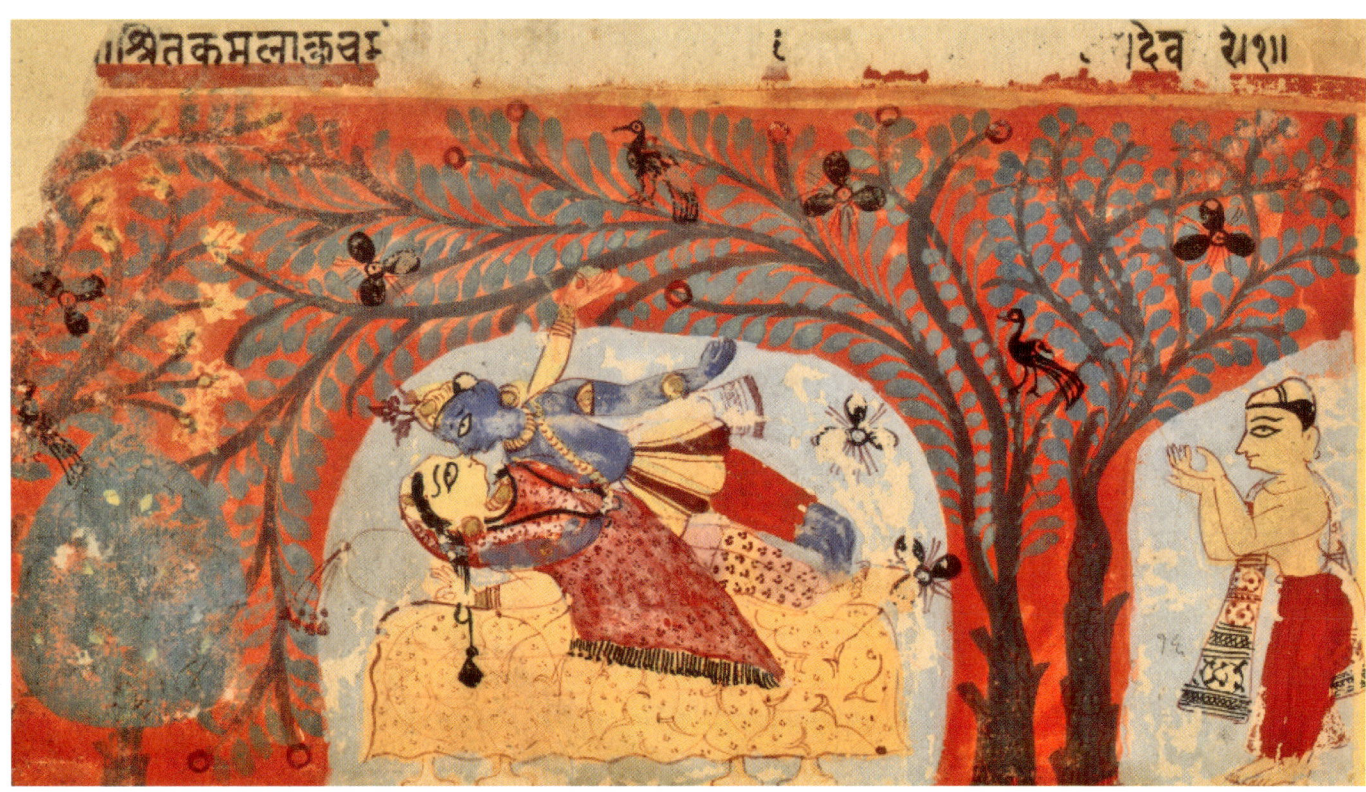

Early Gita Govinda, *16th century, N.C. Mehta Collection, Ahmedabad*

(Page 40-41)
Krishna embracing gopis, folio from Gita Govinda, *Guler Kalam, Pahari Miniature, N.C. Mehta Collection, Ahmedabad*

(Page 43)
'Khajuraho 1', oil and charcoal on canvas, painting by Kanchan Chander

and coast around like a fish in the water.
If anyone needs a head, the lover leaps up to offer his.

Jayadeva's *Gita Govinda*, written in the 12th century, is a highly spiritual work and very much part of Bhakti poetry. It is sung in temples dedicated to Lord Krishna and is quite passionately erotic:

Friend, bring Kesi's sublime tormentor to revel with me!
I've gone mad with waiting for his fickle love to change.
The enchanting flute in his hand
Lies fallen under coy glances;
Sweat of love wets his cheeks;
His bewildered face is smiling.
When Krishna sees me watching him
Playing in the forest
In a crowd of village beauties,
I feel the joy of desire.
Wind from a lakeside garden
Coaxing buds on new Asoka branches
Into clusters of scarlet flowers
Is only fanning the flames to burn me.

42   *Shringara*—the many faces of Indian beauty

*This mountain
Of new mango blossoms
Humming with roving bumblebees
Is no comfort to me now, friend.*

In the domain of *riti kalin* kavya or medieval Bhakti poetry, the feminine has also been adored, loved and worshipped.

*The brilliance of her body
dazzles the eyes.
What is the mirror's gleam, moonlight's glimmer
Or the lustre of the white lily before it?*

From the simplistic yearnings of a lover to the high-pitched longing of the *bhakta*, where both the object and subject are feminine in the form of nayika and *devi*, the exultation of love has been centered on the female form. Women are described as the ecstatic revelation of an external feature—haunting melodies and glorious sunsets, a lovely rustic belle flaunting her robust charms, wearing a necklace of strikingly colourful beads, her dark eyes smeared with kohl.

*Her eyebrows dance with pleasure filled,
Her hips, her waist at last has robbed;
Her voice now agitated is,
and with shyness her eyes do pause:
In movement now she knows no rest,
you may demure to meet her friend,
but youth has made her ripening breasts,
and driven out her ignorance.*
—**Rasikapriya**, Keshavadas

India's classical poetry (kavya), which was probably derived from early ritual theatre, worked explicitly with rasas. The American artist-philosopher John Cage described these emotional flavours as the 'permanent emotions'. And of these, the rasaraja shringara that makes the erotic paramount is definitely the most important.

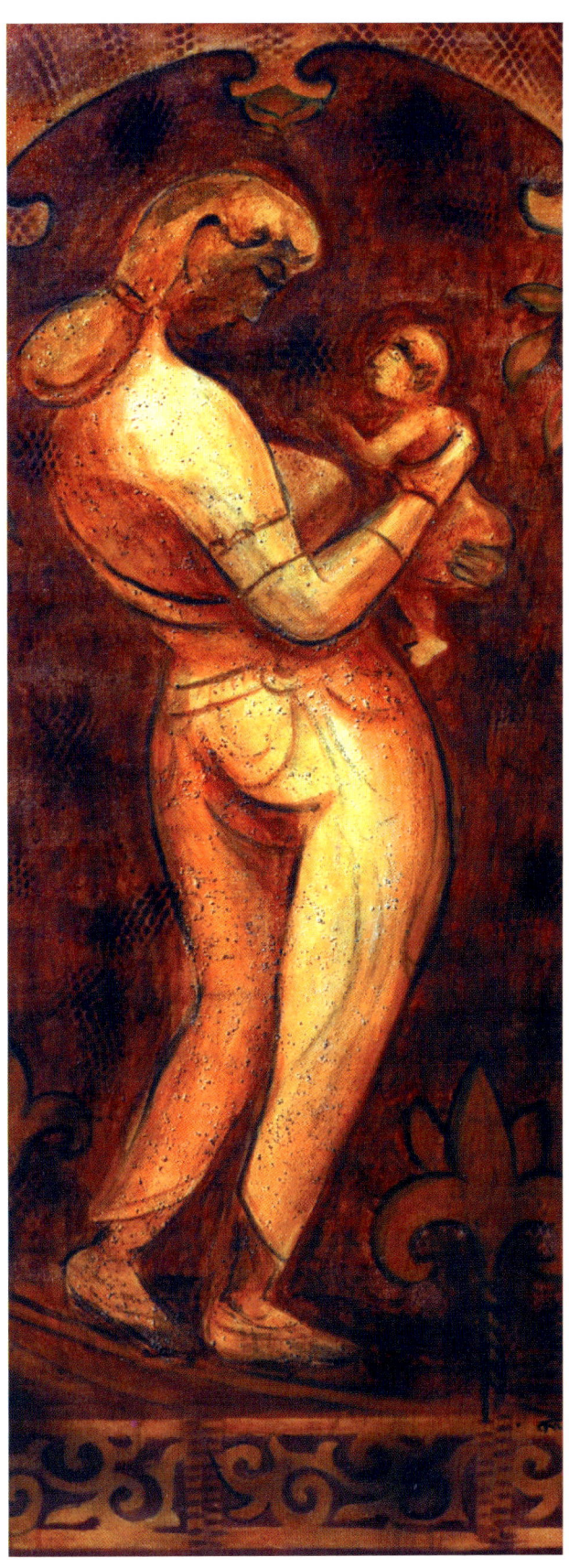

Shringara—the Rasaraja, king of *rasas*

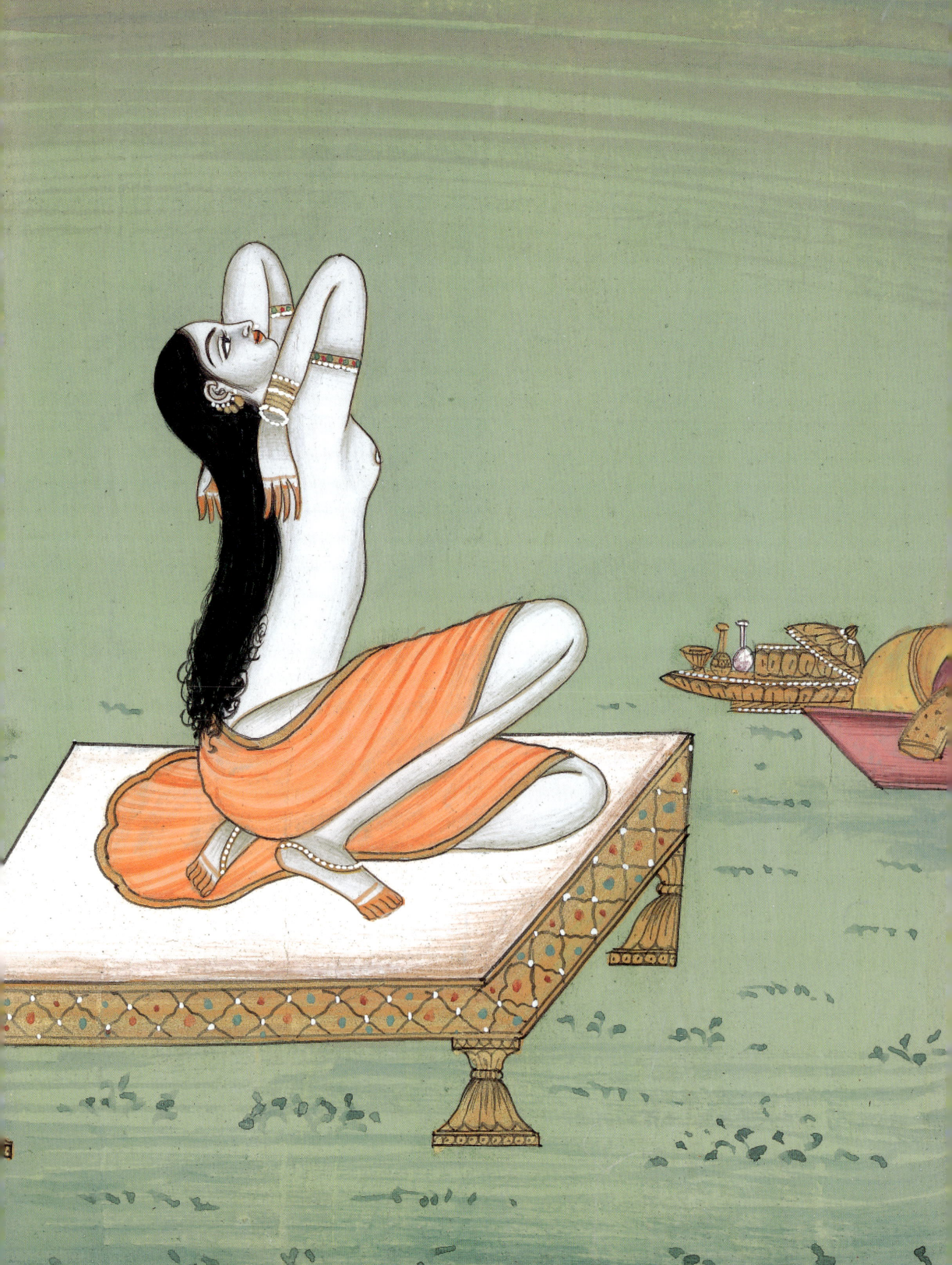

CHAPTER 4

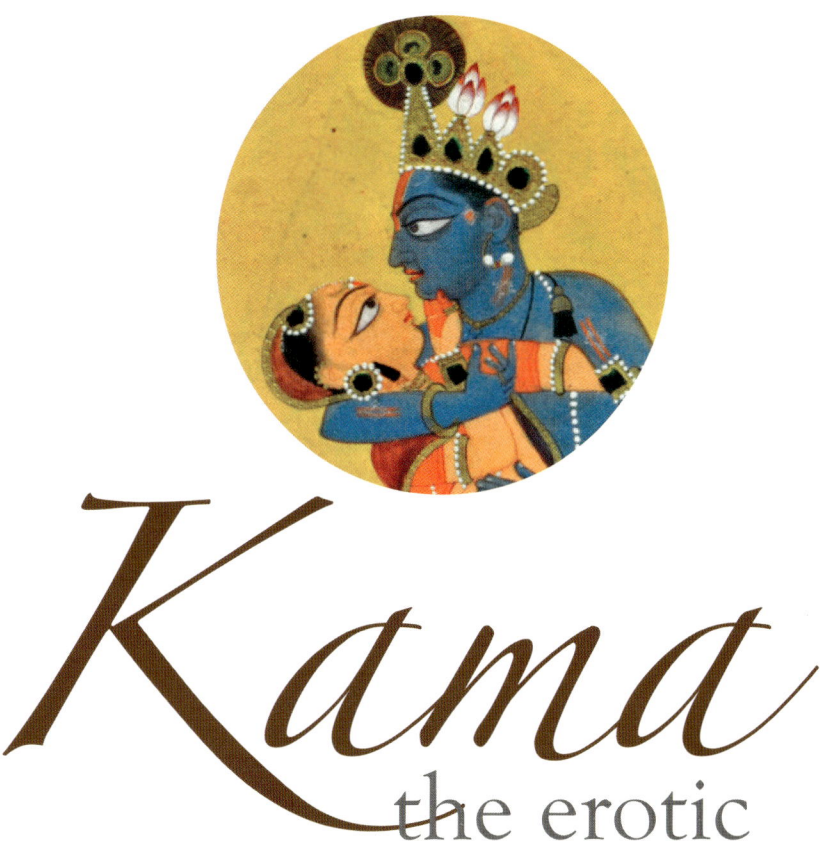

Kama
the erotic

There is no matter for numerical lists
Or textbook tables of contents.
For people joined in sexual ecstasy,
Passion is what makes things happen.

KAMASUTRA, VATSYAYANA

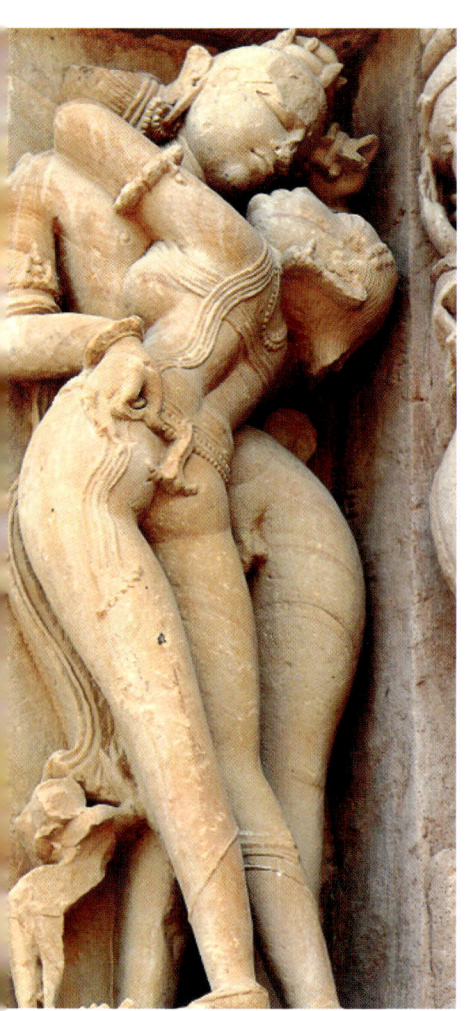

(Page 44)
The 'Nayika' at her toilette, the delicacy of the female form is sensitively nuanced in the contemporary representation of the modern miniature painting from Rajasthan

(Below)
Lovers, Chitragupta Temple, Khajuraho

Kama or the Indian god of love has been integral to the Indian ethos from the dawn of civilization. In *Atharva Veda*, Kama is exalted as the supreme god and creator. In *Taittriya Upanishad* of *Yajur Veda*, space is created out of stillness through Kama and he is responsible for all creation, because without desire there can be no creation. Kama, the Sanskrit word for desire, is not merely sexual love but all desire that stirs the mind. *Bhagvad Gita* explains that kama is located in three places: the mind, the senses and the intellect. Desire begins by an enticement of the senses and it breeds a sense of incompleteness. Kama is that which is amatory, stimulating and sexual. It lies between the romantic and the purely carnal. Kama is that which evokes the shringara rasa and leads to the vilasam bhava (pleasure), which in turn leads to maithuna (the sexual act) and ultimately to the state of ananda (bliss).

In traditional Indian art the sensual and the erotic is intertwined with daily life and has been treated in the same way in the arts. The grandest and most sensual of all rasas, shringara, was profusely depicted in painting and sculpture. In the Western aesthetic, especially coloured by later Victorian morality, such work may appear offensive, as the ideals that govern the Indian mind are not taken into account. A true appreciation of Indian aesthetics and artistic representations is, therefore, possible only when there is a complete understanding of the position that sex occupied in the overall Hindu ethos. The sensual element in Indian art is symbolic of the sublime urge for what lies beyond.

More than a religion, Hinduism is a way of life according to the prescribed codes of ancient India. Every Hindu must undergo sixteen rituals or *samskaras* and four stages of life. The final aim of life is salvation or moksha, which is the merging of the individual soul (atma) with the supreme soul (the paramatma). One can attain moksha by following the aims of life or *purushartha*, which are dharma, artha and kama. While dharma signifies duty, social obligations and justice, artha underpins power and material success. Kama represents love, pleasure and sex and, more broadly, the sensual experience in its totality, encompassing all the arts.

A Divine Union

'The Hymn of Creation' in *Rig Veda*, dated around 900 BC, attributes the beginning of creation to sexual desire and calls it 'the primal germ of the human mind'. One of the earliest representations of sexual motifs in art is found in sculptures from the Buddhist period in the form of *dampati* scenes, or depictions of scenes between married partners. Hinduism, the oldest religion in the world, teaches that the literature of sex and love is of divine origin and *Rig Veda* gives prime importance to the pursuit of sexual pleasure. In fact, so broad is the

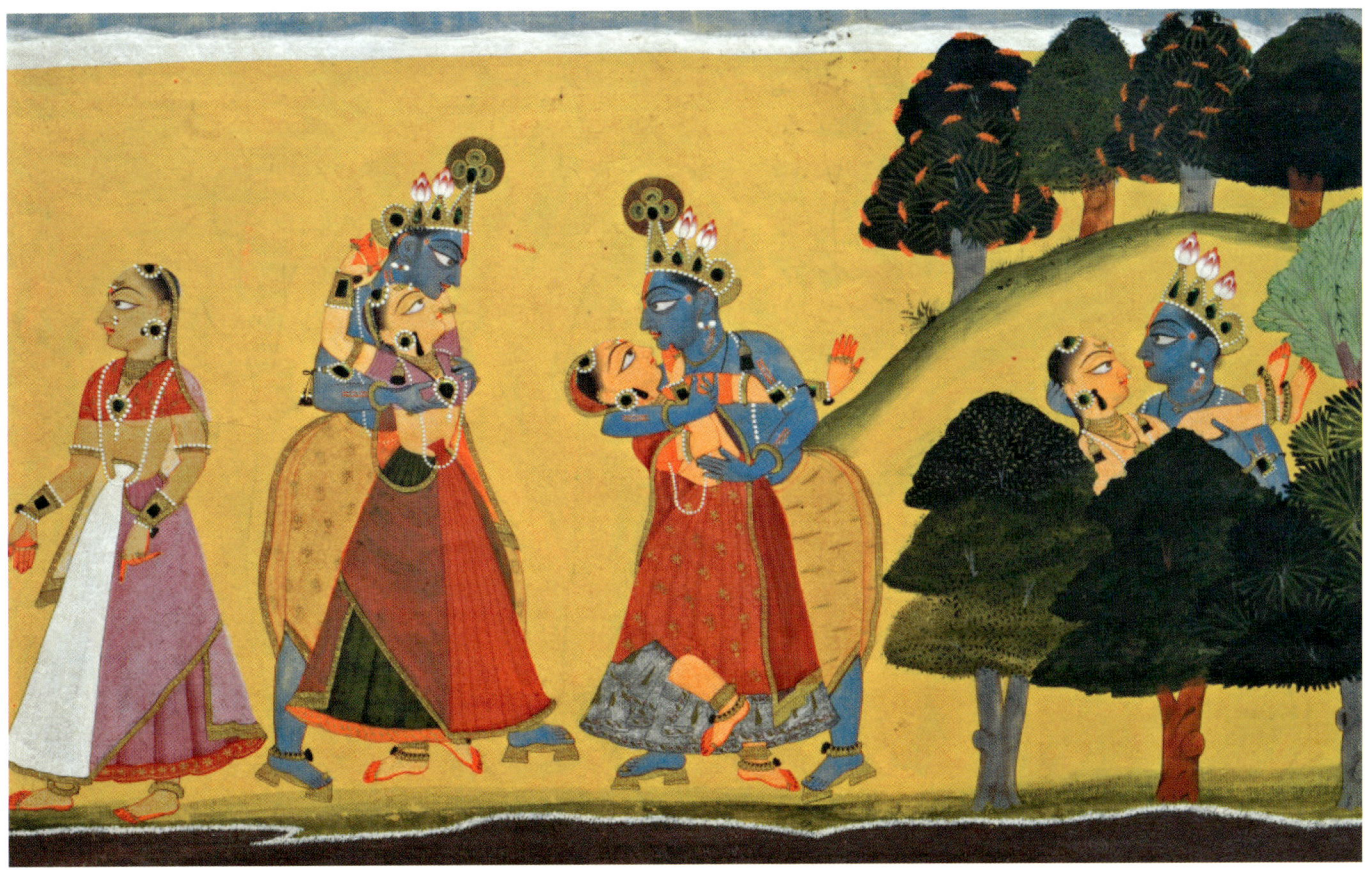

Illustration from Gita Govinda, *Pahari School, Chandigarh Museum*

concept of kama that a very thin line divides the erotic from the esoteric, i.e. the bhakti (devotional) and tantric (ritualistic) traditions.

Erotica was conceived as sacred, a sexual impulse that generated divine pleasure and led to union with the Superior Being. Hindus, in fact, saw creation itself in sexual terms. In the Hindu pantheon, the various aspects of the human and the celestial had existence, reality and the power to manifest itself only when united with its corresponding feminine counterpart, namely, Shakti (power). The uniting of the male and female reproductive organ is the very symbol of the Divine Being's creative potential, as well as the cosmic and physical reality of creation. This union was the beginning and end of existence and the reason for its continuation. Because of its symbolic and creative value, the sexual act was the most important of rituals, an effective means of participating in the cosmic world, and was performed as a rite.

All other rites were but its image and symbolically reproduced the original union. Agni, the god of fire and male principle, burns in the kunda, the altar hearth, or the image of the female principle. Upanishads interpret all aspects of the sacrificial ritual as the various stages in the act of love. Indian

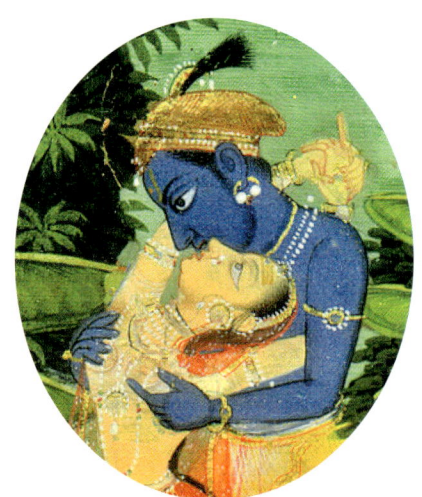

*(Detail & overleaf)
Illustration from* Rasikapriya
*of Keshavadas, Mewar Era,
N.C. Mehta Collection,
Ahmedabad*

mythology is replete with gods leading polygamous lifestyles and indulging in a plethora of sexual activities. The most celebrated deity of the Hindu pantheon, Krishna, is the great lover and had 16,018 wives. But the eternal love of Krishna and Radha (his consort) elevated the sensual and erotic to the state of ananda or heavenly pleasure, and transformed sexual desire from the merely carnal to a oneness with divine and spiritual connotations. Their relationship is, in fact, seen as the highest form of love, a synthesis of passion, spirituality and devotion.

Shiva, the primordial Indian god, is the paramount example of Indian erotica. He is at once the *mahayogi* and *mahabhogi*. Within Shiva lives the strictest ascetic and the most playful lover. While Shiva and his consort, Parvati, epitomize the generative aspect of sex, Krishna and Radha symbolize pure shringara or the recreational aspect of sex.

Tantric Worship

The tradition of the Tantra school of worship is also closely connected to the principle of kama. Highly misunderstood today as a free-love cult, a survival of the psychedelic sixties or a new age spiritual sex therapy, Tantra is a mystical religion aligning man with the universe. Tantrism is so called because its adherents follow scriptures known as tantras. These scriptures contain detailed instructions on a wide range of topics, including spiritual knowledge and science. Although it may appear paradoxical, the tantrics believe that science and mysticism go hand-in-hand. Tantra yoga texts date to the medieval period during the Pala rule in north India (8th to 12th centuries AD).

Several archaeological remains of the yoni and lingam (the female and male organ) from the Neolithic period have led theorists to deduce that 'sex worship', in one form or another, was at the core of the oldest religion in the world. Starting with Vedic literature, the magical aspect of sex assumed an imperative role in everyday life, as witnessed in *Ashvamedha yajna*. This ritual sacrifice was performed over a period of twelve months during which a monarch displayed his power over neighbouring kingdoms by giving his horse free rein to wander through their lands. War resulted if the horse was stopped, but more often than not, the ritual of annexation was peacefully performed. However, copulation and sexual dialogue were important components of the rite and the wives of the king participated; the chief queen being made to lie with the horse while the other queens used abusive language. Another rite stressed restraint as the king was made to lie between the legs of his favourite wife without enjoying her.

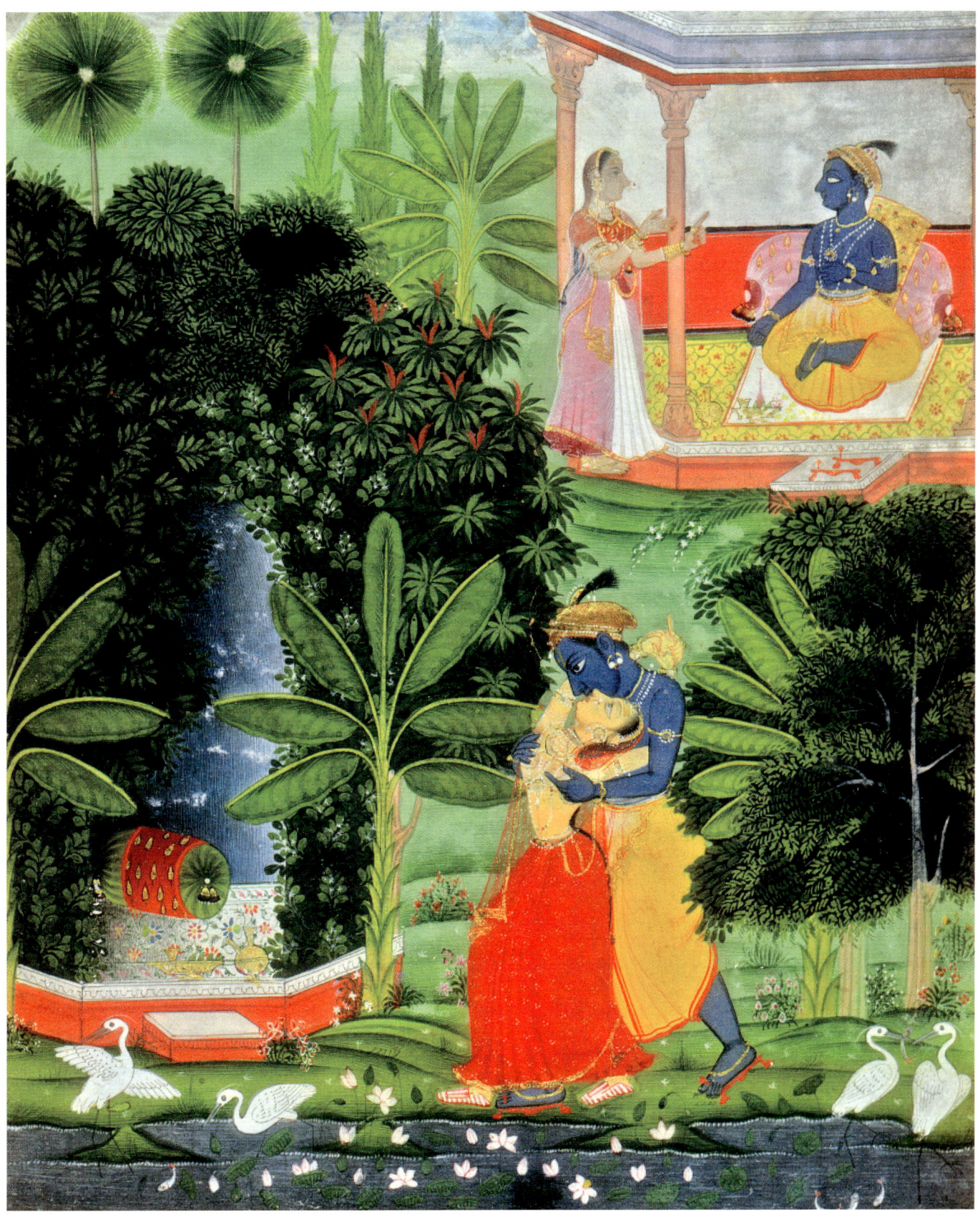

Kama—the erotic 49

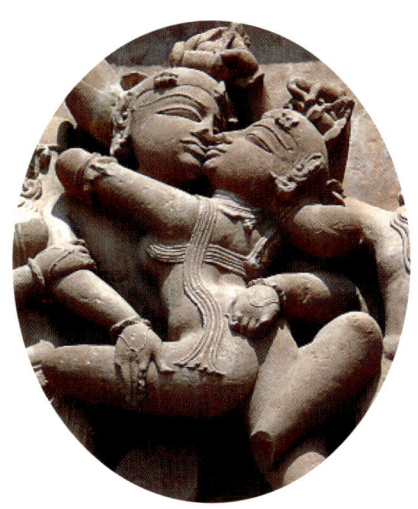

A couple, Lakshmana Temple, Khajuraho

(Page 51)
Kamadeva, Adinath Temple, Khajuraho

The Sacred Tradition

Starting with the 5000-year-old Indus Valley Civilization, India has witnessed an extraordinary evolution in mores, ethnicity and traditions. From the coming of the Aryan tribes in 1500 BC to the early Arabs, Turks and Mughals, and finally the Europeans in the 15th century AD, the country has inherited an extraordinarily amalgamated classical culture. As religion, thought and language began to diversify from region to region, so did art and its varied erotic manifestations.

Beginning with the northern region, the two greatest literary renditions of glorious artistic and philosophical profundity are the Indian epics: Vyasa's Mahabharata and Valmiki's Ramayana, both of which contain several episodes of erotic love. After the Mauryan dynasty fell in 184 BC, the Guptas (3rd to 8th centuries AD) revived the northern empire and ushered in what is today called the Golden Age of Indian Culture. Literature, poetry and drama flourished under the aegis of Chandragupta II. The poet, Kalidasa, lived at his court where he wrote his *Kumarasambhava*. The poem, a celebration of the marriage of Shiva and Parvati whom he regards as the 'primordial parents', is the most intense expression of free love.

Erotic love was always perceived as a manifestation of the divine love of the gods and was, therefore, completely accepted in society and liberated from its conservative imperatives. King Harshvardhan (7th century AD) encouraged Sanskrit writers such as Bana, who wrote *Kadambari*, a masterpiece of erotic prose, that was later completed by his son Bhushana Bhatta. The 11th-century Kashmiri poet, Bilhana, composed the love lyric *Chaurpanchasika*, the final testament of a tutor sentenced to death for falling in love with his pupil, a princess. The poem spans fifty confessional erotic verses written in the first person. This piece of work marks a shift in the depiction of the erotic in this region, with artists giving bolder expression to their imaginative and creative abilities.

In ancient India, the study of the erotic sciences or *kama shastra* was considered as important as the study of *dharma shastra* or religious and social laws, and *artha shastra* or economics and political science. The sacred hymns and chants, the songs and infinite stories, all form part of a tradition that has been passed down the ages in poetry, dance, drama and painting. Vedas, the earliest scriptures of Hinduism, also have several sections devoted to love poetry, making it an inherent part of society and culture. Sex had its significance in the scheme of things for Hindus. They treated it scientifically and objectively. Desire was given equal respect with every other human emotion. From an act of recreation to procreation, sex was not considered profane, nor was it hidden in veils of secrecy.

Shringara—the many faces of Indian beauty

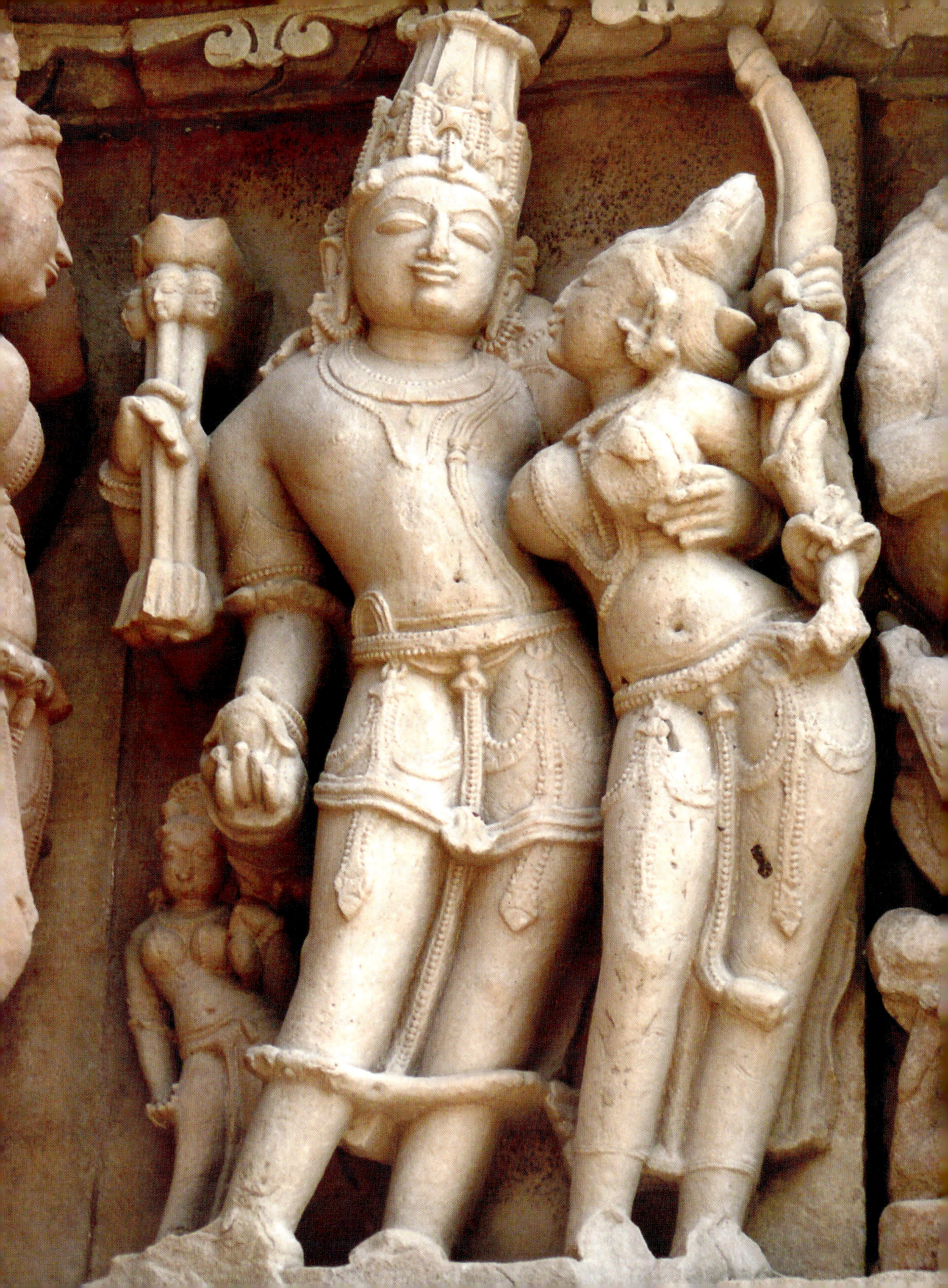

An Act of Creation

In Hindu thought, nature is a coalescence of male and female principles, of Shiva and Shakti; it is the union of these two that creates the world and, to this day, the lingam and yoni, symbolizing Shiva and Parvati, are worshipped. Shringara, the eternal omnipresent cycle of continuity and union, is celebrated as one of the eight essential emotions in Indian dramatic and visual art theory. It covers the depiction of a range of human conditions, from romantic separation and longing, to the visualization of sexual union and ecstasy, and is widely accepted as an allegory for the individual soul's longing for union with the ultimate consciousness, Brahman, or the true reality.

Shringara rasa illustrates particularly clearly the way in which metaphors for complex spiritual ideas stand alongside sensuous imagery in ancient Indian thought, celebrating human beauty, male-female relationships, and the bounty of nature in general. In ancient Indian society, sex was not considered outside

'Longing', Rajput, Bundi, mid-17th century

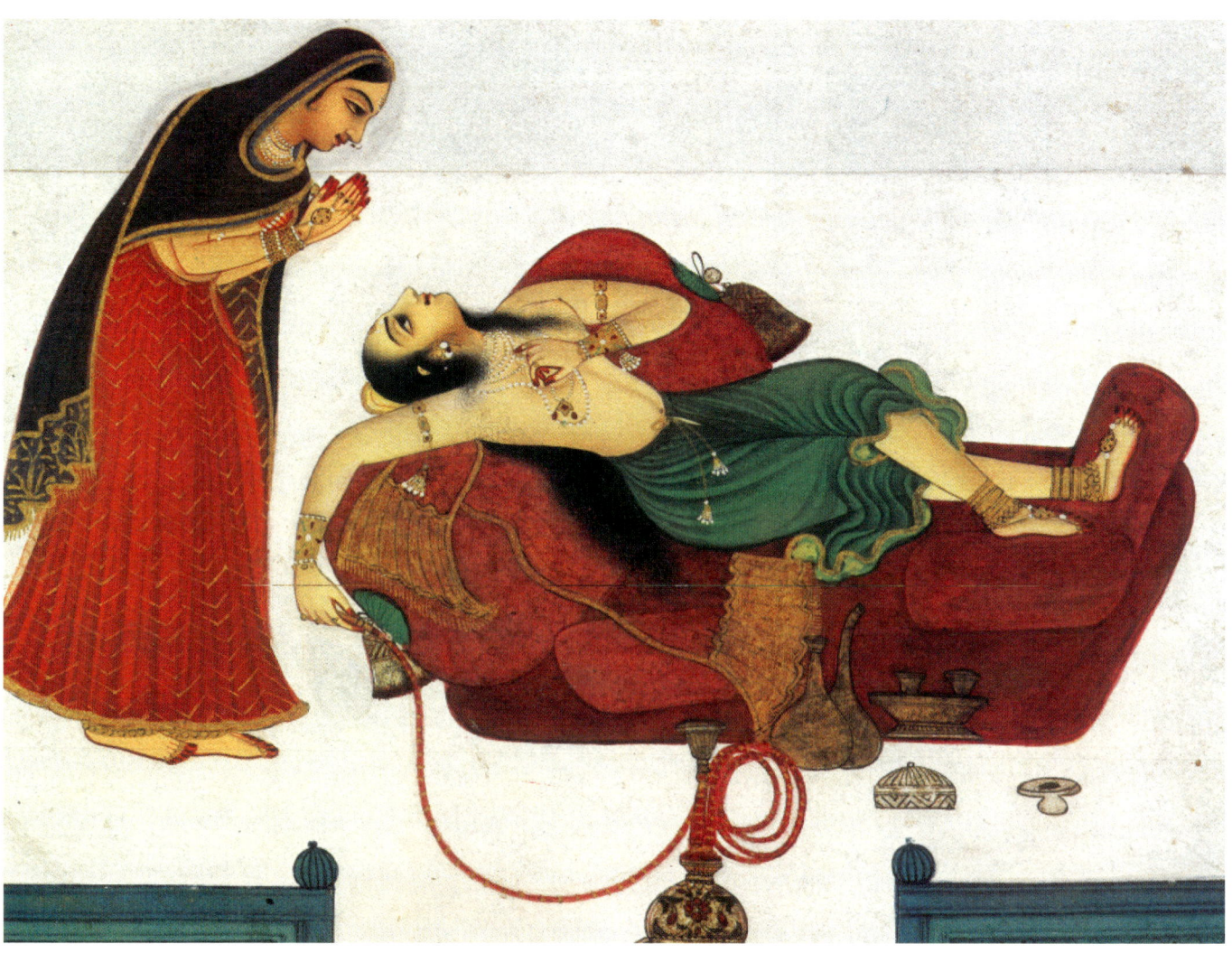

52 *Shringara*—the many faces of Indian beauty

the province of religion; on the contrary, all religious conceptions emphasized the importance of the sexual force. The most appropriate rendition of this is through the visual arts. Interestingly, the erotic manifests itself outside this visual parameter also in a very significant but understated way. The best example would be the metric patterns explained in Bharata's *Natyashastra*. The *Pravara-lalita* metre is described below:

Her body has been scratched by nails, and lips and the cheeks are bitten by teeth,
the head is set with flowers, hair is dishevelled, her gait is languid,
and the eyes are restless.
Ah, a very graceful exploit of love has taken place in a praiseworthy manner.

The female personification of the *lalita* metre is described as:

O lady, hurriedly but gracefully moving, wearing beautiful clothes and with delicate hands and having a blooming lotus-like face, you look charming after the fatigue of love's sports.

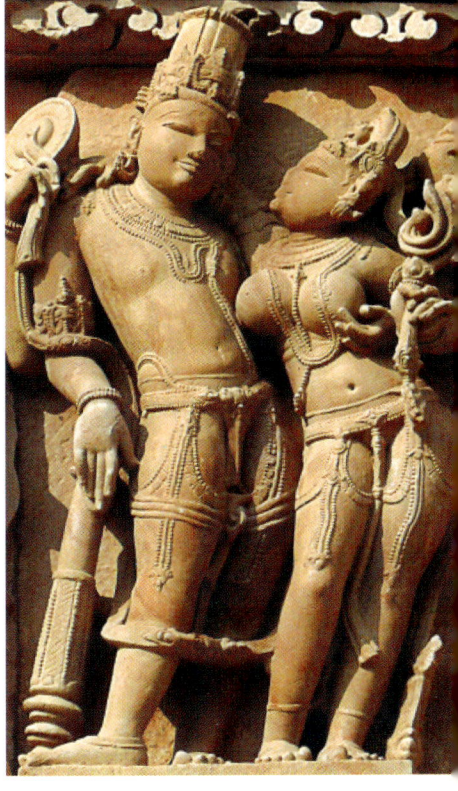

Lovers, Adinath Temple, Khajuraho

In a primarily patriarchal society, the phallus came to symbolize the Supreme Being. From being revered as a cult symbol to an artistic representation of the erotic, the phallus is essentially the emblem or sign of Shiva, the progenitor, who is the cosmic individual. Besides these explicit references to the phallus, it is indirectly and allegorically represented by certain objects or animals: the fish, bird, serpent, bull, the horn, the moon, the foot, thumb, a standing stone or column, and the tree. The arrow evoking the creative organ, that opens in order to fertilize, is linked to the lingam.

The *yajna-kunda*, the hearth hollowed at the top of the altar, represents the yoni. 'Fire obtained by friction, is considered to be the progeny of a sexual union.' (*Histoire des croyances et des idees religieuses*, Mircea Eliade). The concept of fertilization is often represented by the ploughshare penetrating the furrow in the female earth, therefore impregnating the field. It evokes the union of man and woman, the sky and earth. Interestingly, there is a linguistic connect between *langala* (spade) and *lingam* (phallus).

Shaivites consider erotic ecstasy not just as a means of reproduction but also an inherent search for pleasure. According to Sefer Yezirah, the phallus fulfils a function that is not only generational, but confers equilibrium to the structures built by man and the order of the world. The sexual organ, thus plays a dual role, that of procreation as well as the pleasure (ananda).

The phallus is the source of pleasure. It is the sole means of obtaining earthly pleasure and salvation. By looking at it, touching it, and meditating on it, living beings are capable of freeing themselves from the cycle of future lives.

—**Shiva Purana**

The female organ, the yoni, completes the picture of the creative element. It has been variously revered in the scriptures:

The yoni represents the womb of the visible and the subtle world.

—**Yajur Veda**

Because it is the origin of all life, nature is comparable to a womb.

—**Shiva Purana**

When limitless bliss (ananda) *is attained, pleasure* (kama) *no longer has any meaning. Union* (sangha) *gives rise to pleasure, but its goal is joy. Eroticsim is only a means.*

—**Siddhanta, Patel Varige**

Thus metaphors of beauty and erotica in poetry, music, painting, sculpture and other dance forms overlap each other with ease. The artist derives his conceptual ideas from his surroundings. The world and nature provide a visual canvas of ideas, which he renders further into different art forms. The symbolization of these very ideas becomes customary over a period of time. Hence the repetitive mention of erotic metaphors leads to their culturization and they become an inherent part of the society.

Illustration from Gita Govinda, Pahari, *from Lahore Museum now in Chandigarh Museum*

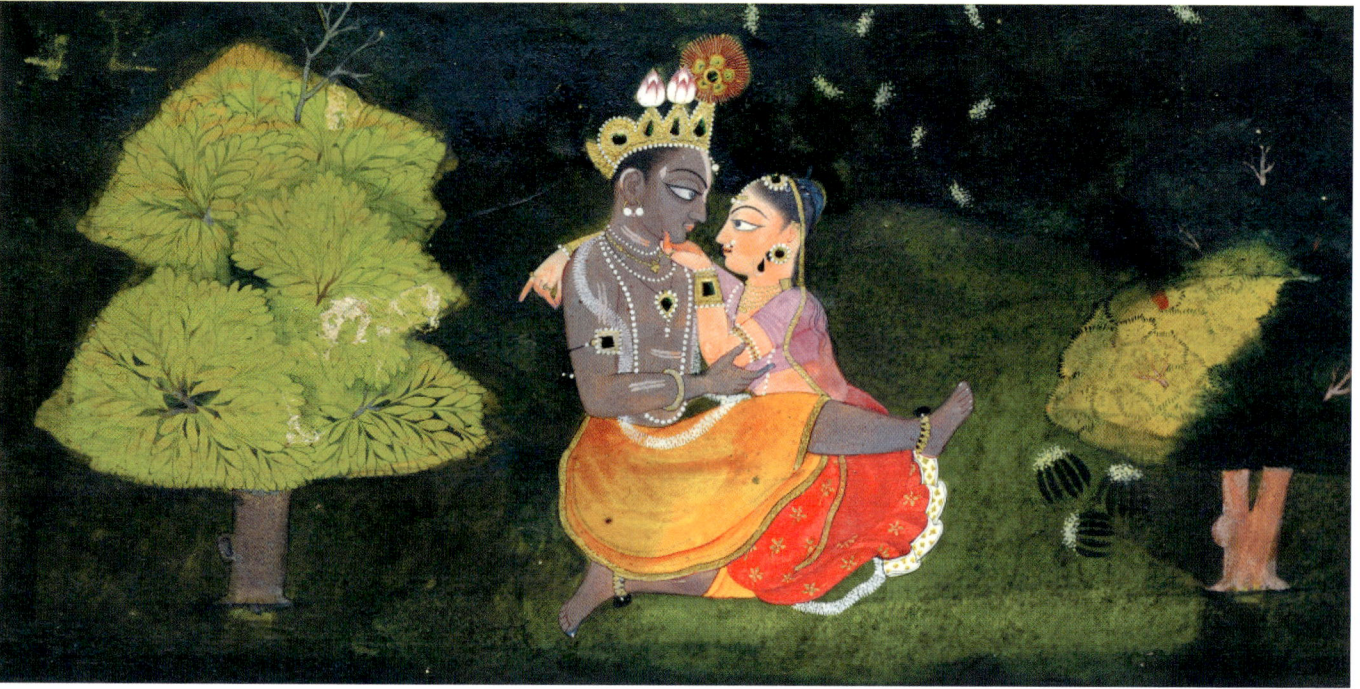

54 *Shringara*—the many faces of Indian beauty

The passage below describes Brahma's directive to Kama on his birth:

In this universe of three worlds, no mobile or immobile beings, including the devas, will be able to protect themselves from your arrows, not to speak of ordinary mortals. Even I Brahma, and Vishnu and Shiva will fall under your control. You will enter the minds of living beings in an invisible form and by creating desire you will assist in the activities of procreation forever. The minds of all human beings will be particularly vulnerable, helpless against the effect of your soft flower arrows. I have assigned to you, Kama, Lord of Desire, the honourable task of facilitating creation.

—A Puranic Version

The Marriage of Kama

Armed with beauty, vanity and confidence, Kama desires a bride. *Shiv Purana* gives a vivid account of the marriage of Kama with the model of eroticism, Rati:

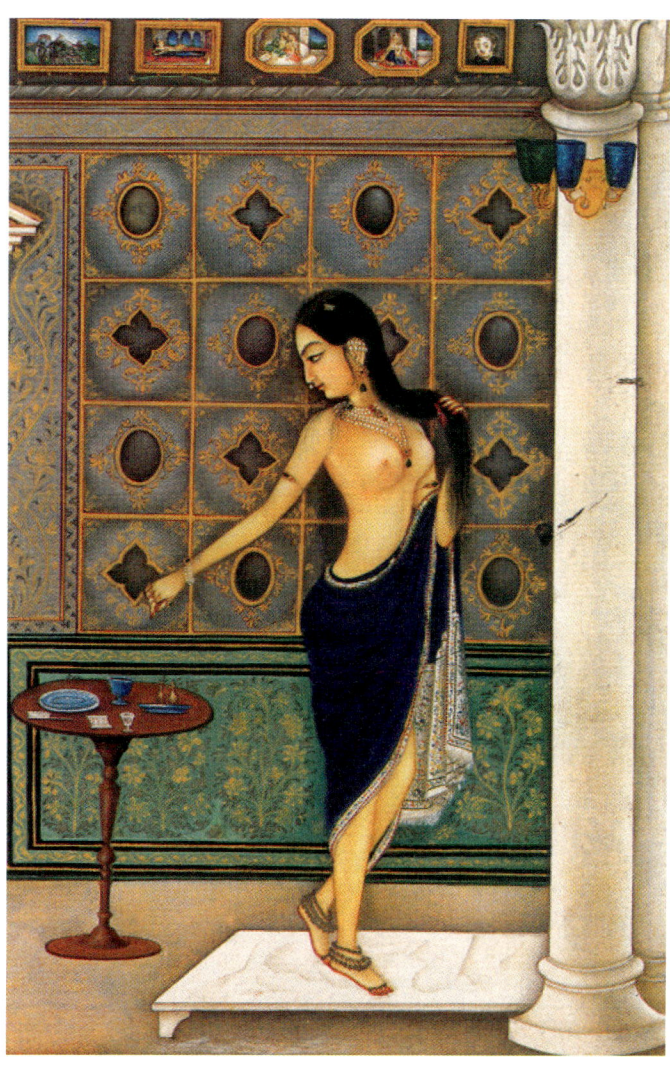

A courtesan at her toilette as represented by a contemporary miniaturist from Rajasthan

Daksha, the mind-born son of Brahma remembered his father's words and said to Kama, 'O Kama, this girl born of my body I give to you in marriage. She is endowed with loveliness and good qualities. She will be a befitting companion to you, take her as your wife and constant co-partner'. Saying this, Daksha presented Kama with his daughter born from his sweat, naming her Rati.

On seeing Rati, Kama was overcome with joy. It was as if he had been struck by his own arrows. His wife had all the prerequisite qualities for his profession. Her complexion was becoming, her fawn-like eyes were large, attentive, gentle and adoring. On surveying her face he could not help but think that her eyebrows were better shaped than his famous bow. Her roving eyes made Kama doubt his own swiftness as an archer. She smelt so sweet that Kama forgot all the wonderful gardens and groves of love that he frequented. Her face was so brilliant that he mistook it for the moon. Her breasts firm and tapering like golden lotuses, with dark nipples like bees hovering around them.

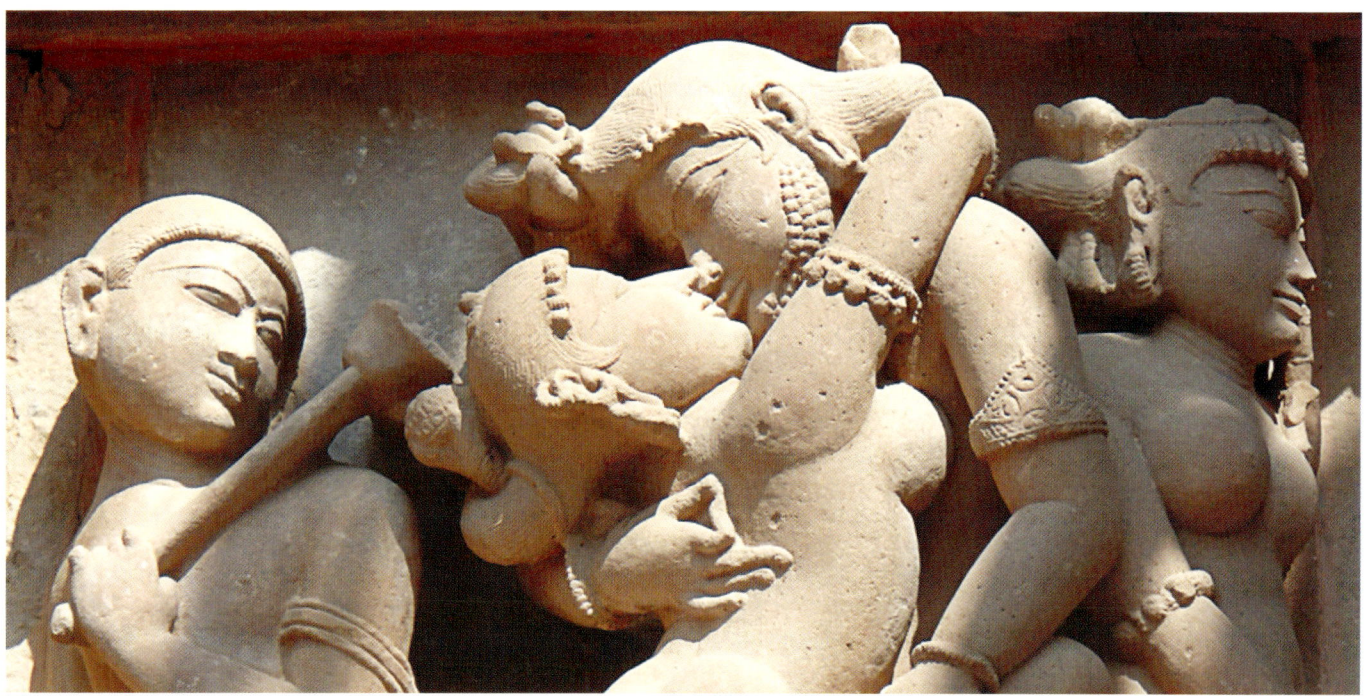

Kamasutra, Lakshmana Temple, Khajuraho

The splendid well-proportioned lady was indeed a match for his playful amorous activities. Her slender waist, golden hue, her thighs smooth and firm as plantain stalks were inviting and seductive. Her heels and fingertips were tinged with pink, the sign of health and vigour. Her arms were as silky and supple as lotus stems with elegant expressive fingers. She carried a disc and lotus in her hands. Her loveliness was as playful as the sea, her eyebrows, reacting to every stimulus, rippled like the waves; her glances rose and ebbed as the gentle tide. Her glimmering eyes had the brilliance of the dark blue lotus and her hair was dark, with the soft fullness of a rain cloud. She was dressed in exquisite jewellery, peacock feathers and flowers. She was skilled in the art of lovemaking and uncanny in her use of the sixteen amorous gestures. Rati was so gifted she charmed the whole world and illuminated the entire universe with her radiant aura. When Kama learnt that, by the grace of Brahma, his job was to instill desire in the mind of all, to sustain creation, and that no one would be able to protect themselves from his arrows, he was overjoyed. Kama thought to himself that he must make a fitting start to his career. Since Brahma and his sons were present, they would be witness to the beginning of Kama's illustrious debut.

He then set about testing his prowess and skill. Brahma and the sages were standing near at hand; so was Sandhya, Brahma's mind-child. Bending in the correct position, Kama held out his bow and drew the string. A fragrant breeze enveloped everyone and they were charmed by the graceful archer. Brahma and the sages fell under the spell of Kama's flower arrows and, staring at Sandhya, passion rose in their depraved minds. Though they were her father and brothers, they began to lust after her. Kama did not stop his onslaught till all of them had lost their sense and wisdom. He was delighted at the repercussions and grew unduly proud and daring.

—**Kama's Debut**, *Divine Ecstasy*

According to *Kamasutra*, sexual enjoyment complements the moral, material and spiritual well-being of a person. It was regarded as natural as sight and scent, not something to be hidden in shame and then brooded on with guilt. Texts like *Kamasutra* and visual art as seen in the temples of Khajuraho, served to educate, regulate and help man become proficient in matters of sex, not to become a slave to it. Despite its basic theme, *Kamasutra* actually lays down instructions dealing with several aspects of life, covering pleasure as well as duties.

Nowhere in the world has the feminine form been so celebrated as in Khajuraho. From gorgeous *alasya kanyas* to women at their toilette, the female form is represented in its full abundant glory. In Ajanta, however, scantily-clad beautiful women are embodiments of the spiritual domain. Indian art and culture celebrate femininity in paeans sung in verse, the haunting melodies of stringed instruments, the gentle nuances of dance or the delicately coordinated visual feats of painting. Behind the din of masculine sagas, sacred Hindu literature is filled with themes of feminine emotion, dreams and fury. There are tales of goddesses who strike their children with fever, nymphs who seduce sages, celestial virgins who run free

Kamasutra, Lakshmana Temple, Khajuraho

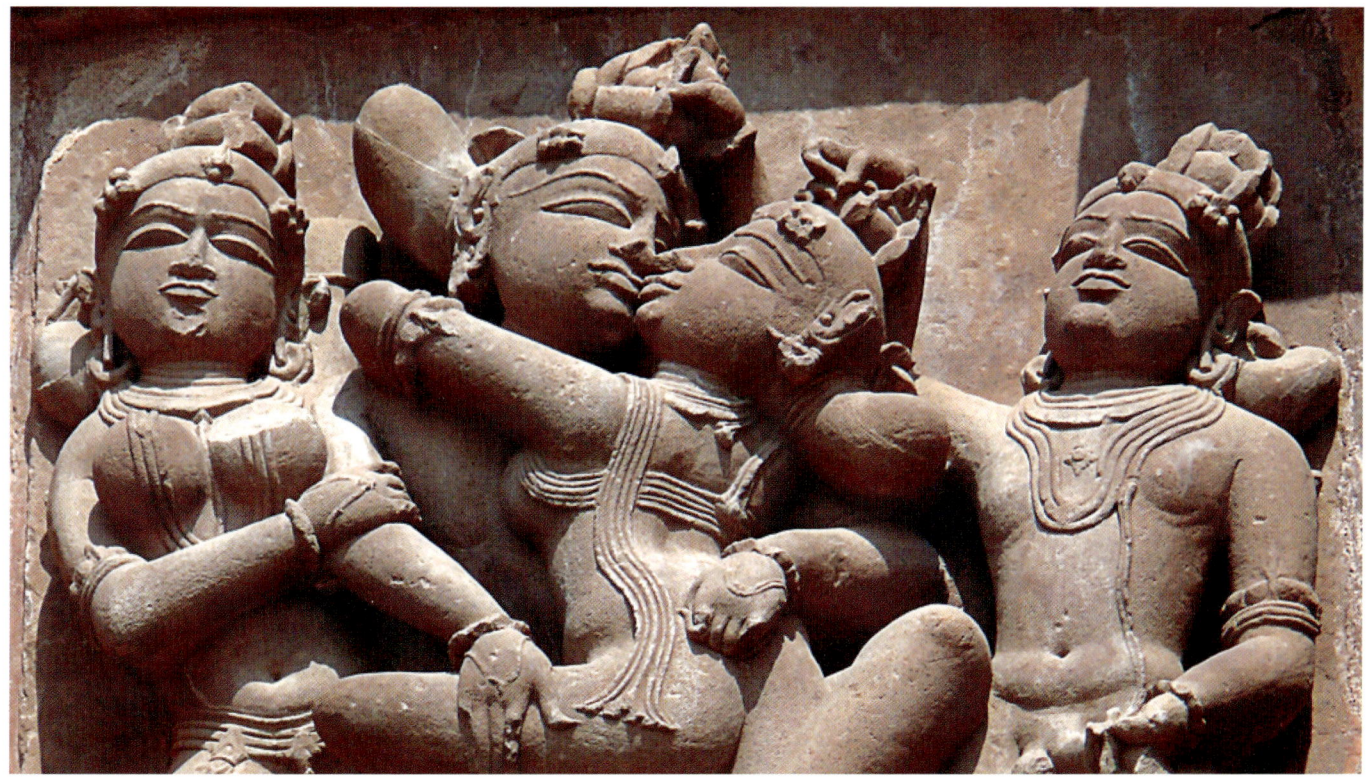

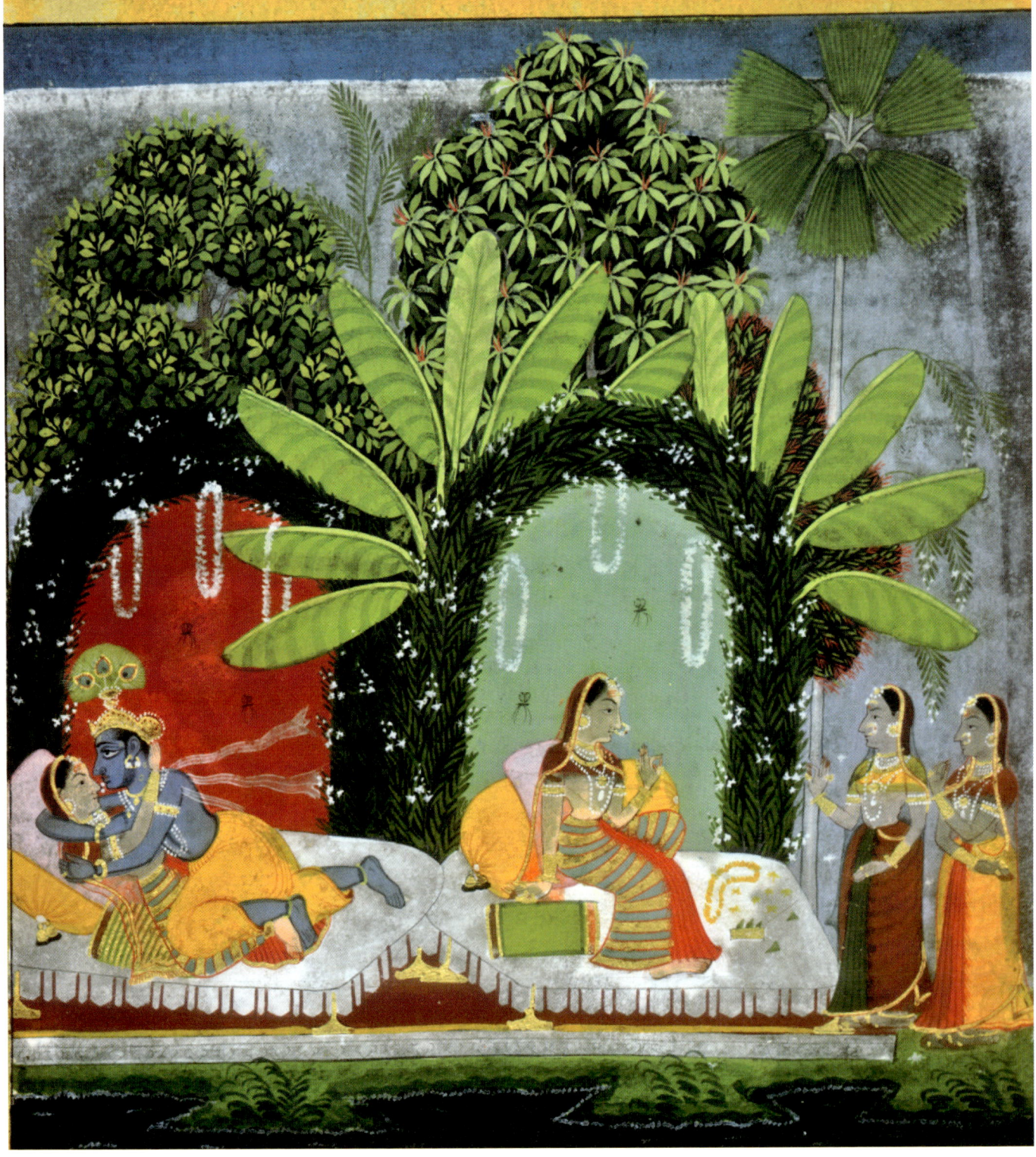

58 *Shringara*—the many faces of Indian beauty

in forests, and chaste wives who fling themselves on funeral pyres to become guardians of feminine virtue. Painting and sculpture stand testimony to the ease with which sex and sexuality in all its manifestations, ranging from auto-eroticism to homo-eroticism, bestiality to orgies, the sexual acts of gods and men, all found expression and representation without taboo or apology for thousands of years.

It should be kept in mind that the word Hindu in this discussion refers to 'Indian' in the broader sense. The parallel between sexuality and spiritualism and the possible access of power through meditation and asceticism, where sexual pleasure gets sublimated into spiritual power, were common strands running through all three religions—Hinduism, Buddhism, and Jainism—each one an integral part of the cultural tradition and ethos of India.

As mentioned earlier, traditional scriptures lay down the four goals of life for an Indian householder as: desire (kama), attainment of material means (artha), observance of social and religious obligations (dharma), and finally, liberation from the chain of rebirth (moksha). Mahabharata, the great Indian epic, is also seen as a philosophical treatise and a book of rules to live by. It contains an interesting debate between the five Pandava brothers on artha, dharma and kama, and which is the most desirable goal. Bhima, one of the Pandavas, says:

> *Without kama a man has no wish for worldly profit (artha), without kama a man does not strive after the good (dharma), without kama a man does not love; therefore kama stands above the others. For the sake of kama the rishis even give themselves up to asceticism, eating the leaves of trees, fruits, and roots, living on the air and wholly bridling their senses, and others bend all their zeal to the Vedas and lesser Vedas, making their way through the whole of the holy study, as also to ancestral offerings, and sacrificial acts, to alms giving and alms-taking.*
>
> *Traders, husbandmen, herdsmen, craftsmen, as also artists, and those that carry out actions consecrated to the gods, give themselves up to their works because of kama. Others, again, take to the sea filled with kama. No being ever was, or is or will be, higher than the being that is filled with kama.*
>
> *It is the innermost core (of the world), O king of righteousness; on it is founded dharma and artha...*
>
> —**Sexual Life in Ancient India, Johann Jakob Meyer**

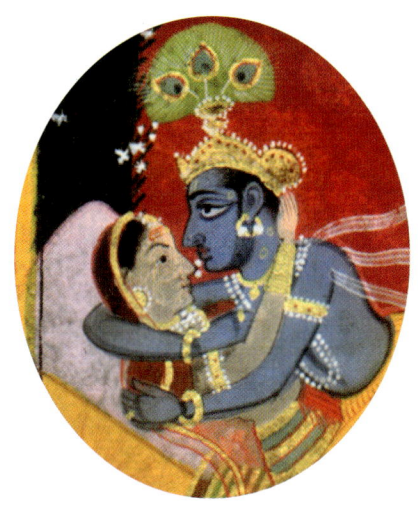

(Detail & overleaf) Illustration from Bihari's Satsai, *Mewar, AD 1719, Attri, N.C. Mehta Collection, Ahmedabad*

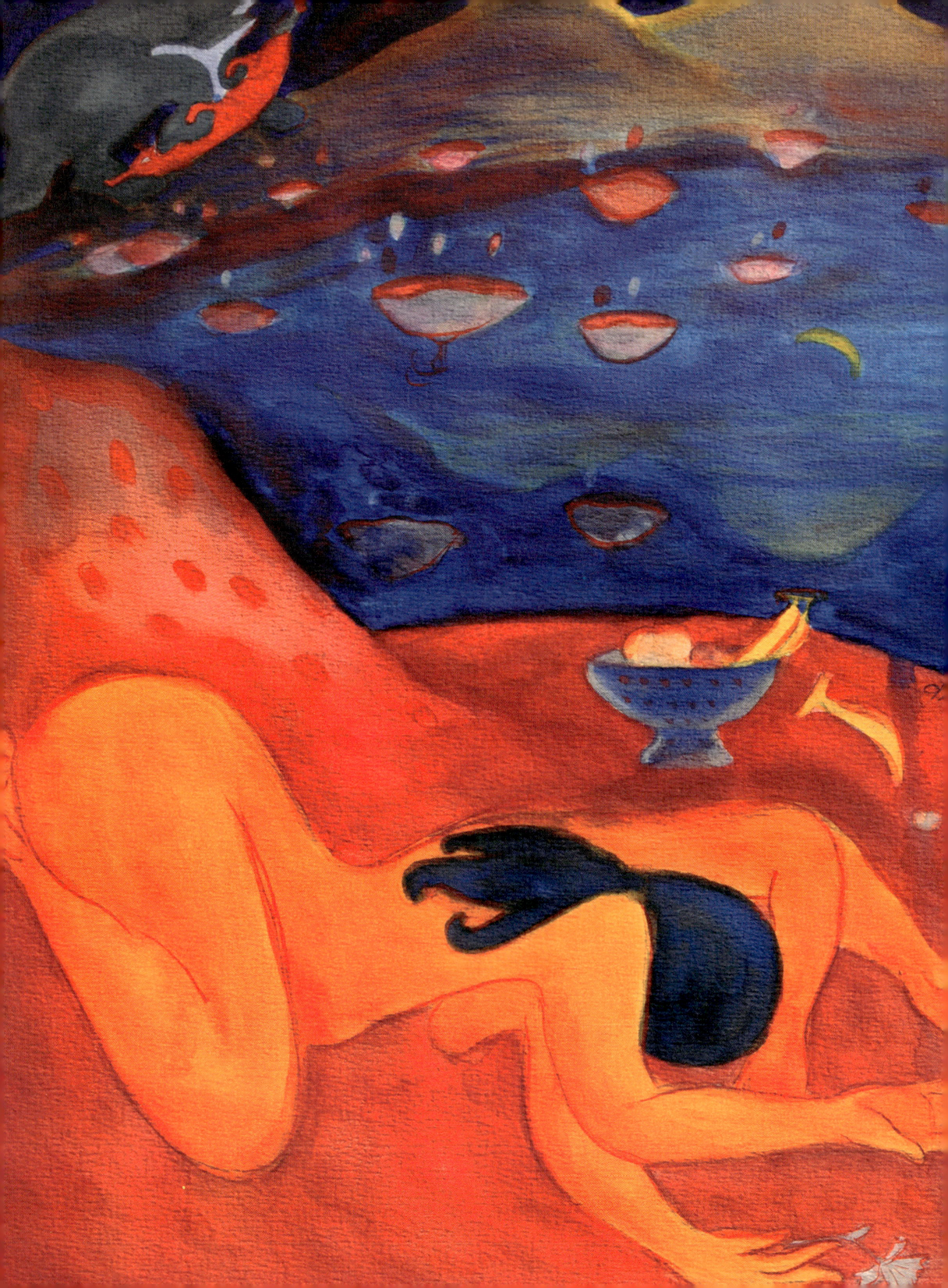

CHAPTER 5

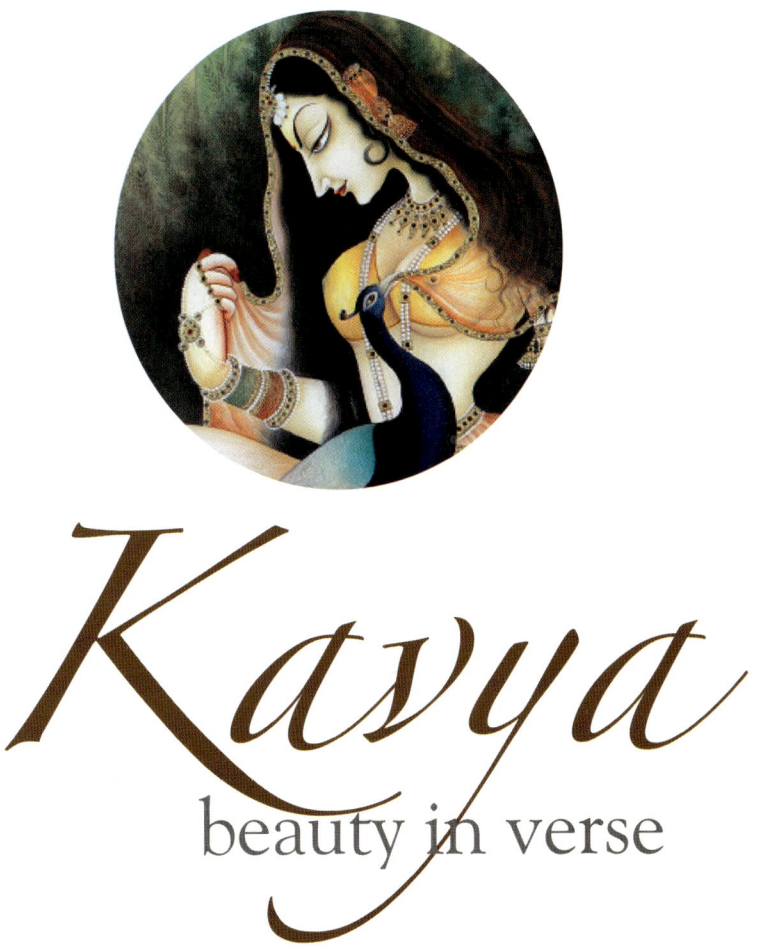

Kavya
beauty in verse

*On the swing with quivering eyes
she is ashamed of the stirrings in the region of her loins;
with a smiling face she looks
all round at the sounds of the doves;
The dishonest one does not ask for the touch of the tips
Of the thorns in the pleasure grove:
The slender one's age is ready, by dismissing innocence,
To become a friend of the sensitive.*

JALHANA AND SARANGADHARA
INDIAN KAVYA LITERATURE, ANTHONY KENNEDY WARDER

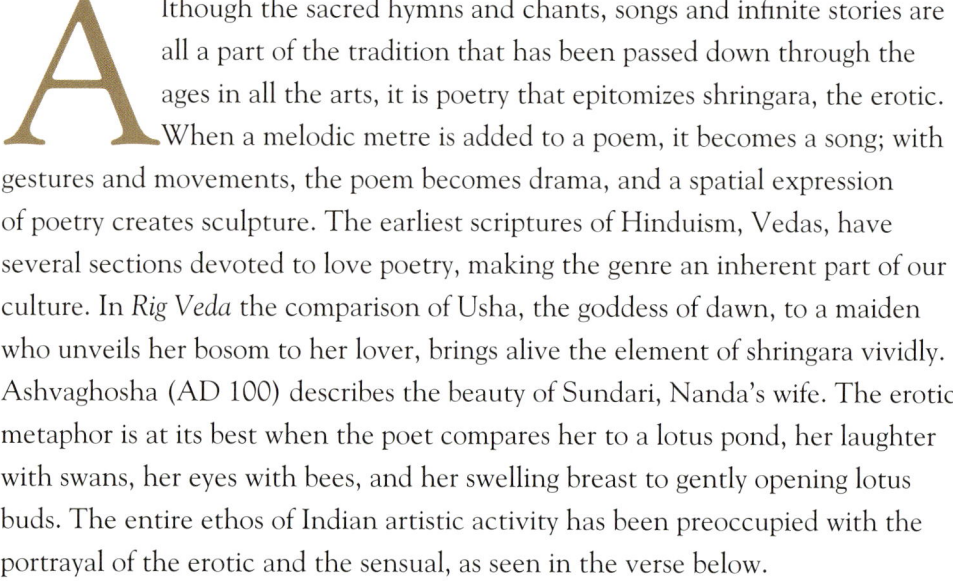

(Page 60)
*'Gathering scattered petals',
painting by
Kanchan Chander*

*(Below)
The lotus, a divine symbol of
purity, non-attachment and
beauty*

Although the sacred hymns and chants, songs and infinite stories are all a part of the tradition that has been passed down through the ages in all the arts, it is poetry that epitomizes shringara, the erotic. When a melodic metre is added to a poem, it becomes a song; with gestures and movements, the poem becomes drama, and a spatial expression of poetry creates sculpture. The earliest scriptures of Hinduism, Vedas, have several sections devoted to love poetry, making the genre an inherent part of our culture. In *Rig Veda* the comparison of Usha, the goddess of dawn, to a maiden who unveils her bosom to her lover, brings alive the element of shringara vividly. Ashvaghosha (AD 100) describes the beauty of Sundari, Nanda's wife. The erotic metaphor is at its best when the poet compares her to a lotus pond, her laughter with swans, her eyes with bees, and her swelling breast to gently opening lotus buds. The entire ethos of Indian artistic activity has been preoccupied with the portrayal of the erotic and the sensual, as seen in the verse below.

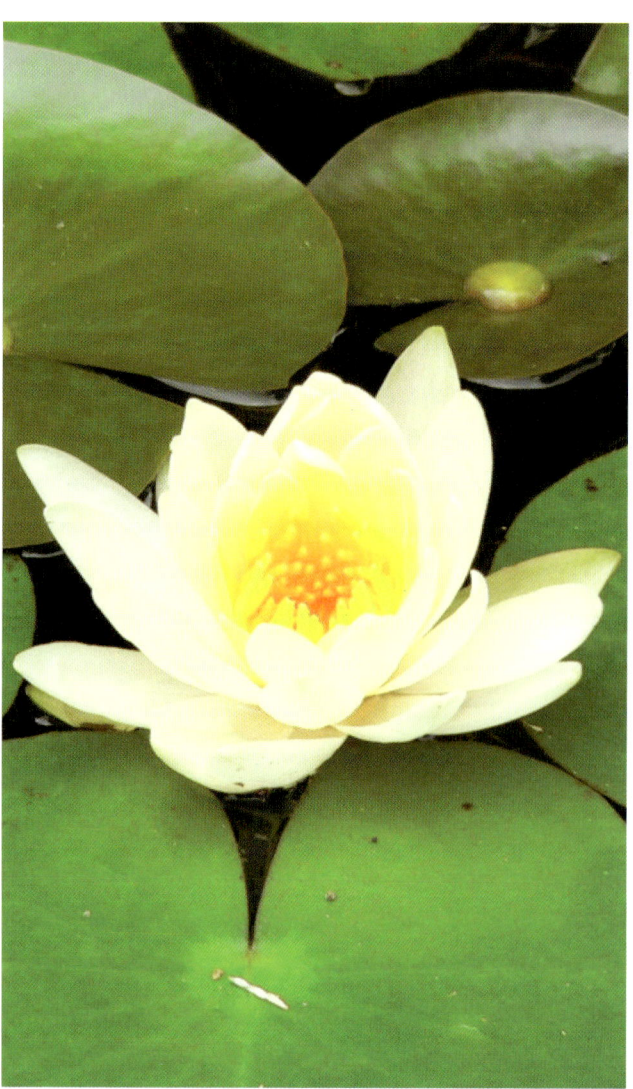

*How can I describe his relentless flute
that pulls virtuous women from their homes
and drags them by their hair to Shyam
as thirst and hunger pull the doe to the snare?
Chaste ladies forget their lords
Wise men forget their wisdom
And clinging vines shall lose from their trees
Hearing that music
Then how shall a simple dairymaid withstand its call?*
—Chandidas, 15th century Bengali poet
*The Sword and the Flute: Kālī & Kṛṣṇa: Dark Visions
of the Terrible and the Sublime in Hindu Mythology* by
David R. Kinsley

Lessons in Lovemaking
The literature of love aimed to educate in two ways—first, by instruction to the senses, where the etiquette or rules of a certain culture resided; and second, by instruction in art, where the idea of love was depicted in classical patterns seen in painting, drama or sculpture. In Bharata's *Natyashastra*, the doctrine of rasa or the aesthetic experience is compared to the tasting of food. A nagarka or a refined, sophisticated person 'tastes' in his mind the various sentiments of love, sorrow, pain and pleasure that are hidden in a work of art, as he would taste the different spices that flavour food.

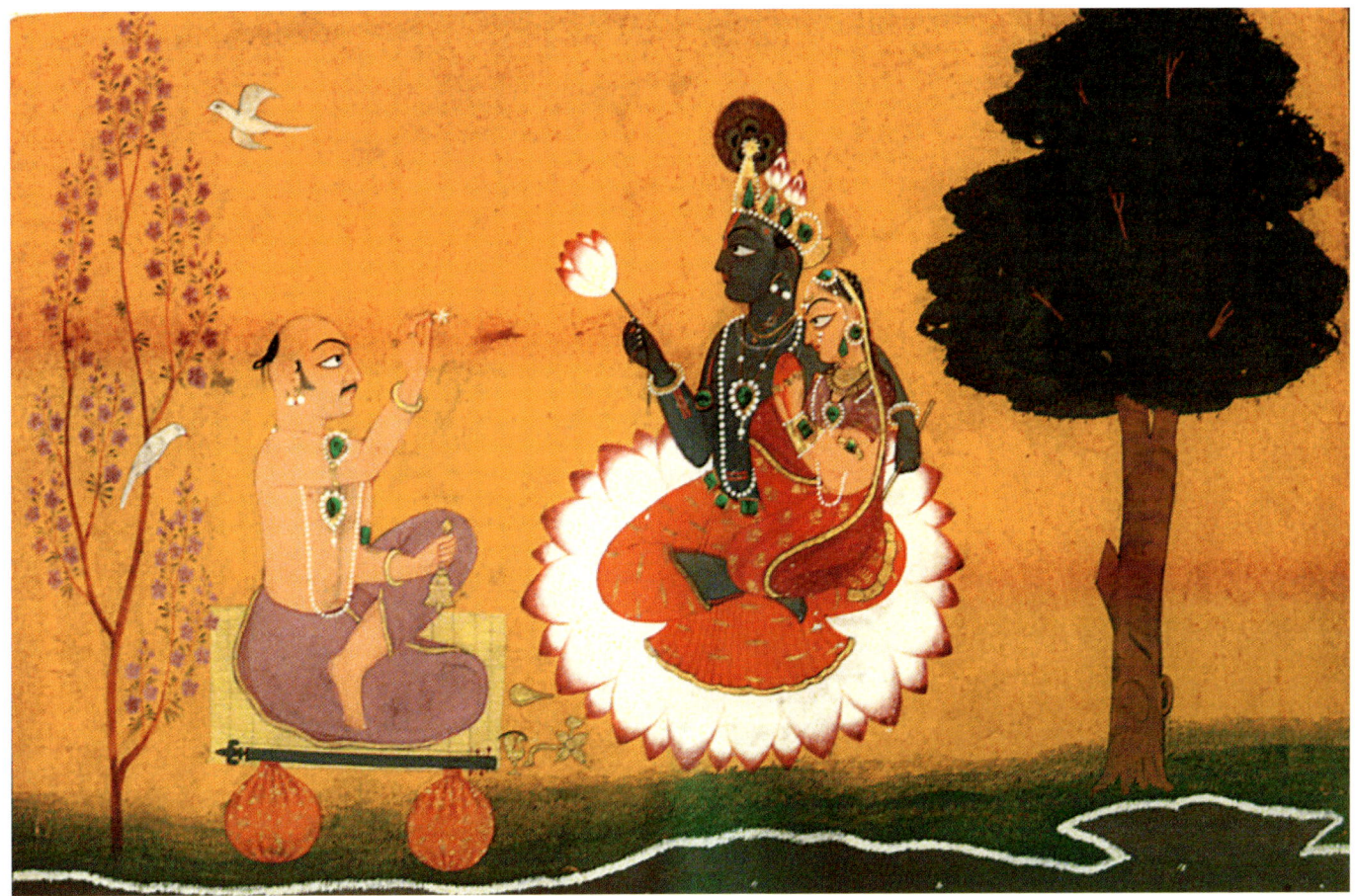

The poet Jayadeva worshipping Radha and Krishna, Miniature painting, National Museum, New Delhi

The book mentions eight rasas: shringara (erotic), hasya (humourous), karuna (pathetic), raudra (anger), vira (heroic), bhayanka (fearful), bibhatsa (repugnant) and adbhuta (amazing). In poetry the shringara rasa with its underlying essence of love or desire finds expression in the pastoral setting—flowers, gardens and all things associated with love and lovemaking. The *Natyashastra* also classifies men and women as nayak and nayika, heroes and heroines, or lovers and sweethearts, based on their emotional and physical characteristics.

Poets drew their inspiration from love and nature, expressed through panegyric, moral debates and story-telling. Legends of the gods were common but deep religious feelings in courtly literature were comparatively rare. Bhartrihari (c. 400) wrote occasionally on religious themes with the intensity of deep faith, but for all its mythological trappings and polite invocations to the deities, classical Sanskrit poetry remained predominantly secular. When the gods made an appearance they usually had the characteristics of superhuman beings.

According to the Indian tradition there are three kinds of literary genres: *shruti* which is received or heard, *smriti* which is derived from memory and *vaak* which

Kavya—beauty in verse 63

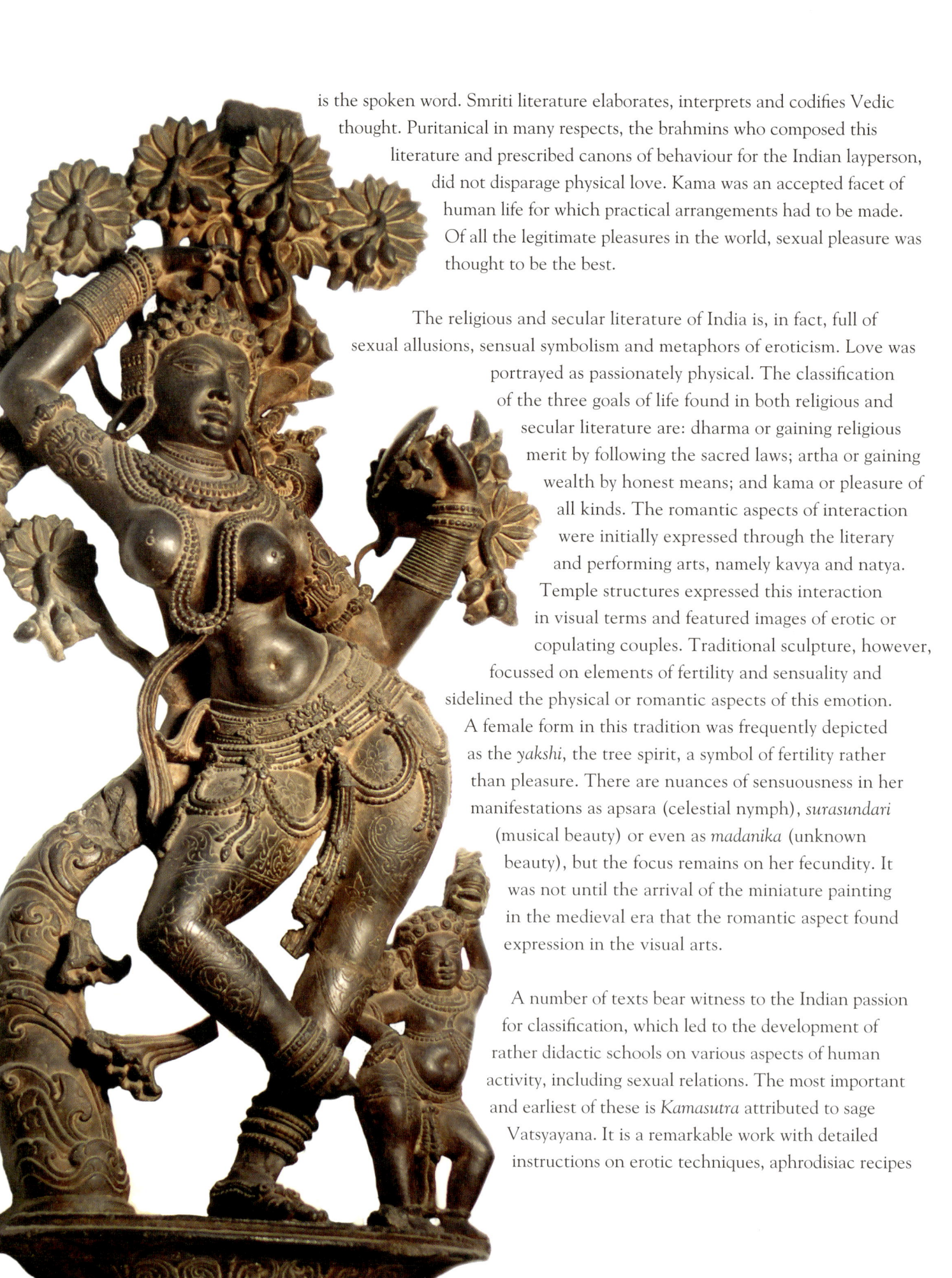

is the spoken word. Smriti literature elaborates, interprets and codifies Vedic thought. Puritanical in many respects, the brahmins who composed this literature and prescribed canons of behaviour for the Indian layperson, did not disparage physical love. Kama was an accepted facet of human life for which practical arrangements had to be made. Of all the legitimate pleasures in the world, sexual pleasure was thought to be the best.

The religious and secular literature of India is, in fact, full of sexual allusions, sensual symbolism and metaphors of eroticism. Love was portrayed as passionately physical. The classification of the three goals of life found in both religious and secular literature are: dharma or gaining religious merit by following the sacred laws; artha or gaining wealth by honest means; and kama or pleasure of all kinds. The romantic aspects of interaction were initially expressed through the literary and performing arts, namely kavya and natya. Temple structures expressed this interaction in visual terms and featured images of erotic or copulating couples. Traditional sculpture, however, focussed on elements of fertility and sensuality and sidelined the physical or romantic aspects of this emotion. A female form in this tradition was frequently depicted as the *yakshi*, the tree spirit, a symbol of fertility rather than pleasure. There are nuances of sensuousness in her manifestations as apsara (celestial nymph), *surasundari* (musical beauty) or even as *madanika* (unknown beauty), but the focus remains on her fecundity. It was not until the arrival of the miniature painting in the medieval era that the romantic aspect found expression in the visual arts.

A number of texts bear witness to the Indian passion for classification, which led to the development of rather didactic schools on various aspects of human activity, including sexual relations. The most important and earliest of these is *Kamasutra* attributed to sage Vatsyayana. It is a remarkable work with detailed instructions on erotic techniques, aphrodisiac recipes

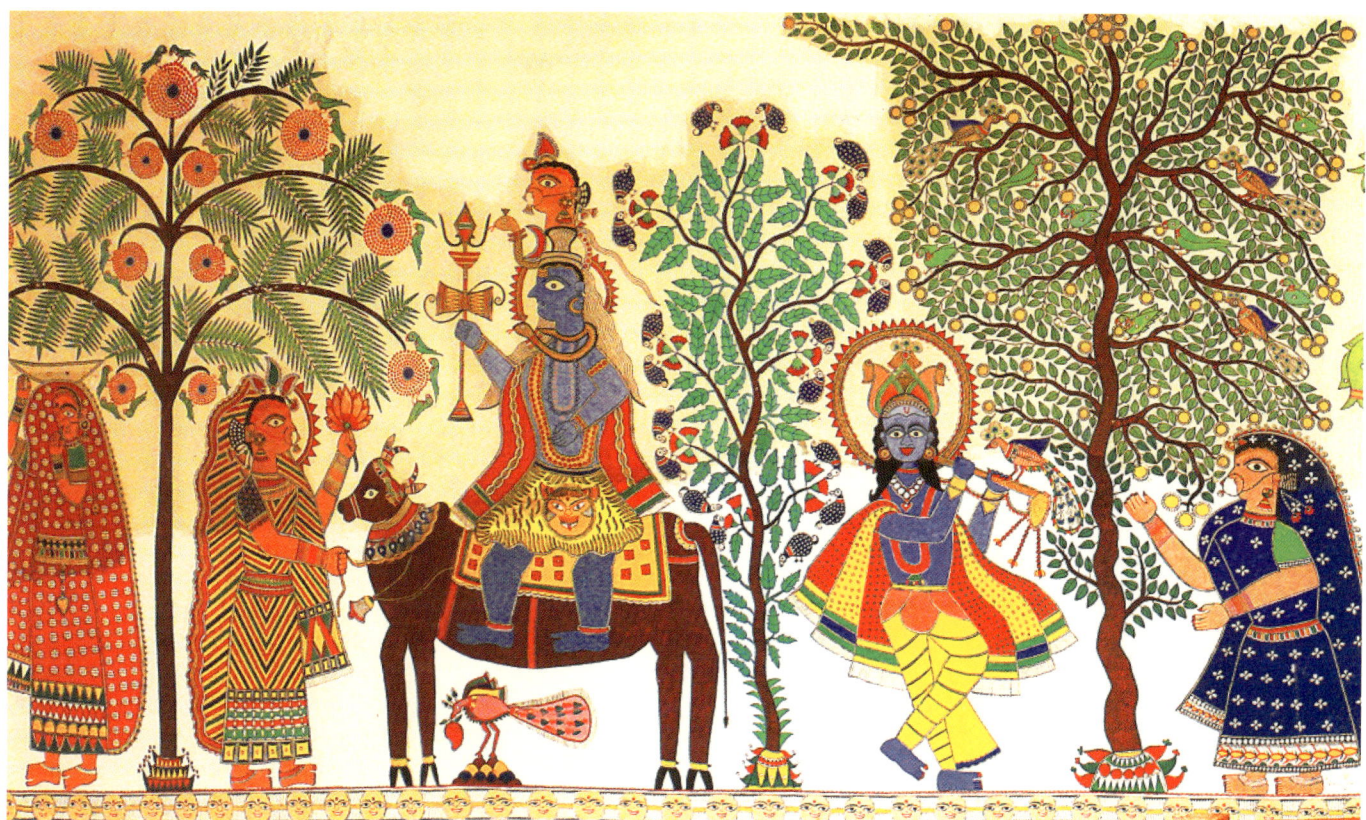

Madhubani painting, Crafts Museum, New Delhi. An art predominantly practiced by women, Madhubani paintings mostly depict Hindu motifs, deities and themes

(Page 64) Mohini, an enchantress in Hindu mythology, bronze, Western Chalukya, Karnataka, 11th century, National Museum, New Delhi

and charms, and incidentally, valuable information about society in ancient India. Sexuality was regarded as a refined mutual relationship for the satisfaction of both the partners involved. *Kamasutra* advises the sophisticated townsman, for whom it was written, to consider the satisfaction of his mistress as well as his own, for she is as passionate as him. Her pleasure in sex, according to the author, is greater than his. Foreplay is classified in detail and *Kamasutra* defines sixteen types of kisses. Displaying scratches, bruises, tooth marks and other signs of passion to friends is considered to be a favourite poetic convention.

The ideals of feminine beauty in ancient India differed from the Greek and European: in India a beautiful woman was expected to have broad hips, a slender waist and heavy breasts. The poets loved to describe their heroines in terms of luxurious opulence, while at the same time observing conventional restraints. The gentler side of Indian sensual expression can be seen in this extract from *Kamasutra*:

> *On the evening of the tenth day (after the wedding) the husband should speak gently to his wife...to give her confidence...Vatsyayana recommends that a man should at first refrain from intercourse, until he has won over his bride and gained her confidence, for women, being gentle by nature, prefer to be won over gently. If a*

Kavya—beauty in verse

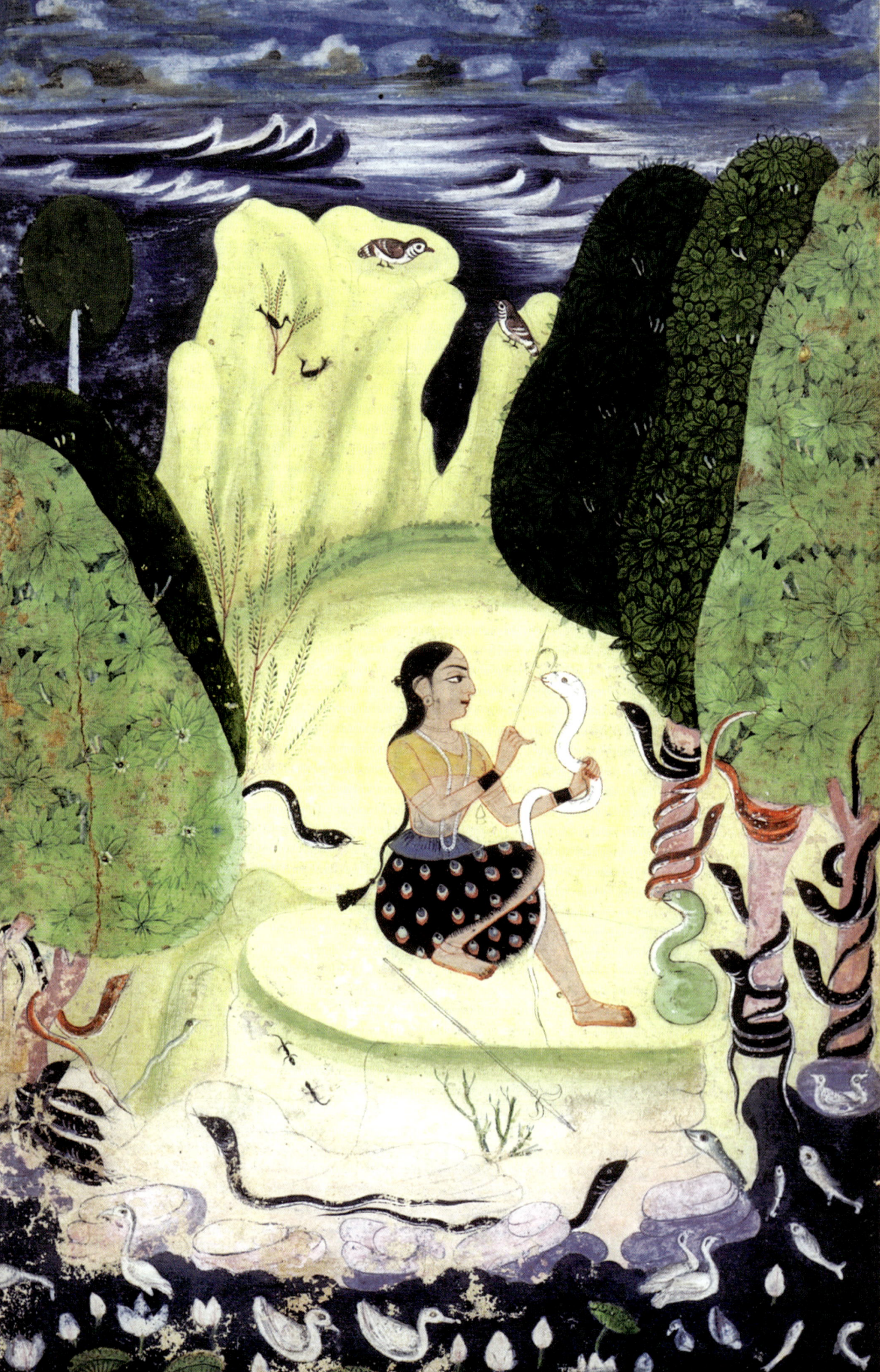

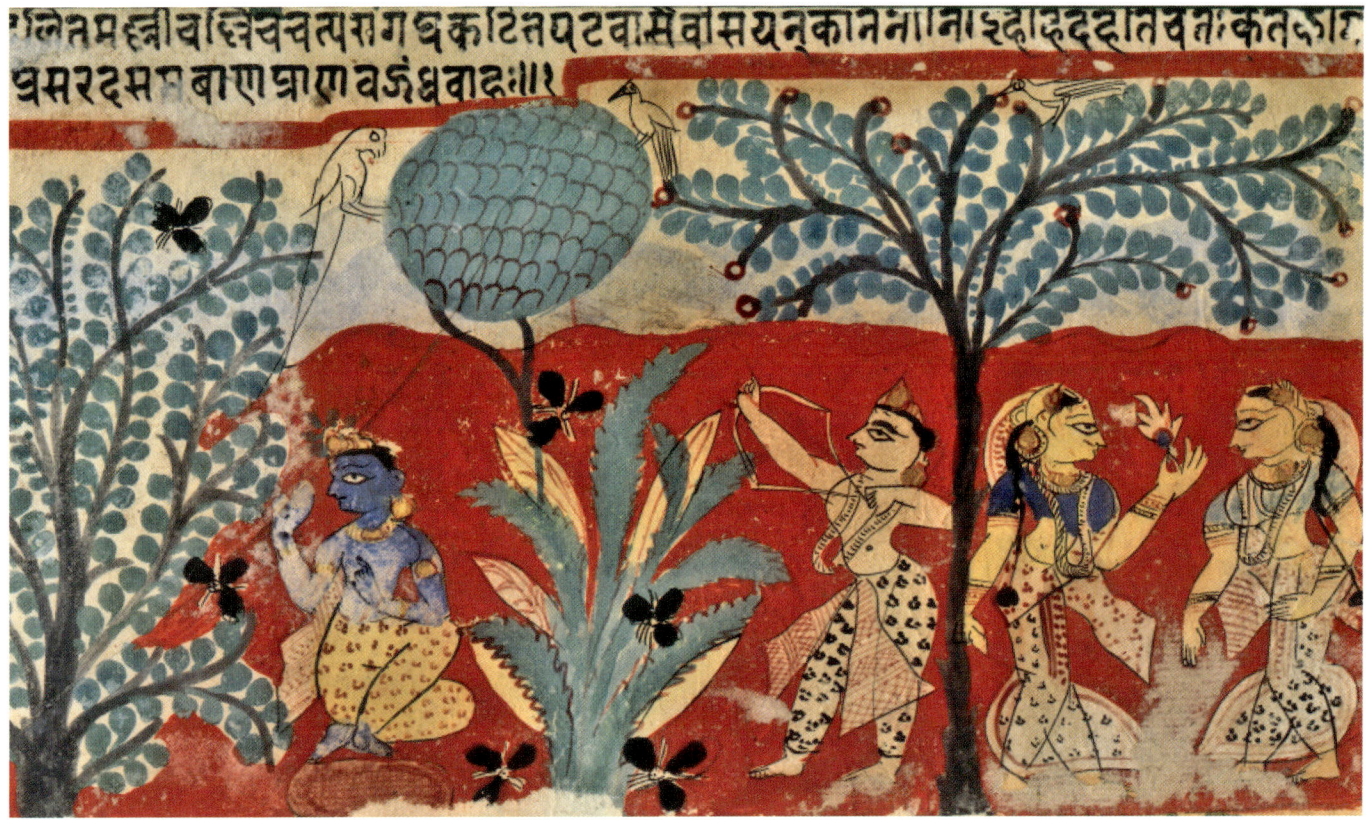

woman is forced to submit to rough handling from a man whom she scarcely knows she may come to hate sexual intercourse, and even to hate the whole male sex…or she may grow to detest her husband in particular, and may then turn to another man.
—**An Introduction to Indian Thought, A.L. Herman**

Metaphors from Nature

The phenomenon of the seasons, day and night, the birds, beasts and flowers, were used to frame human emotions, or were used to personify human subjects. A deep love for nature runs through all ancient Indian literary works and is found most particularly in the works of Kalidasa (5th century AD). In his monumental work *Ritusamhara* (garland of seasons) he gives a vivid account of the seasons, while establishing a sensual connection between the erotic and nature. The erotic metaphors are taken to their heights and repeated parallels are drawn with the world of nature—the rising moon awakens love in the hearts of women seeking their lovers; the lovelorn heroine is sad when the mango flower blossoms, and sheds tears in remembrance of her beloved. In *Kumarasambhava* Kalidasa writes a detailed description of the lovemaking between Shiva and Parvati. The goddess, though shy and tentative, arouses and satisfies her husband as they come together in union.

Early Gita Govinda, Gujarat, 16th century, N.C. Mehta Collection, Ahmedabad

(Page 66) Ragini Asavari, Bundi, Rajasthan, 18th century, N.C. Mehta Collection, Ahmedabad

Kavya—beauty in verse

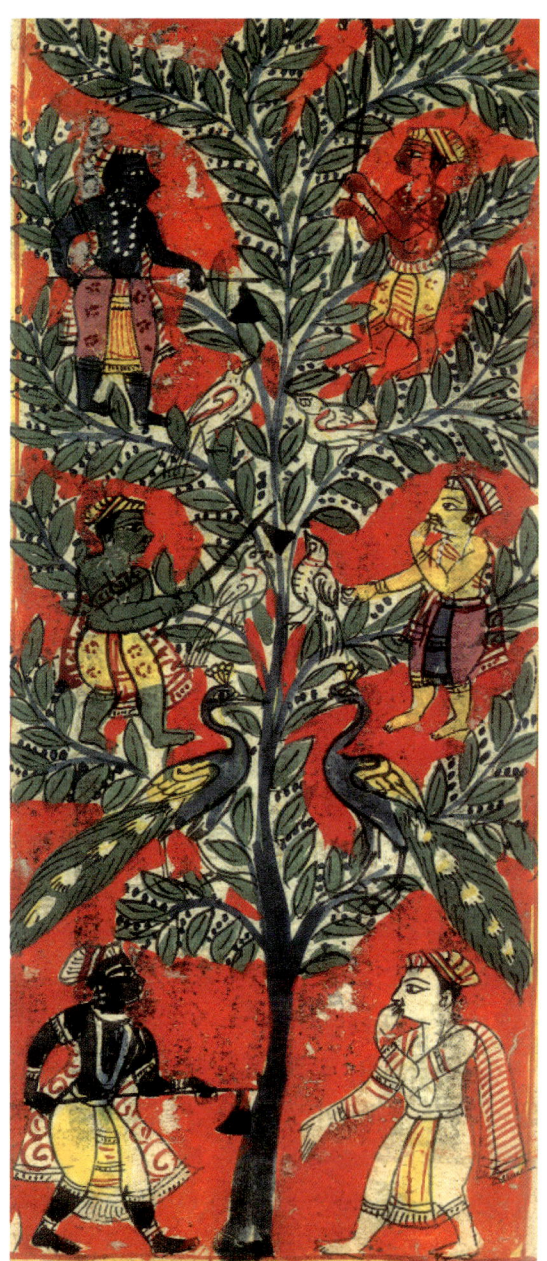

Folio from Sangrahani Sutra, *western India, N.C. Mehta Collection, Ahmedabad. The Sangrahani Sutra is a illustration, cosmological text in Sanskrit*

(Page 69)
Vamana Temple, Khajuraho

Addressed she could not answer;
When he touched her gown she sought to leave him;
With head averted she clung to her couch;
Yet nonetheless did she delight Shiva.

Ritusamhara describes the six seasons of the Hindu year in relation to shringara. *Meghadutam* (the cloud messenger) is full of imagery and word pictures that contain the essence of the culture of those times. It relates the story of a *yaksha* dwelling in the divine city of Alaka. Having offended his master, Kubera, he has been banished for a year to the hill of Ramgiri. Separation from his beautiful wife is the worst aspect of his exile. On seeing a large cloud passing northward to the mountains, he pours his heart out to it. He describes in beautiful verses the lands, rivers and cities over which it should pass:

Stay for a while over the thickets haunted by the girl of the hill-folk.
Then press on with faster pace, having shed your load of water,
And you will see the Narmada River, scattered in torrents,
by the rugged rocks at the foot of the Vindhyas,
Looking at the plastered pattern of stripes on the flank of the elephant.

Kalidasa further evokes the shringara rasa by his description of the city:

Where the wind from the Sipra River prolongs the shrill melodious cry of the cranes,
Fragrant at early dawn from the scent of the opening lotus,
And, like a lover, with flattering requests,
Dispels the morning languor of women, and refreshes their limbs.

Love can be broadly classified as *rati* or love between man and woman, *vatsalya* or love between mother and child, and *bhakti* or devotion towards god. An individual experiencing such an emotion is completely immersed in it and forgets the world around him as well as his own existence.

In verses evoking shringara, the poet Bhartrihari often expresses an undercurrent of dissatisfaction as though trying to convince himself that love is not a futile waste of time after all. In the midst of his amours, he is seen to use words with religious connotations:

68   *Shringara—the many faces of Indian beauty*

Your hair self-denying, your eyes understanding the whole of scripture
Your mouth full of groups of naturally-pure Brahmans,
Your breasts lovely from the presence of emancipated souls
Slim girl, your body, though free from passion, disturbs me.

Amaru's 8th century works epitomize shringara rasa. His stanzas on love, although often voluptuous, are humorously tender at times:

'I'll see what comes of it,' I thought, and hardened my heart against her.
'What, won't the villain speak to me?' she thought, flying into a rage.
And there we stood, sedulously refusing to look one another in the face, until at last I managed an unconvincing laugh, and her tears robbed me of my resolution.

The King of Love Poetry

Written in 12th-century Bengal, Jayadeva's *Gita Govinda* is in a class of its own. It describes the love of Lord Krishna and Radha in a series of dramatic lyrics mainly intended for singing. While it is without doubt a passionate rendition of the shringara rasa in which the line between devotion and passion gets blurred, the spirituality of the interaction is not compromised in any way. Through the medium of passionate union, *Gita Govinda* illustrates the search for the divine and the submission of the human soul that attains fulfilment only through complete surrender.

You rest on the circle of Sri's breast,
Wearing your earrings,
Fondling wanton forest garlands.
Triumph, God of Triumph, Hari!
The sun's jewel light encircles you
As you break through the bond of existence -
A wild Himalayan goose on lakes in minds of holy men.
Triumph, God of Triumph, Hari!
You defeat the venomous serpent Kaliya,
Exciting your Yadu kinsmen
Like sunlight inciting lotuses to bloom.
Triumph, God of Triumph, Hari!
—***The Love Song of the Dark Lord: Jayadeva's Gita Govinda,*** **Barbara Stoler Miller**

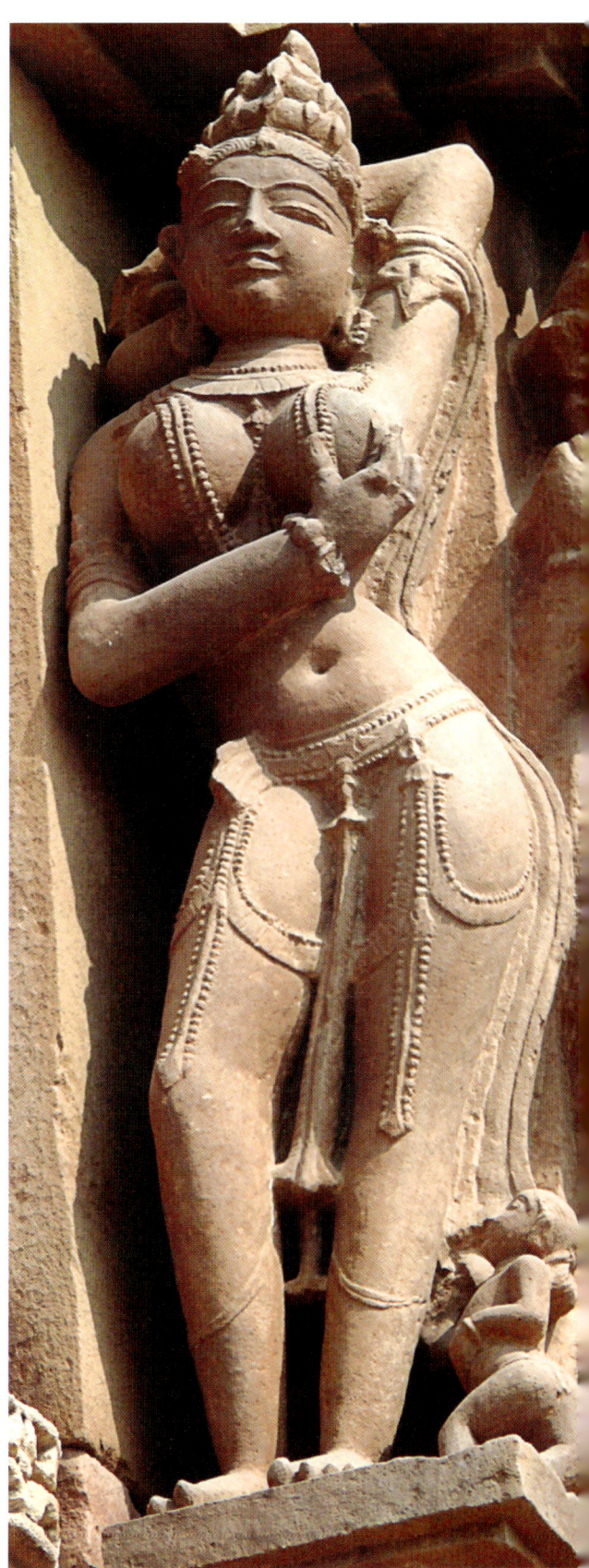

Kavya—beauty in verse 69

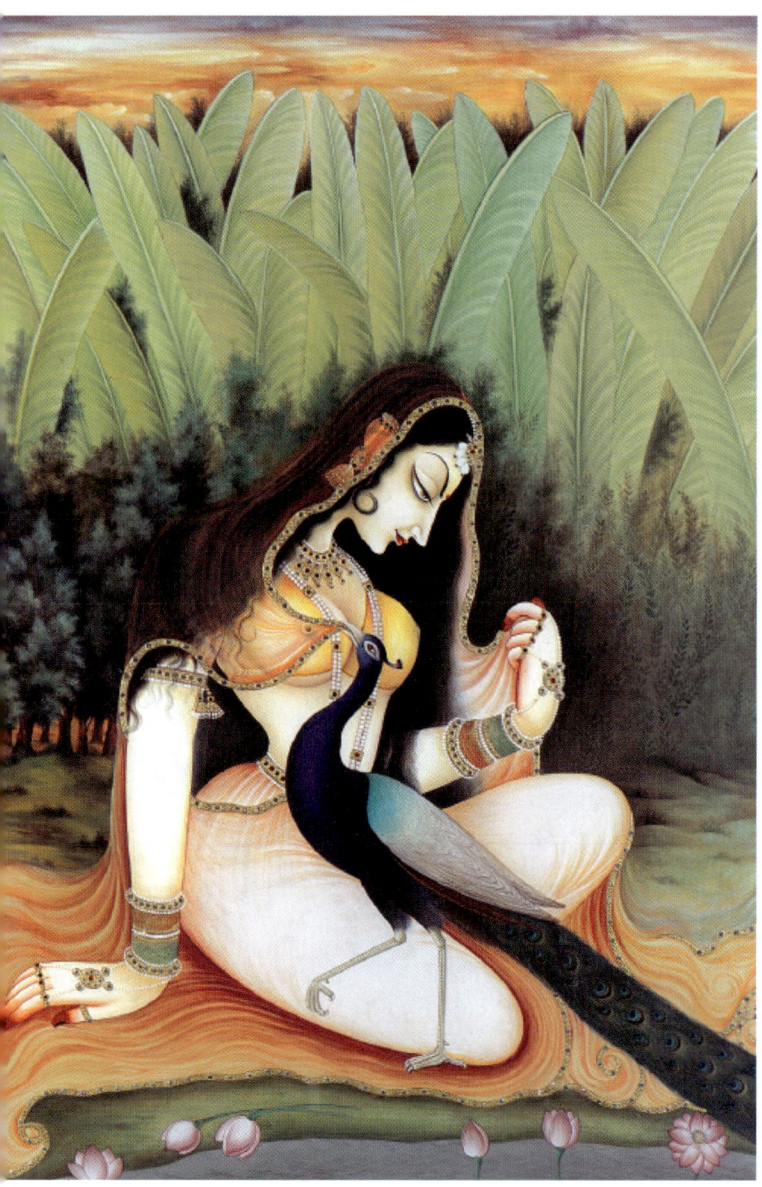

The nayika, at play with the peacock, Kishangarh/Rajasthan style of painting

*(Page 71)
Bharatnatyam dancer
Lakshmi Viswanathan*

The naming of the twelve *sargams* or songs of *Gita Govinda* aptly describes the moods of the Lord in love-play. They are:
* The joyful Krishna (*Saamoda Daamodara*)
* The careless Krishna (*Aklesa Kesava*)
* The bewildered Krishna (*Mugdha Madhusoodana*)
* The tender Krishna (*Snighdha Madhusoodana*)
* The lotus-eyed Krishna longing for love (*Saakanksha Pundarikaksha*)
* The indolent Krishna (*Kunta Vaikunta*)
* The cunning Krishna (*Naagara Naarayana*)
* The abashed Krishna (*Vilakshya Lakshmi Pati*)
* The languishing Krishna (*Manda Mukunda*)
* The four quickening arms (*Chatura Chaturbhuja*)
* The blissful Krishna (*Saananda Daamodara*)
* The ecstatic Krishna (*Suprita Peetambara*)

Although Jayadeva stood out as the undisputed leader of medieval romantic poetry, the 15th century poet, Bhanudatta, carried the tradition further with his *Rasamanjari*. His work elaborated on the classification of the romantic heroines of Nayikabheda and illustrated sensually the various moods and seasons of love and their effect on the nayaks and nayikas.

The Different Strands

In the next few centuries following Jayadeva, two significant movements established themselves through the length and breadth of the country. These were Ritikavya and Bhaktikavya. Ritikavya dealt with the sensuous aspects of romantic love between Radha and Krishna, whereas Bhaktikavya was more devotional in character. However, the elements of spirituality and sensuality were conspicuous in both forms, making them two fibres of the same fabric. Indian literature in the medieval period emerged from many different strands. Regional court poets composed poems in praise of kings and warriors; many poets produced works based on themes from the Sanskrit epics and Puranas; and the Persian-speaking Muslim court introduced elements of Islamic culture to India.

The spread of Hinduism, in particular, produced large amounts of religious literature, often dedicated to the deities Rama and Krishna. This was the

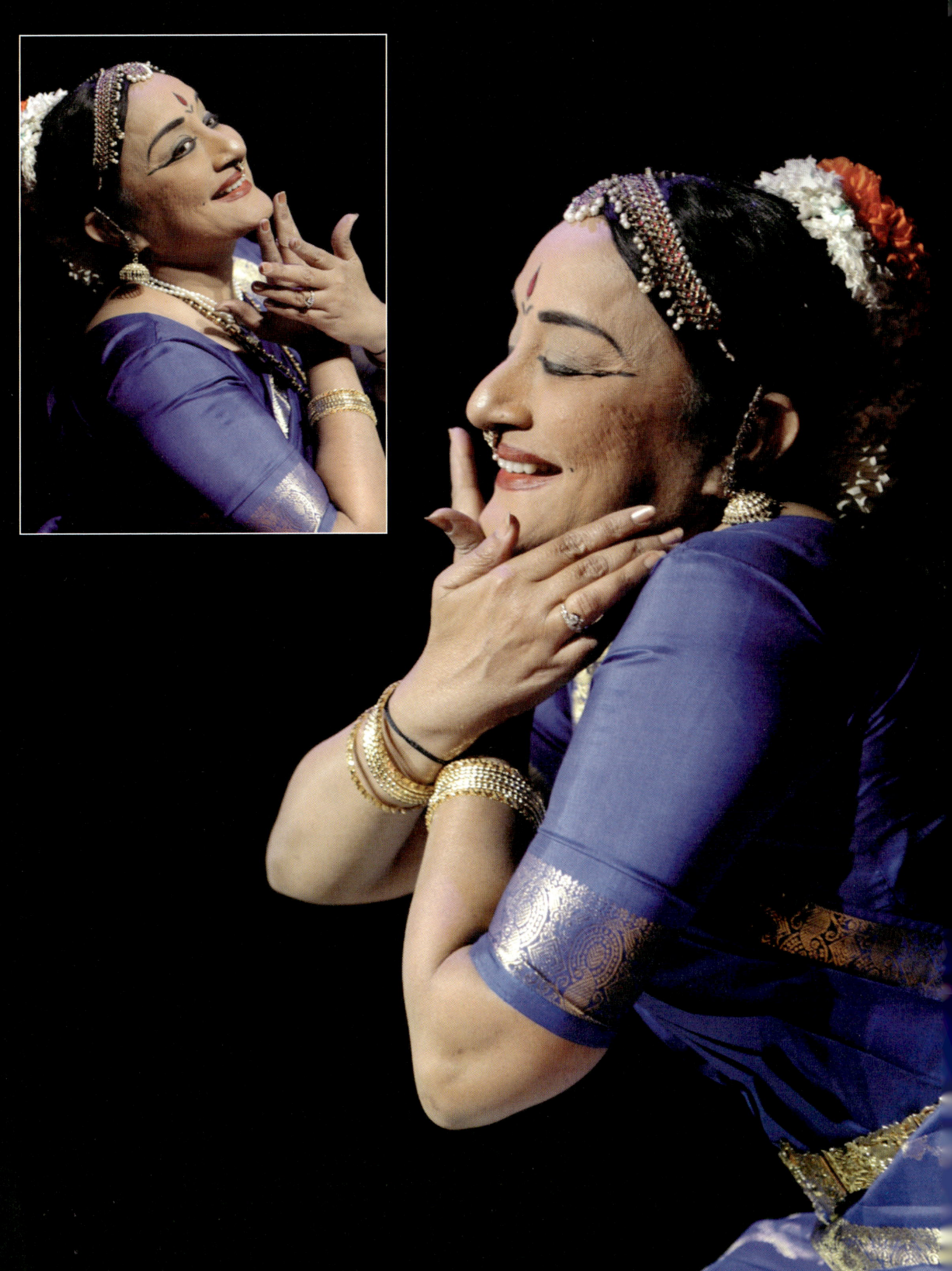

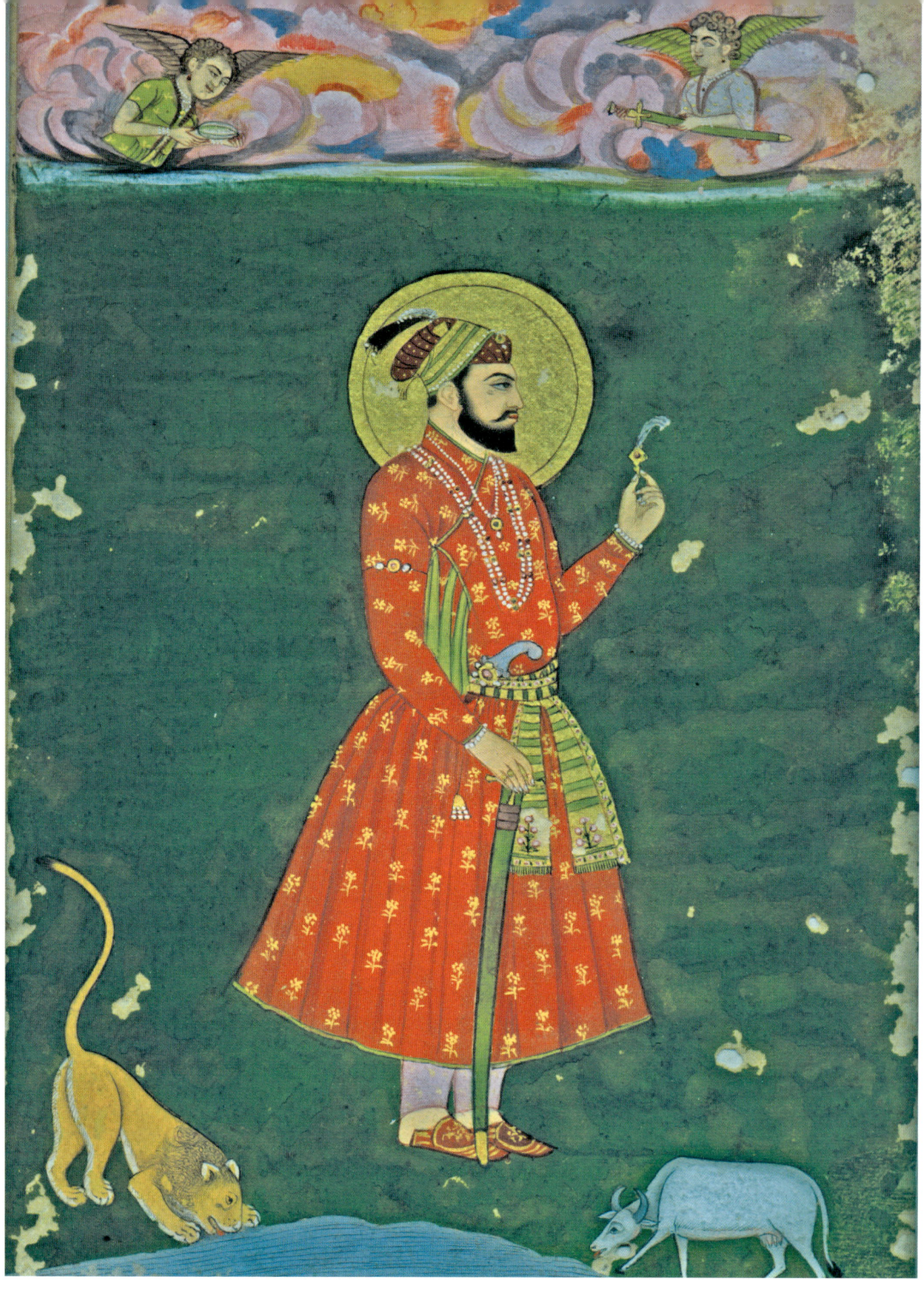

72　*Shringara*—the many faces of Indian beauty

literature of Bhakti (devotional religion), based on the importance of a loving relationship between the worshipper and God. Meanwhile, folk poetry, celebrating the seasons and festivals, was passed down from generation to generation and continues to be part of the rural repertoire.

During the medieval era the expression of shringara in art and literature went through a significant change. The explicit mention and celebration of shringara in poetry and literature, particularly in the Mughal period, served either as a visual aphrodisiac to otherwise prudish rulers, or as a surreptitious attempt to whet the baser appetites of society. Though there was a resurrection of the earlier erotic texts like *Kamasutra*, their expression was somewhat inhibited. *Rati Rahasya* (mysteries of passion) better known as the *Koka Shastra* was one such work, written by Pandit Kukkoka in the 12th century to please his overlord, Vendutta, who was perhaps a king.

Koka Shastra is almost identical in its content to *Kamasutra* and contains nearly 800 verses divided into 10 chapters called Panchivedas. But there are some subjects treated in this text that find no mention in *Kamasutra*. These include a classification of women into four groups, namely Padmini, Chitrini, Shankini and Hastini. Koka's enumeration of the days and hours during which women of different classes become subject to love is also written about for the first time. The division between the spiritual and the secular was finally becoming blurred through these texts.

Kalayanmalla, the 15th century poet, stated the purpose of writing his book *Anang Ranga* (Theatre of the Love God) as: 'No one yet has written a book to prevent the separation of the married couple and to show them how they may pass their life in union. Seeing this I felt compassion and composed this book.'

It is evident that this was written for a society that had changed from one of gay abandon to a more sedate one. Romance had taken a backseat and the woman's place was rooted in the house. Men and women no longer met socially and pre-marital courtship was unheard of. *Anang Ranga* is a manual for marriage and not a lover's handbook, and is based on the premise that sex in marriage, while losing its passion, gains in spiritual mystery. It covers the usual subjects, but adds a description of the eight nayikas and an elaborate section on palmistry.

(Page 72)
Portrait of Farrukhsiyar, Mughal School, N.C. Mehta Collection, Ahmedabad

Sri Devi, Vijayanagara, National Museum, New Delhi

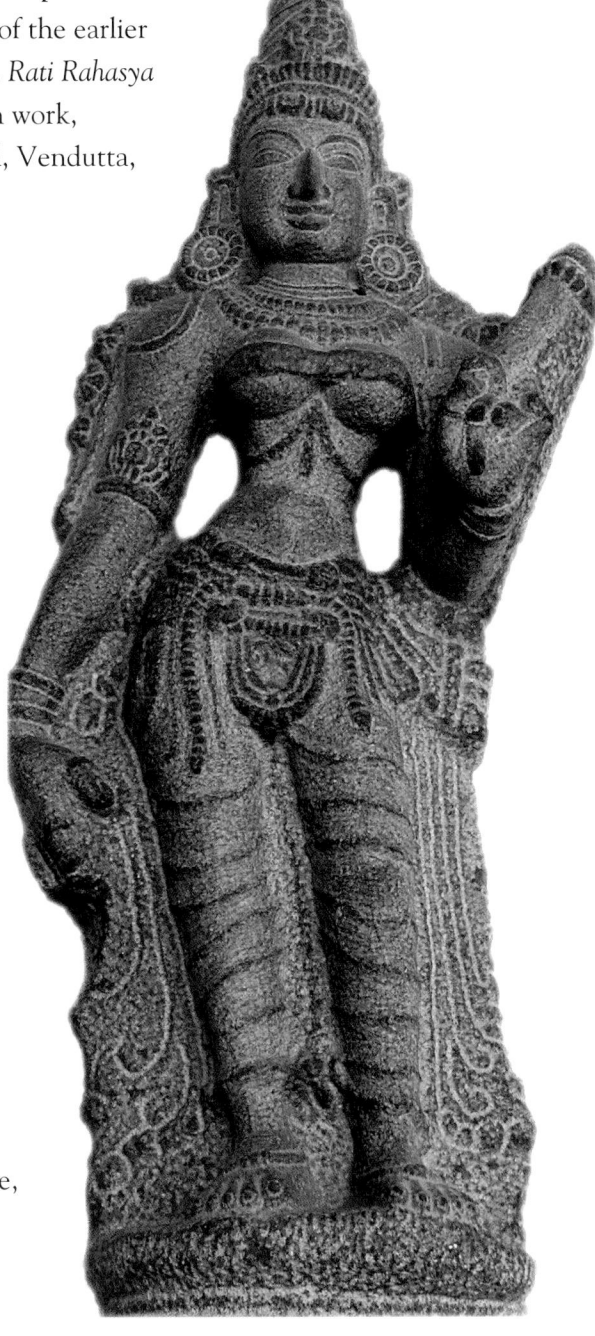

Kavya—beauty in verse

Ecstatic Devotion

With the spread of the Bhakti movement, shringara was expressed as an outpouring of love towards a personal and intimate God. Bhaktikavya held a strong grip over northern India and the eternal love of Radha and Krishna was extensively portrayed in literature and art. The movement later spread to the eastern provinces of Bihar and Bengal. Drawing inspiration from the Aham poetry of the ancient Tamil country, Bhakti songs were sung in temples by Tamil singer-saints, the Alvars and Nayanmars, who assumed the persona of the female lover of God. The movement developed essentially as Krishna bhakti with the poets portraying Krishna as the romantic hero while blending bhakti and shringara.

Bhakti literature developed in Avadhi and Braj, the dialects spoken by the best-known of its devotees and singer saints: Tulsidas, Kabir, Surdas and Mirabai. Tulsidas's *Ramacharitmanas* was written in Avadhi, while Tulsidas's *Vinay Patrika* and Surdas's *Sur Sagar* were written in Braj. Kabir, however, preferred to write his dohas in Sadhukaddi, yet another dialect spoken in north India. Mirabai's family were devotees of Vishnu and her poems are devoted to the god in his incarnation as Krishna whom she calls Girdhara (he who carried the mountains). Devoted to Krishna from an early age, she asks in one of her poems:

O Krishan, did you ever rightly value my childhood love?
In the calm of the night
I will rise and go to him,
And return at dawn.
Night and day I will remain engrossed
In communion with my lord.

Deeply immersed in the Bhakti movement, the blind poet and mystic, Surdas, composed beautiful songs in praise of Krishna. He was a proponent of the Shuddhadvaita school of Vaishnavism also known as Pushti Marg, a philosophy based on the spiritual metaphors of Radha-Krishna lila. In his most famous *Sur Sagar*, he compares the company of Krishna and the milkmaids to a beautiful lake that submerges the shringara rasa:

Krishna shines in the group of young Braj-ladies, which appears like a lake.
Their eyes are the lotus flowers. Their earrings are the moving fish.
Their breasts are the Chakravaaka birds, which are looking at the moon,
Their pearl-made necklaces are the band of noisy cranes on the bank.

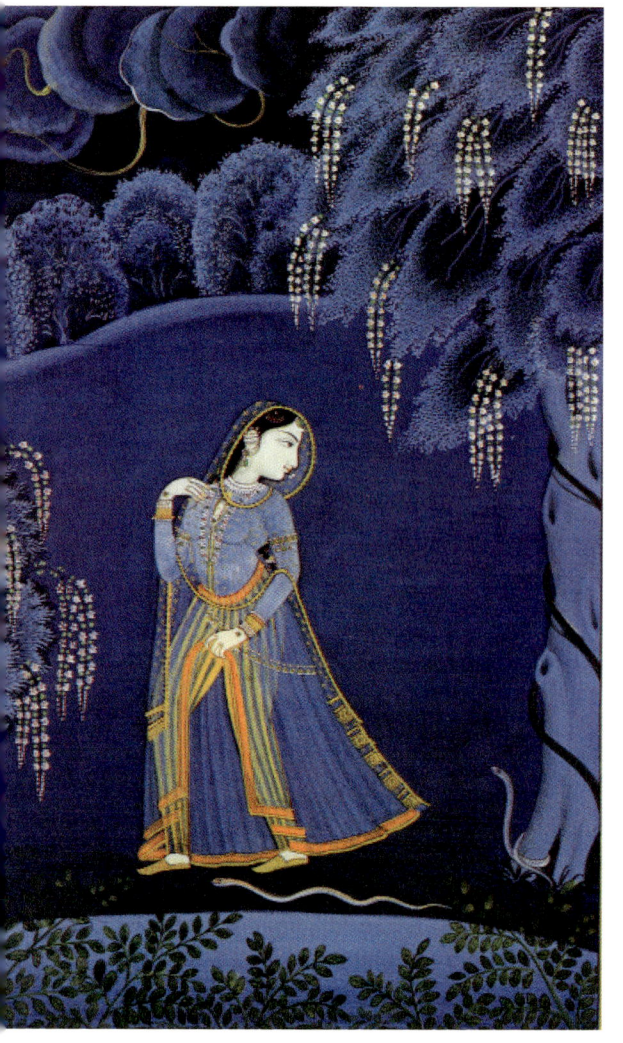

Braving all odds to meet her beloved the 'Abhisarika' nayika walks in the dark forest and encounters serpents in her path

*The basil garland is the group of
beautiful swans, peacocks, and parrots,
sitting on the tuft of grass.*

On Radha and Krishna making love,
he writes:

*...With garlands of pearls and flowers
decked
he takes her to the Yamuna bank
and there makes love; even Kama
is envious to see them dally thus.
And when the sweet notes of his pipe
resound, all her passion dies,
and with love's rapture she thrills.
Says Surdasa, the Lord sports thus and
fills her with love-making's first delight.
He held her in a tight embrace
as she came, thrilling with delight,
love fulfilment suffused her face
with joy, her passion satisfied.*

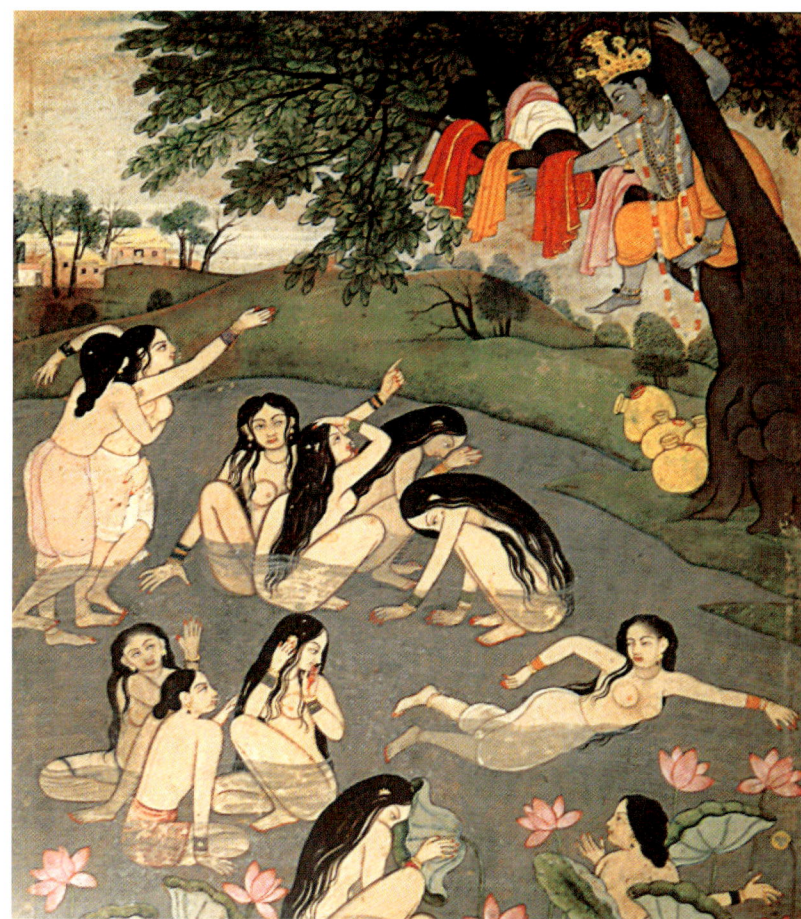

Krishna teasing the gopis in the popular theme of 'Vastraharan', Pahari School, National Museum, New Delhi. The Pahari School of art emphasized the emotions of women, and their main theme was love, a primary source of inspiration with the Krishna legend at its centre

Kabir wanted to unite the *Jivatma* and
Paramatma, or the human soul with the Divine. According to him it was the constant, intense pursuit of the devotee for his ideal love that qualified him to attain enlightenment. G.N. Das, a well-known Kabir scholar, quotes some poignant and passionate verses:

*Tell me, Brother, how can I renounce Maya?
When I gave up the tying of ribbons, still I tied my garment about me;
When I gave up tying my garment, still I covered my body in its folds.
So, when I give up passion, I see that anger remains;
And when I renounce anger, greed is with me still;
And when greed is vanquished, pride and vainglory remain;
When the mind is detached and casts Maya away, still it clings to the letter.
Kabir says, 'Listen to me, dear Sadhu! The true path is rarely found.'*

—***Songs of Kabir*, Rabindranath Tagore**

Bhagavata Purana established the romantic tradition of *bhakti shringara* or ecstatic devotion. This tradition saw the metaphorical manifestation of the innocent

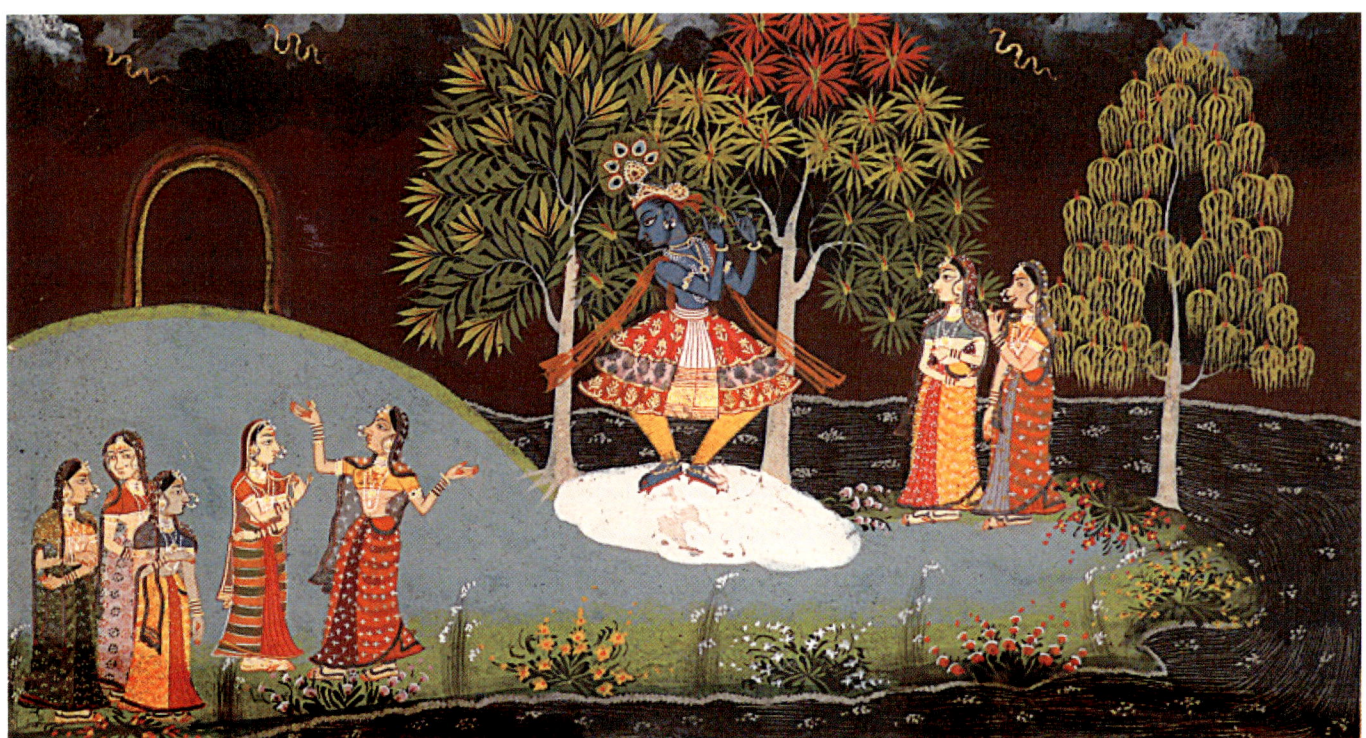

Krishna playing the flute, Mewar School, National Museum, New Delhi

dedication and surrender of the gopis to Krishna. The creations of *Bhagavata Purana* rose out of the fusion of bhakti shringara and Aryan ritualism found in the northern Puranic tradition. The most significant section of the Purana is the tenth chapter that highlights the *rasa lila* of Lord Krishna with the gopis. This became the ultimate inspiration for love poetry for centuries thereafter. The ambiguity between the two personae of Krishna was interpreted in myriad ways, but was essentially understood as an allegory for the relationship of Jivatman with the Paramataman.

The Kashmiri poet, Bilhana, established a significant shift with his sensual yet secular composition, *Chaurapanchashika*, written in the 11th century. The work was a collection of fifty verses held together by the repeated refrain *adyapi*, a word that means 'reminiscence'. The work has a certain sonorous and sensuous quality to it. Steeped in shringara rasa, it is a feast for the senses, redolent of the fragrance of musk and sandalwood, night-blossoming jasmine and lotus pollen. Soft arms clinging around the neck like vines, wine-smeared lips, a lotus bed of passion, kohl-blackened eyes, vermilion lips, hot red blood from bites on the lips… the text is replete with colourful verses describing moments of passion.

Bhakti literature is the most important creative contribution of the medieval period. Krishna and Rama, the two main incarnations of the god Vishnu, were widely worshipped. Temples dedicated to these two deities abounded, and their worshippers

76 *Shringara*—the many faces of Indian beauty

were divided into a number of different sects, each one following a particular spiritual teacher. Much of Bhakti literature was written in the form of hymns, sung until today, praising these two deities and their deeds, or humbly asking for their help.

While Krishna the playful lover is worshipped in romantic songs and verse, Rama is revered as an ideal and heroic king, and his wife, Sita, is the model of Hindu womanhood. The monkey god Hanuman, faithful henchman of Rama in the war against Ravana, appears as the ideal devotee.

The Sufi Tradition

Islamic mysticism was also evolving around the same time as the Bhakti movement. The Sufis sang about their own personal experience of divine love, thus distancing themselves from the dogmatic conformity of the Shar'iah. They believed that *ishq-i majazi*, worldly love, was only a bridge to reach *ishq-i haqiqi*, divine love. The homoerotic metaphor found expression in Sufi literature, as many Sufis believed that only same-gender love could transcend sex. The Radha-Krishna tradition of bhakti had a great influence on Sufi poetry and this can be seen in the many folk tales and love stories, among which are Heer-Ranja and Sohni-Mahiwal, along with the Central Asian Laila-Majnu, Shirin-Farhad, Yusuf-Zulaikha and Mahmud-Ayaz.

The introduction of the ghazal in Urdu poetry was by far the finest expression of the erotic in Islamic culture. Literally a love song, the ghazal became the most popular form of poetry in the later Muslim era. Various Muslim dynasties ruled much of India, from their arrival in the 1100s upto the 1800s. Most of them spoke Persian or Turkish, used in a slightly Indianized form for the business of government and the court.

Malik Muhammad Jayasi, Raskhan and Rahim, among other Muslim poets, wrote Sufi and Vaishnava poetry. Bulleh Shah, the most famous Muslim Punjabi poet, popularized Sufism through Punjabi *kafi* (a verse form). Shah Laatif, a Sindhi poet, wrote *Risalo*, an important Sufi text. Amir Khusrau (1253-1325), the legendary Sufi poet who was one of the early proponents of India's unified culture, composed verses in Urdu, a language that evolved out of a fusion of Persian and Hindi. The poetry written in Urdu has largely followed Persian forms and metres. The poet Sauda (1706-81) gave rigour and versatility to Urdu poetry, while Dard (1720-85) and Mir Taqi Mir (1722-1810) gave it maturity, ushering in the modern period of literature.

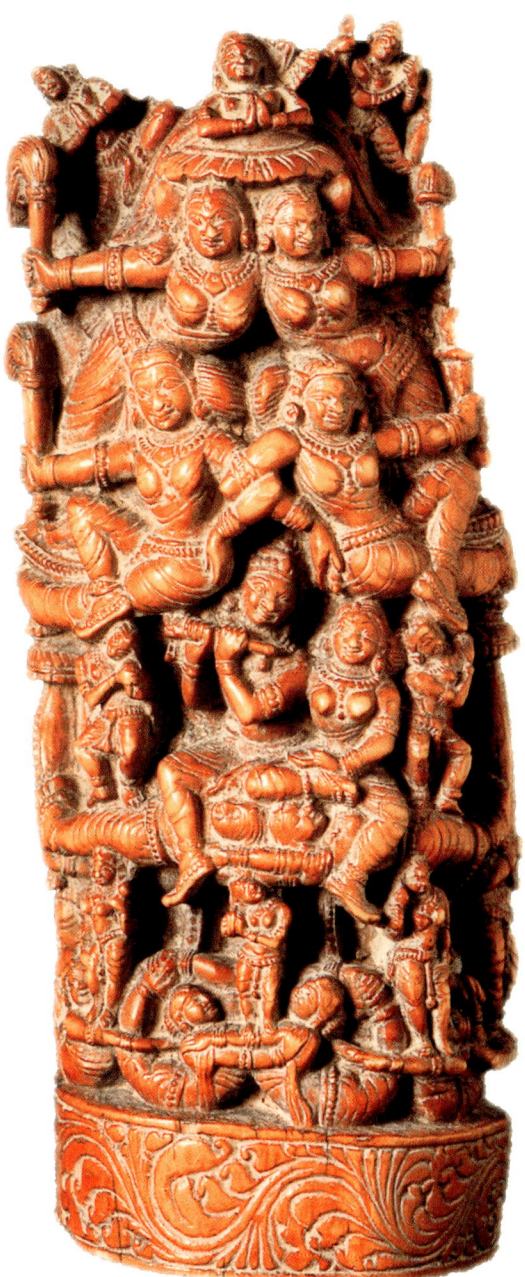

Krishna and Radha surrounded by female figures in wood, South India, Crafts Museum, New Delhi

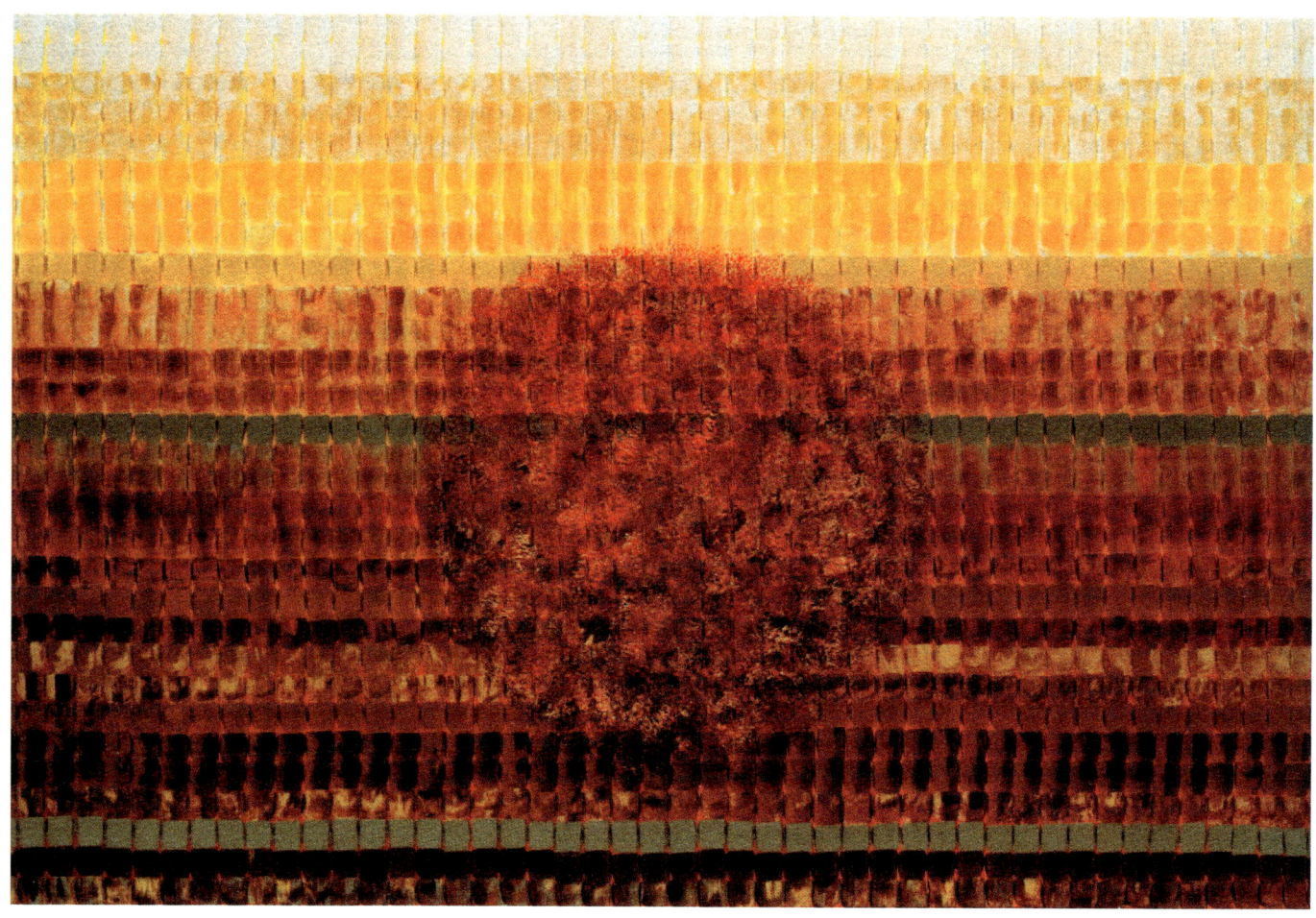

'Fire', acrylic on canvas, painting by Kalpana Shah

The Epitome of Shringara

Ritikavya was the other genre of romantic poetry in Indian literature which, as opposed to bhakti kavya, added a worldly and sensuous dimension to the earlier devotional Radha-Krishna poetry. Radha in the hands of the Riti Kal poets became the epitome of shringara. In the Indian tradition, Radha is not an individual; rather she is a universal figure who has become depersonalized, and stands for every woman who is in love.

Ritikavya was redolent with courtly elegance and splendour. Instead of portraying a love story, it elucidated the romantic moments of courtly love. The gopis of the earlier poems were restructured into a new urban and elite social order; this allowed a free personal and intimate interaction with the nayak and the nayika, who were mostly courtly nobles. However, Ritikavya also took poetry out of the courts and into the lives of common men, thus giving birth to a rich folk music tradition. The important poets of this genre are Vidyapati, Keshavadas, Bihari and Ghanananda. Radha occupies centre stage in Vidyapati's works, as against Jayadeva, who was basically a devotee of Krishna.

The Riti poetry reached great heights with the works of the 16th-century poet Keshavadas. His *Rasikapriya* is a celebrated treatise on erotic love. It describes how Krishna would offer to an angry Radha flowers 'longing to become fragrant by the touch of her breasts', or an ivory necklace 'yearning to fulfil its destiny by going on a pilgrimage to her bosom'. The book deals with different kinds of nayaks and nayikas, their lovemaking, their moods, emotions and sentiments. Accounts of lovers in different situations—sometimes 'hidden' and sometimes 'manifest'—are also illustrated.

The expression of shringara comes to the fore in the poet's description of the nayika: 'O Sakhi, the Nayika resembling the flame of a lamp ran to hide herself in the grove of sandal trees entwined by lovely clove creepers of undimmed leaves where she conceals the lustre of her limbs in her blue garment. Startled on hearing the sound of wind, water, birds and animals, she looks around with eagerness of union with her beloved. Waiting for Krishna in the bower she looks like a caged bird.'

In another verse, the poet describe the union of the quarrelsome nayika:

> At first obstinate she did stay,
> And sulkingly got up and went,
> This act of hers I saw, my friend,
> But you could not; Shri Krishna then chased
> And caught her; then she or herself
> In his arms sought to be embraced;
> He held her and her breasts did crush
> Most savagely; and so essayed
> To hurt her by his teeth and nail,
> As one his enemy would treat,
> But soon offered her betel-leaves;
> Dear friend, what strange love he did make!

Keshavadas's work is quite close to the Puranic tradition where mortals share the same love celebrated by the gods and

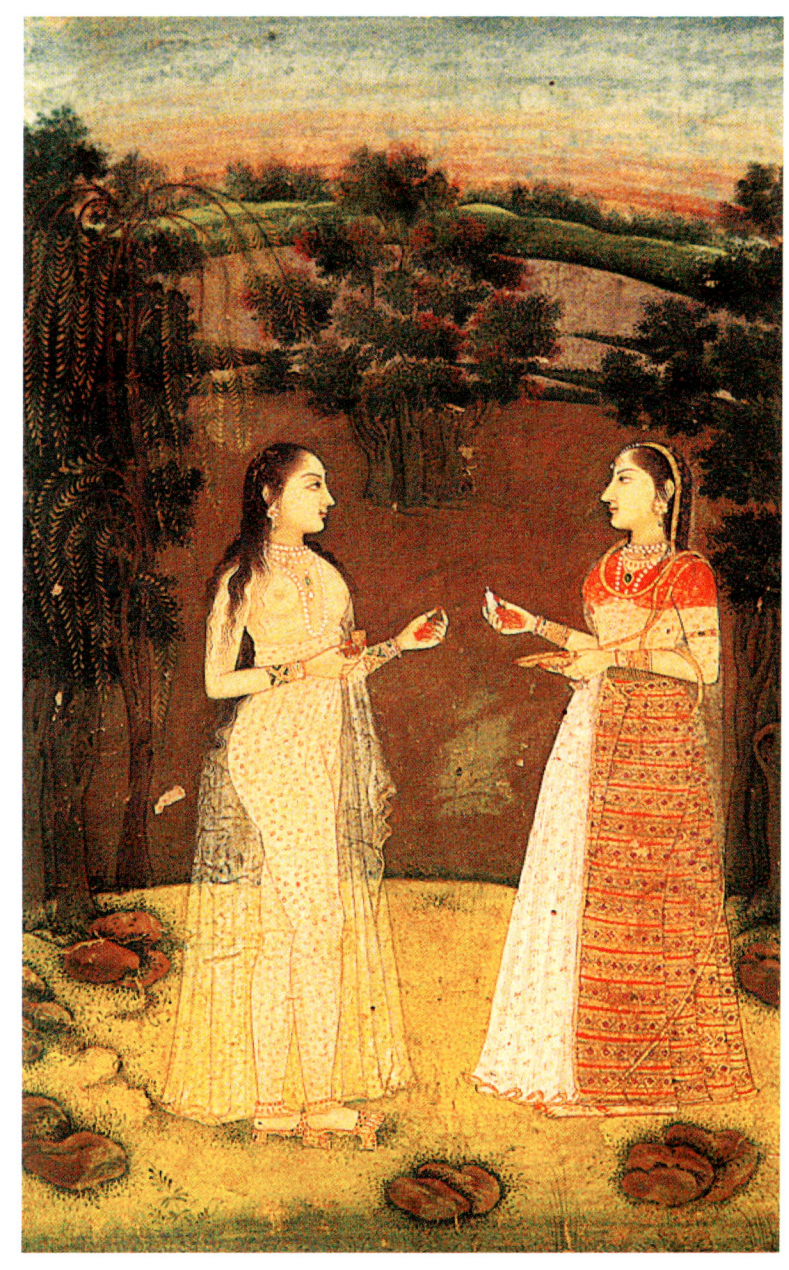

The nayika being adorned by the hand maiden as she prepares to meet her lover, Mughal Period, National Museum, New Delhi

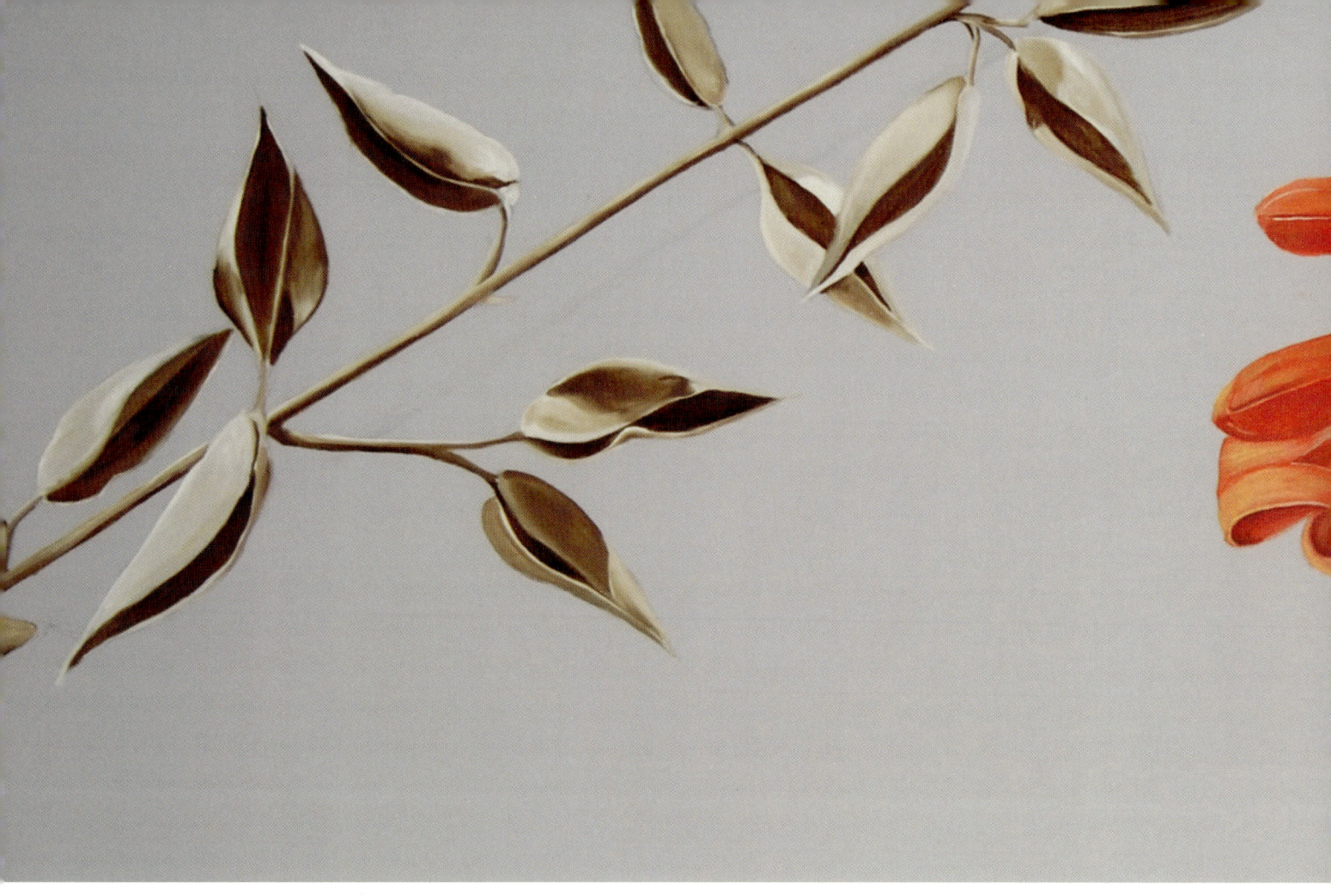

'Inveigle', painting by Rajita Schade

goddesses. As he says, 'When eyes speak and minds are united, bodies also wish to unite.'

The 16th century witnessed yet another revolution brought about by Vallabhacharya who founded the sect of Vaishnavism, whose most important proponent was Surdas. His monumental work *Sur Sagar* added a missing element of shringara rasa to *Bhagavata Purana* and lent a new dimension and meaning to Krishna bhakti.

A very important class of poetry that flourished all through this period was the *barahmasa*, or seasonal poetry of the twelve months. *Shadrituvarnam* or the depiction of six seasons, *vasanta, grishma, varsha, hemanta, shravan,* and *shishira* is an important part of kavya literature in Sanskrit. However, while Sanskrit did not have a barahmasa tradition in itself, the oral forms of this poetry became an integral part of secular verse, as well as Hindu, Jain and Sufi religious poetry.

With the advent of the British colonialist, and the influence of Victorian morality at the turn of the century, sexuality and eroticism in Hindu culture and literature was frowned upon. In the late 19th century, social reformers in Andhra Pradesh

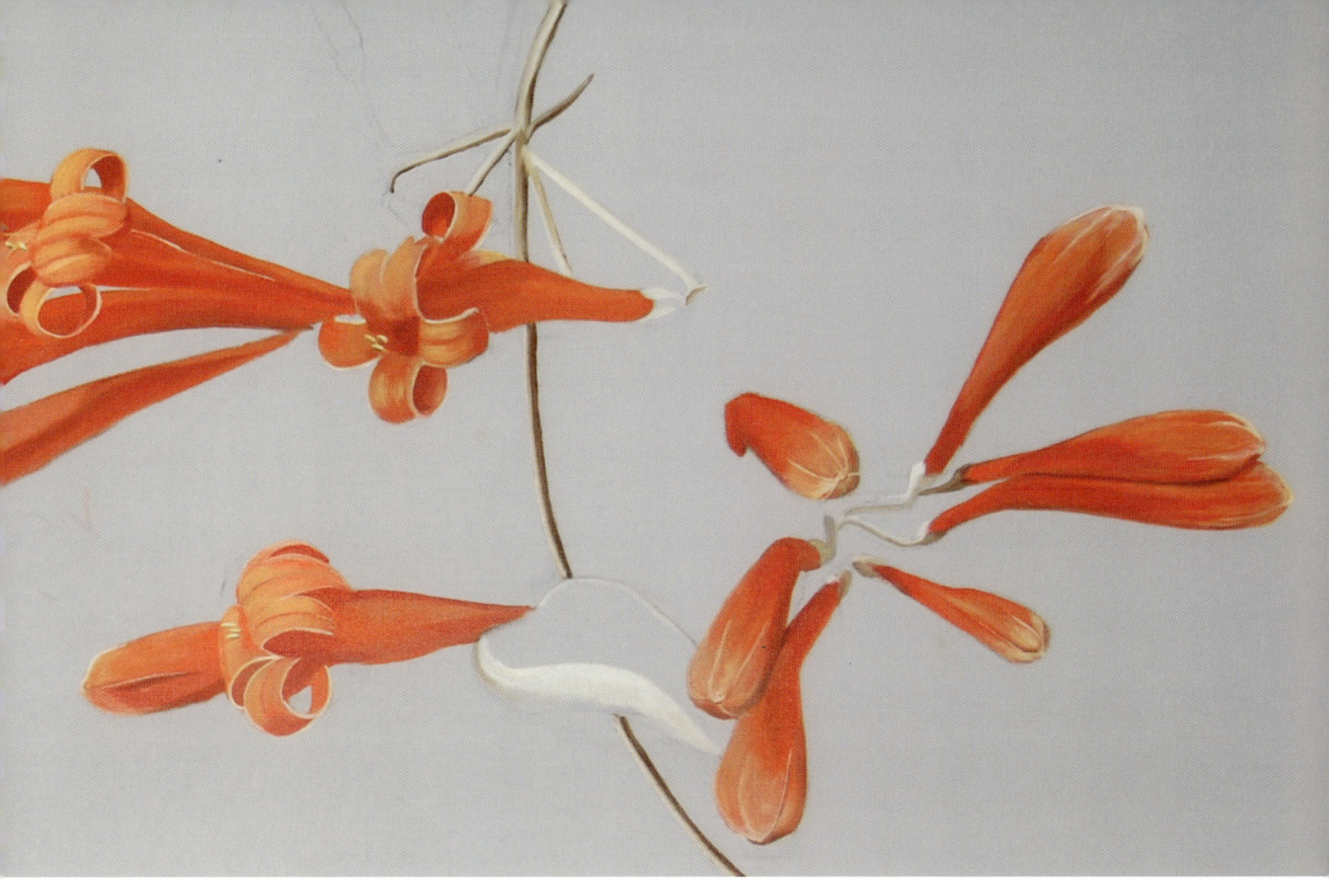

opposed the activities of the courtesans who had so far played a major role in the development of poetry. The *ganikas* or courtesans were highly esteemed because of their beauty, intelligence, knowledge of poetry and expertise in music and dance. *Kuttanimata*, a poem written by Damodaragupta in the 8th century, described the qualifications of a ganika: among her many accomplishments, she was adept in the art of arranging beds, the art of dressing, wearing jewels, perfuming the hair and braiding it. Skilled in playing musical instruments, dancing and singing, she could also read a man's character in his features. She was also well versed in etiquette and in the art of paying compliments. But the social reformer, Kandukuri Viresalingam (1848-1919), started the anti-nautch movement, which advocated that respectable men should not patronize courtesans. The growth of the arts suffered a severe blow, since it was only the courtesan, among women, who enjoyed as much freedom as a man, and was given the same honour as court poets.

The love play between Radha and Krishna, which was the leitmotif in romantic Indian literature, became part of the religious genre that suffused the collective consciousness of society. The gradual change from religious to secular literature resulted in an obvious shift towards individual expression, which found different forms of expression in poetry of the 20th century.

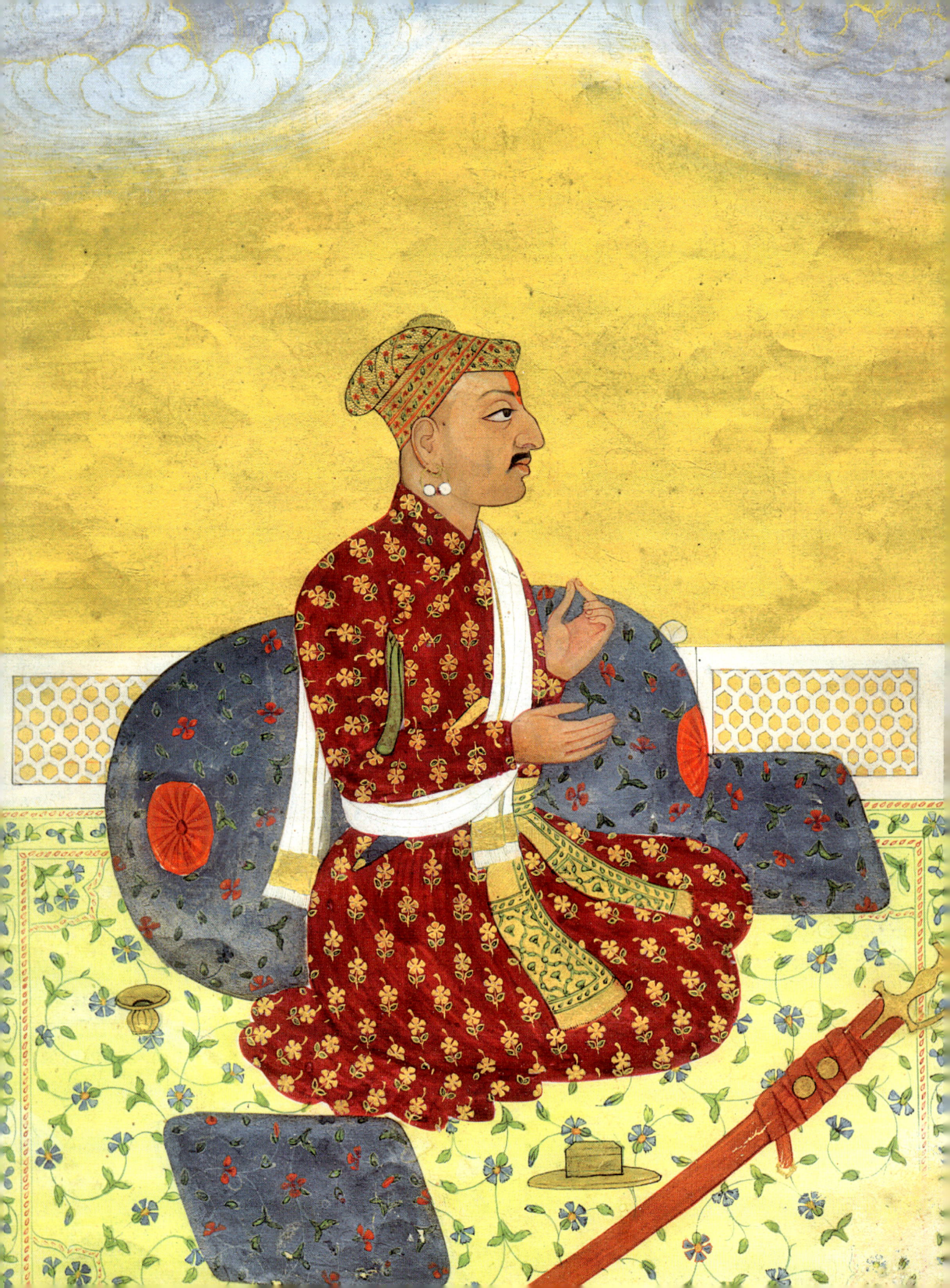

CHAPTER 6

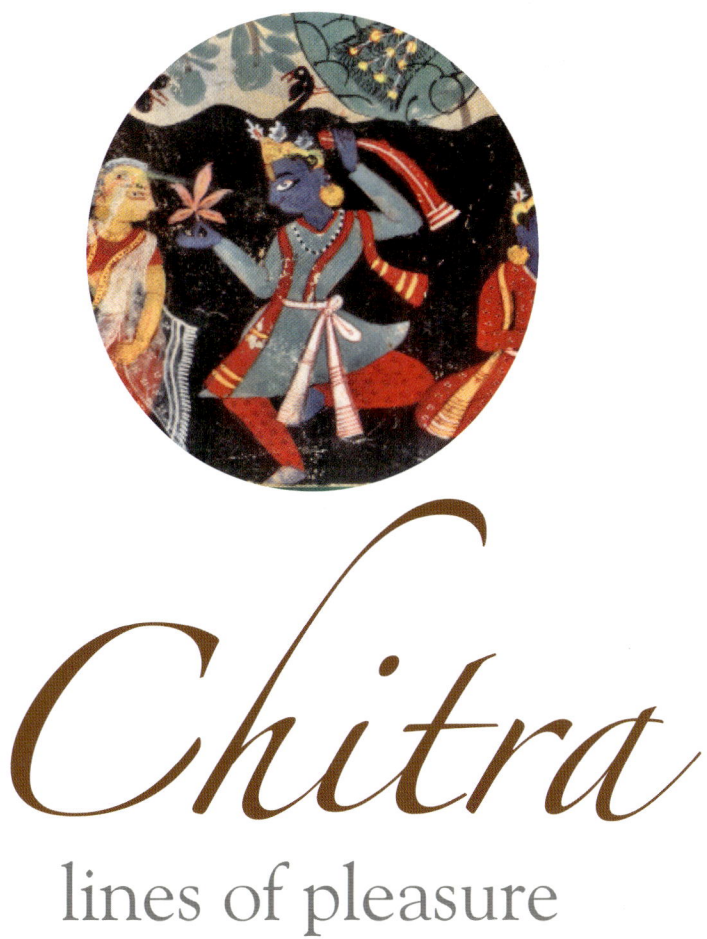

Chitra
lines of pleasure

The whole basis of Indian artistic creation is directly spiritual and intuitive… and its highest business is to disclose something of the Self, the Infinite, the Divine.

SRI AUROBINDO

Indian painting traditions go back to antiquity, as is evident from the murals of Ajanta and Ellora, Bagh, and Badami. Ancient texts outlining theories of colour and aesthetics and social commentaries suggest that it was not uncommon for households to paint their doorways and outer walls, or even the walls of guestrooms. Cave and temple paintings from Ajanta, and the cave art of Bagh and Sittanvasal testify to a love of naturalism, both in the human form and in the depiction of nature. The earliest testimony to this is found in the red, blue and white paintings in the Bhimbetka caves, that go back more than 2,000 years, and are considered by many to be the root of Indian painting.

An Unbroken Tradition

Indian art is witness to a common thread right from early civilization to the present times. It finds its roots in the traditional forms such as the Buddhist palm leaf manuscripts, the Jain illustrated texts and the various schools of miniature painting. The beginnings of the miniature form can be found in the evolution of the written record from the spoken word, a change pioneered by the Buddhists and Jains who recognized its importance and were the first to create illustrated

(Page 82)
Raja Dilip Singh, 1770, Guler Kalam, Pahari, N.C. Mehta Collection, Ahmedabad

(Below)
Folio from Chaurapanchasika Series, N.C. Mehta Collection, Ahmedabad. This series of paintings is based on the love poem 'Chaurapanchasika', written by Bilhana, in the 11th century

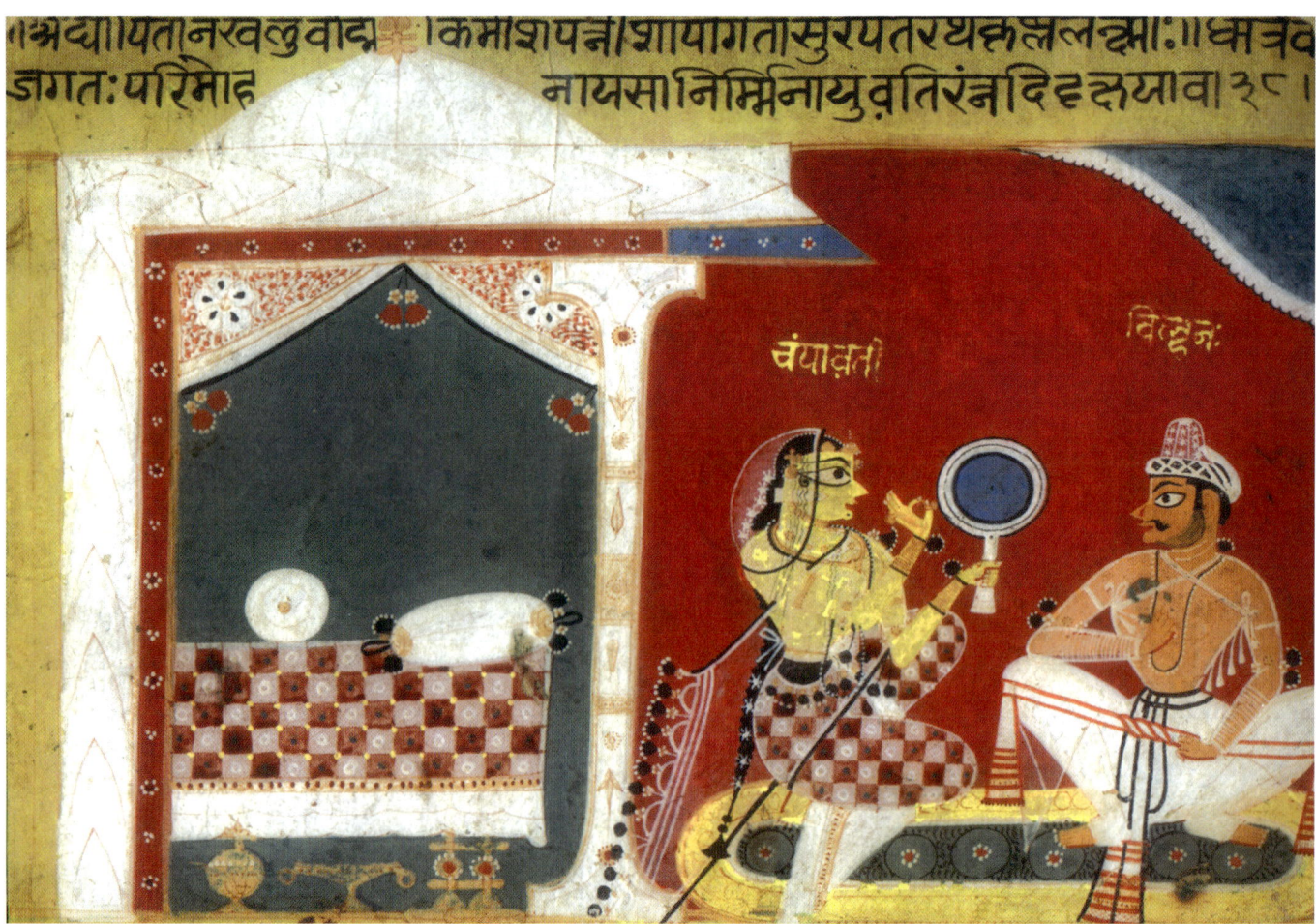

Shringara—the many faces of Indian beauty

manuscripts describing their traditions and beliefs. *Bhujra Patra* were the earliest Buddhist manuscripts to be illustrated. They belong to the Pala dynasty situated in what is now West Bengal (8th to 12th centuries) and are perhaps the precursors of the miniature form, painted in delicate colour schemes. The Jain manuscripts of the 13th to 15th centuries, on the other hand, were characterized by brilliant hues of red, blue and green.

The long history of Indian art falls naturally into two periods. The first and classical period, begins with Emperor Ashoka's conversion to the Buddhist faith in the 3rd century BC. The second phase begins with the invasion and occupation by the Muslim powers of north India in the 13th century and the Deccan in the 14th century.

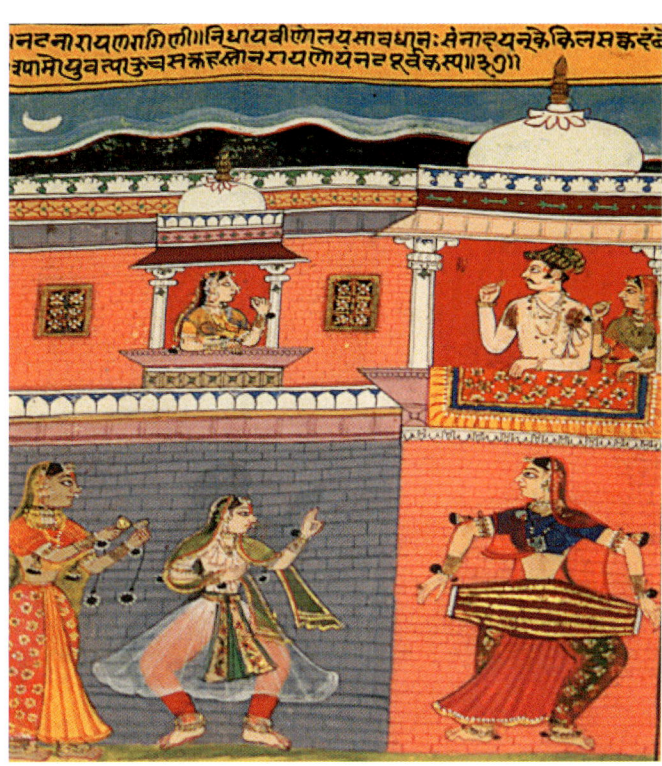

Ragini Natanarayana— Raga Megh, Deccan, National Museum, New Delhi

From the earliest times, Indian art has not only been preoccupied with, but also in many ways, obsessed with erotica. From the secular to the non-secular, from Advaita to Tantric philosophy, from Buddhist to Islamic, and from folk to tribal, erotica is a dominant motif. Starting from the 7th century, an opulent collection of works exists, in which shringara or erotica attains a high level of visibility. Ajanta, Konark and Khajuraho are brilliant examples of the erotic sentiment in the visual arts. Of course, *Kamasutra* holds pride of place amongst the many erotic texts written. In classical theory, the body was transformed into a geometric ideal of beauty, popularized by Tantric thought that had a wide following and practice from the 10th century onwards. Tantric philosophy spilled over to the Indian miniature painting tradition, particularly in the Rajasthani and Pahari miniature schools.

Nitya-Lalita—The Divine Enchantress

The 12th century poet Jayadeva's *Gita Govinda* was the muse for a number of miniature painters. The cosmic love between Radha and Krishna served as an important inspiration for court painters and folk artists alike, all of whom were unabashed in their depiction of the erotic, often showing the divine couple in amorous dalliance. The origins of the erotic cult based around god Krishna are not directly related to Tantric philosophy. Many thinkers believe that the personification of Krishna, the ideal lover of the gopis of Brindavan, is in fact the representation of the highest female form, Nitya, also known as Lalita, the great

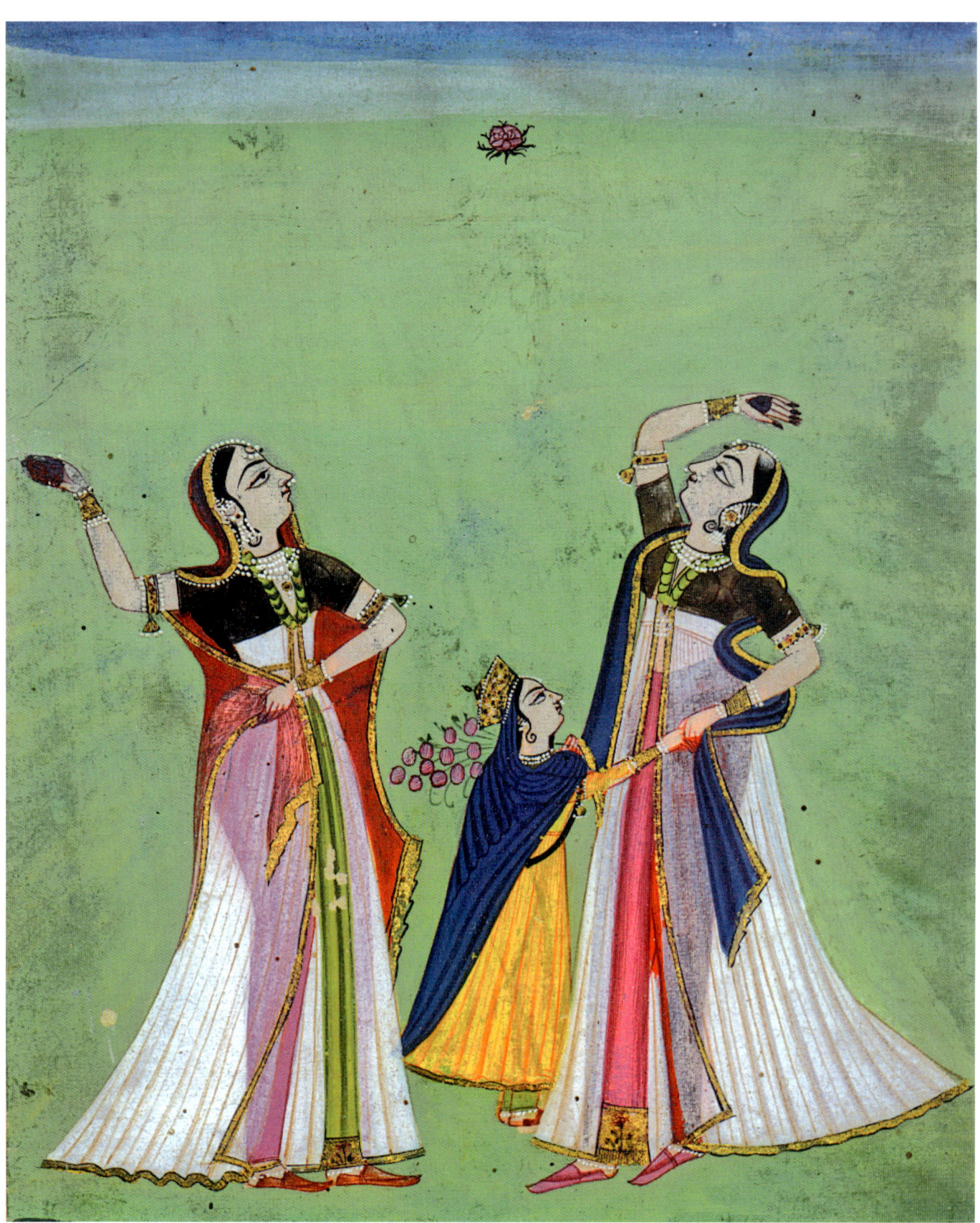

goddess herself, embracing all women and entrancing the world. This female principle of Nitya-Lalita, is also believed to be Parvati, the wife of Shiva. Krishna thus becomes the dominant erotic symbol in the whole of Indian culture.

The love between Radha and Krishna represents transfigured desire seen in different perspectives. Literary texts give detailed descriptions of the acts performed by the divine lovers and the postures they achieve. The visual imagery, in fact, moves a step further by depicting the divine lovers in the most intimate and ecstatic erotic detail, promoting 'an endless transcendent desire fanning the inner fire of bhakti' (*Tantra: The Indian Cult of Ecstacy* by Philip Rawson).

The Magic of the Miniature

The late 16th and early 17th centuries saw the rise of the miniature schools of painting in Rajasthan and the hill states. Mewar, Bundi-Kota, Kalam, Jaipur, Bikaner, Kishangarh, Basholi, Bilaspur, Chamba, Guler, Mandi and Kangra were the principal centres where this art flourished. The most popular themes depicted were from nature—hills, valleys, gardens, birds, flowers and trees; scenes of life in the royal court, religious processions, festivals; and depictions of Radha, Krishna, Shiva and Parvati.

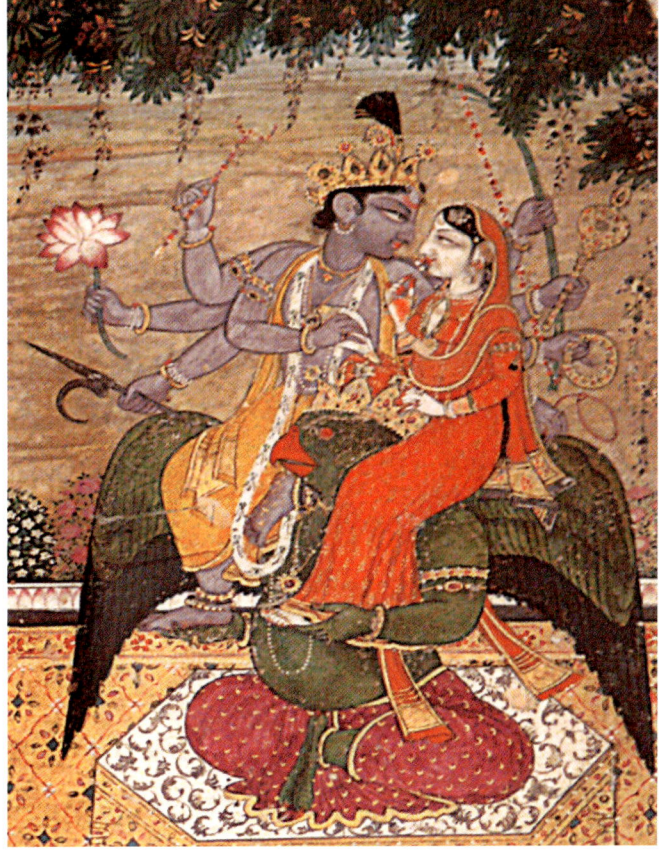

(Page 86) Nayikas playing with a flower, Jodhpur, early 18th century, N.C. Mehta Collection, Ahmedabad

Vishnu-Lakshmi, Kangra, National Museum, New Delhi

Many artists also produced works based on Indian classical music. They personified the different ragas in pictorial images, conveying a specific mood and sentiment, and thus a new category of miniature paintings, the Ragamala, emerged. Apart from the Ragamala, other significant bodies of work were based on classical texts such as *Bhagavata Purana*, Ramayana, *Rasikapriya* and *Amarusataka*.

There were many schools of Rajput painting, all with their own particular distinctive styles and features. It was, however, the Kangra School in the Punjab hills that went well beyond the Rajput tradition. In the Kangra School, the natural element takes precedence over the human. Thus the nayika is placed in a natural landscape that reflects her inner longings and desires, the intention being to bring out the mood of each particular rasa. This school is among the best known and its paintings the most sensuous and ecstatic among the Pahari tradition.

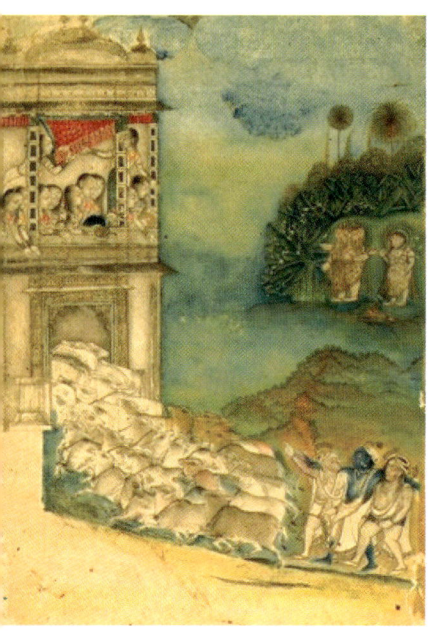

'Godhuli', Rajasthani Miniature

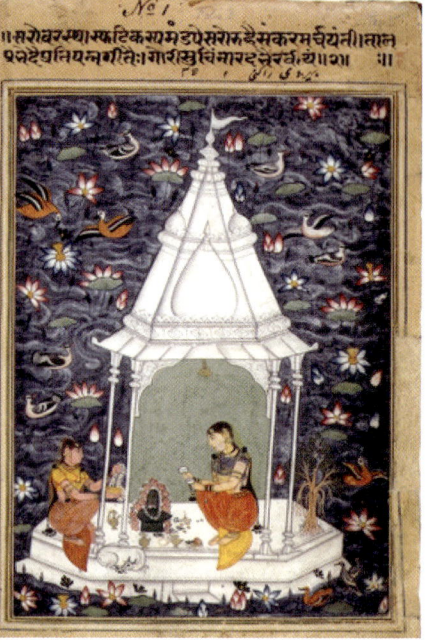

Bhairavi ragini, 1610, Rajasthan

(Page 89)
'Bliss', painting by Kanchan Chander

The earliest Kangra paintings appear in the reign of Ghamand Chand (1761 to 1774) and reach their peak of excellence under Sansar Chand (1765 to 1823). The artists excelled in the use of vivid colours and depiction of slim and aesthetic human figures placed in surroundings etched out in fine detail: tall and almost bare trees, small houses in the distance, robust lines attenuated by a hint of shading in which the gentle landscape is used to frame amorous moonlit scenes.

The Bundi School of Rajput painting also gained tremendous popularity during this time. It reached its peak under the Hara family in the 18th century. While maintaining its own distinct style, especially in terms of representing nature, the Bundi artists adopted certain characteristics of the Mughal School. This included a certain glossy pallor, a profusion of foliage, and the use of shadowy outlines, all of which merged with the predominant use of green and orange to create an effect of exotic beauty. The freehand treatment of natural forms and the iconographic compositions made the Bundi style unique and aesthetically accomplished.

In the 16th century, painters in the Deccan developed a new style that brought about a fusion of Indian with Persian and Turkish painting traditions. Known as the Deccan School, it flourished in Ahmadnagar, Bijapur, Golconda, and Aurangabad.

The Eternal Nayika

The nayika (heroine or beloved) is one of the core elements found in miniature paintings of the north. Keshavadas classifies the nayika in his work *Rasikapriya* (1590), based on a number of physical and aesthetic attributes of the goddess Durga, with her fierce and sometimes violent character. The eight manifestations are:

1. Ati-Chanda
2. Chamunda
3. Chanda
4. Chandanayika
5. Chandavati
6. Chandroga
7. Prachanda
8. Ugrachanda

Different manifestations of the nayika are to be found in the miniature schools.

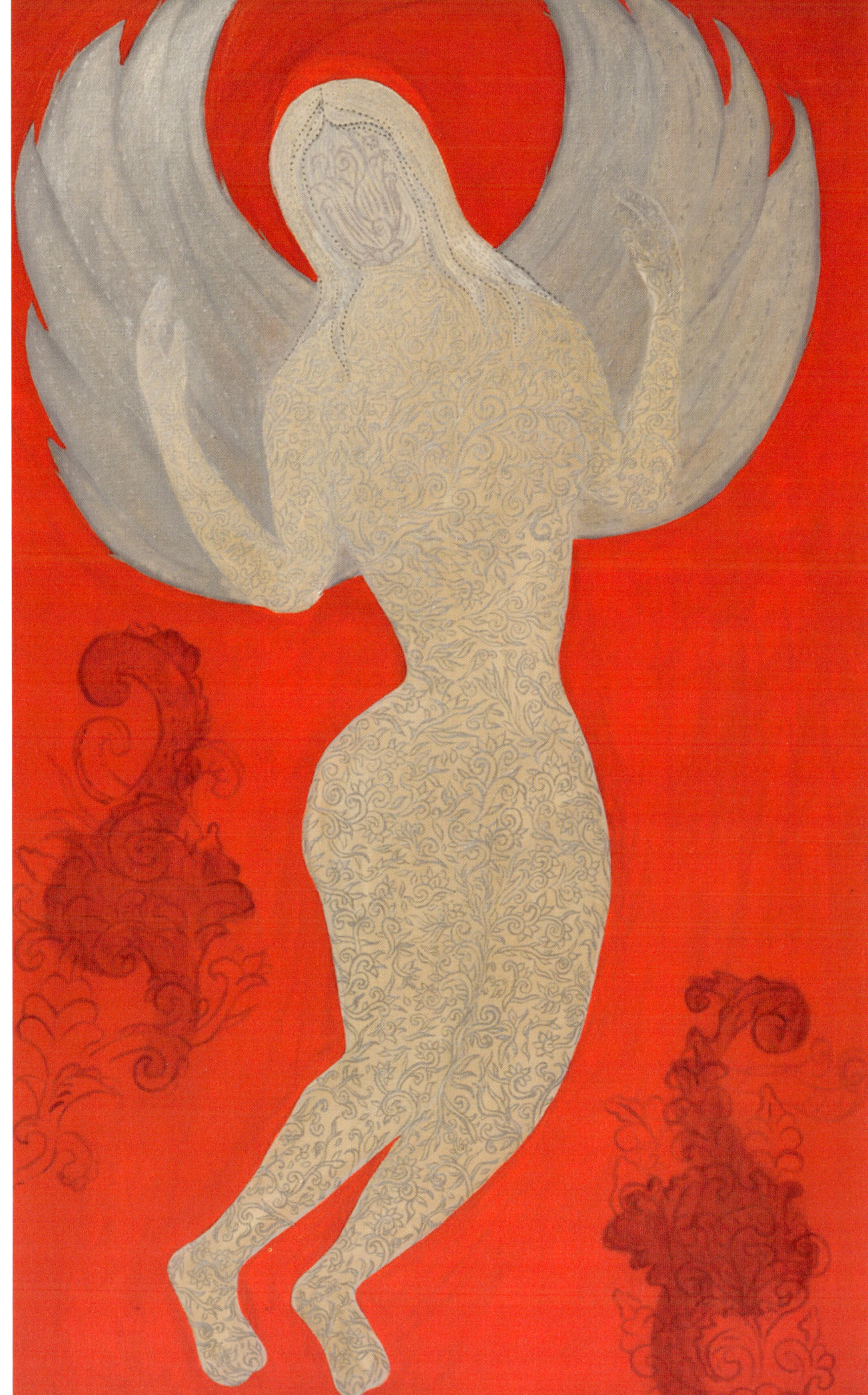

*(Page 91)
Radha and Krishna
sheltering from the rain,
Bikaner, National Museum,
New Delhi*

*Raga Sri, 1590-1600,
Bijapur School, Bikaner*

Musical Moods

The Ragamala style was one of the most original forms of painting to develop at the beginning of the 17th century in the Kangra, Rajput, as well as the Bundi schools. The Ragamala were a set of illustrated paintings depicting the garland of ragas or the melodic moods of Indian classical music. According to traditional musical theory, the ragas are infused with certain inherent features that connect them to a particular season and the atmosphere that prevails at that time. The basic aim of the Ragamala paintings was to express the moods of the different seasons associated with a particular raga. This was done in a skilful manner through varied colour combinations and the imaginative use of subject matter in a painting.

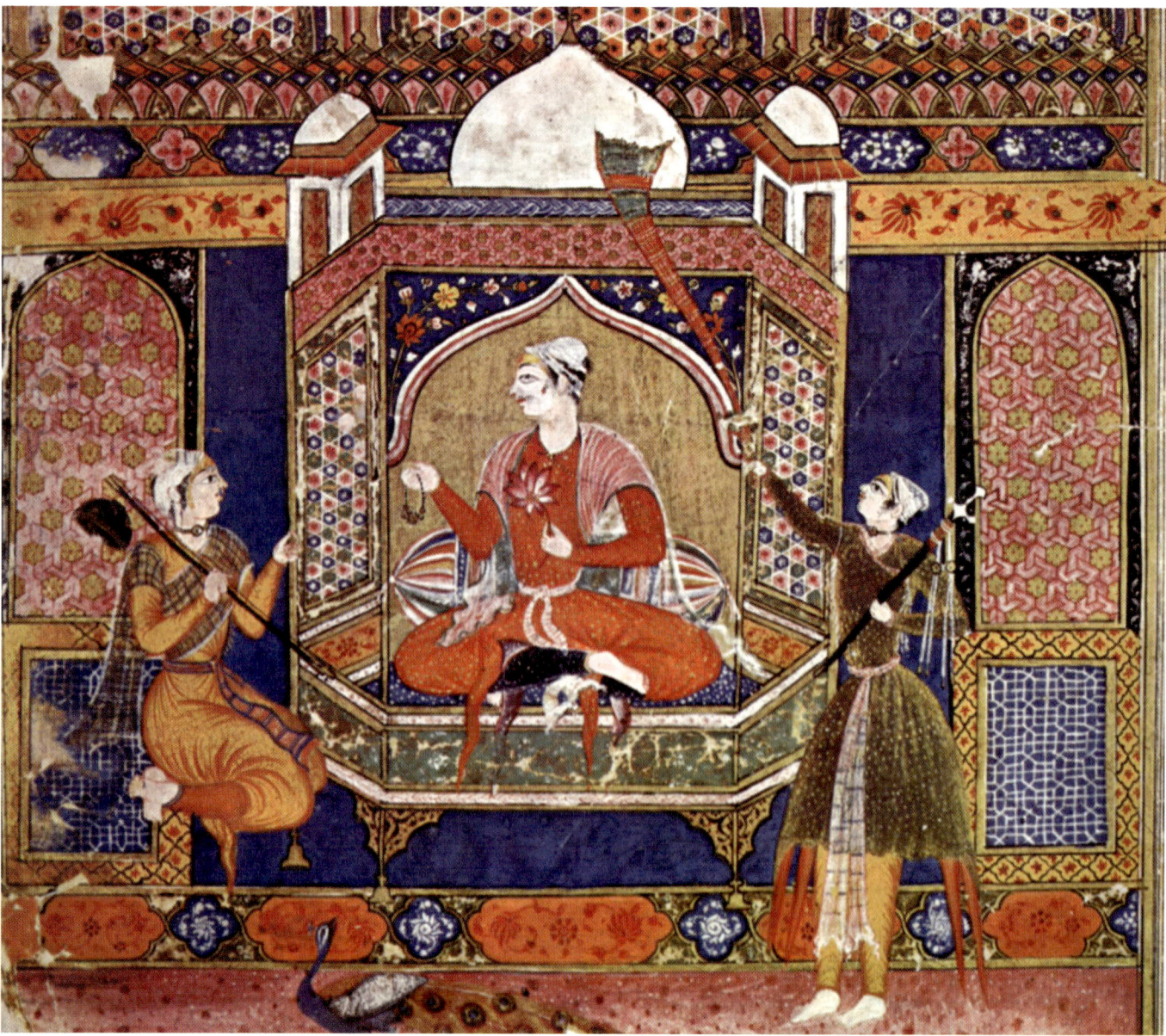

90   *Shringara*—the many faces of Indian beauty

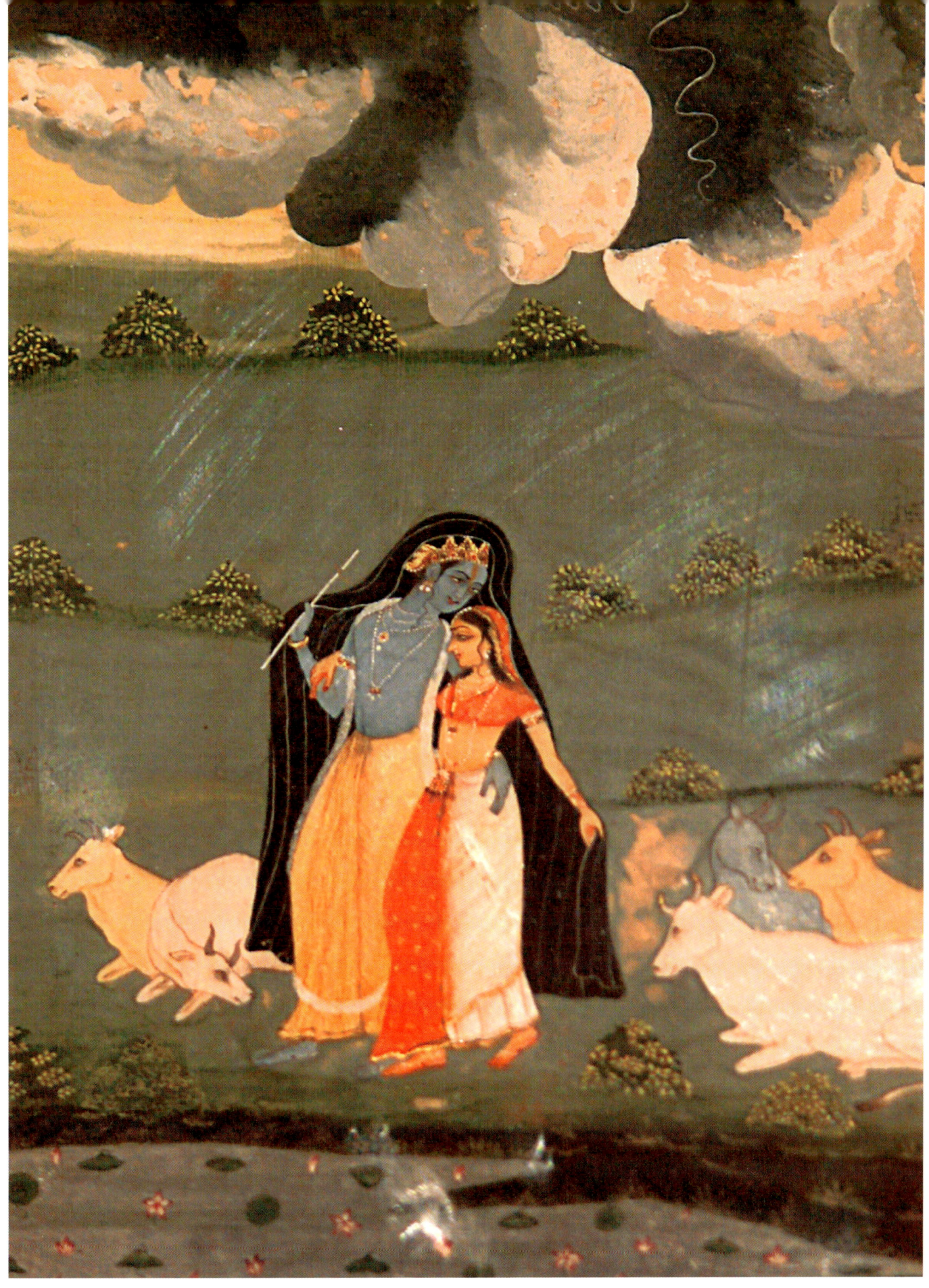

Chitra—lines of pleasure 91

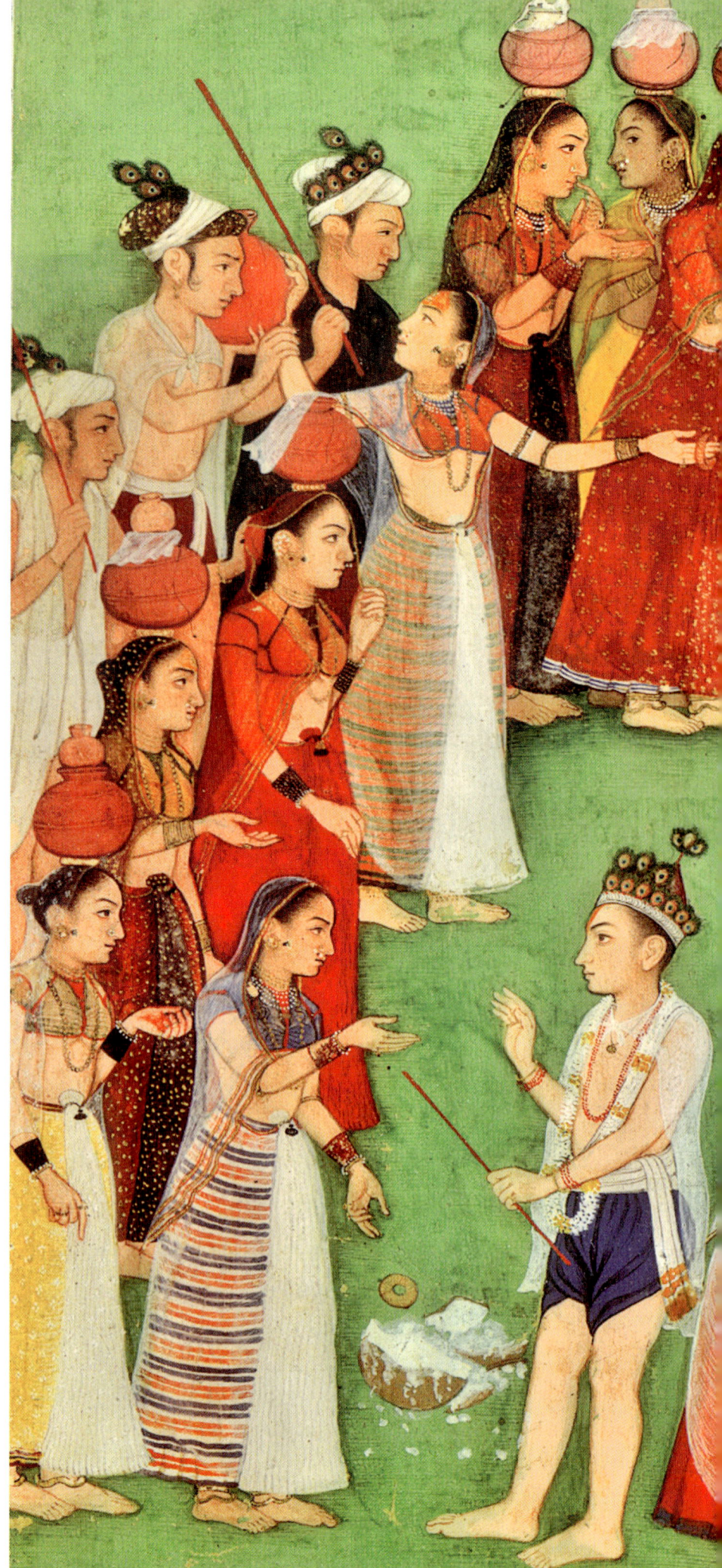

*'Toll of curds', Bikaner,
late 17th century,
N.C. Mehta Collection,
Ahmedabad*

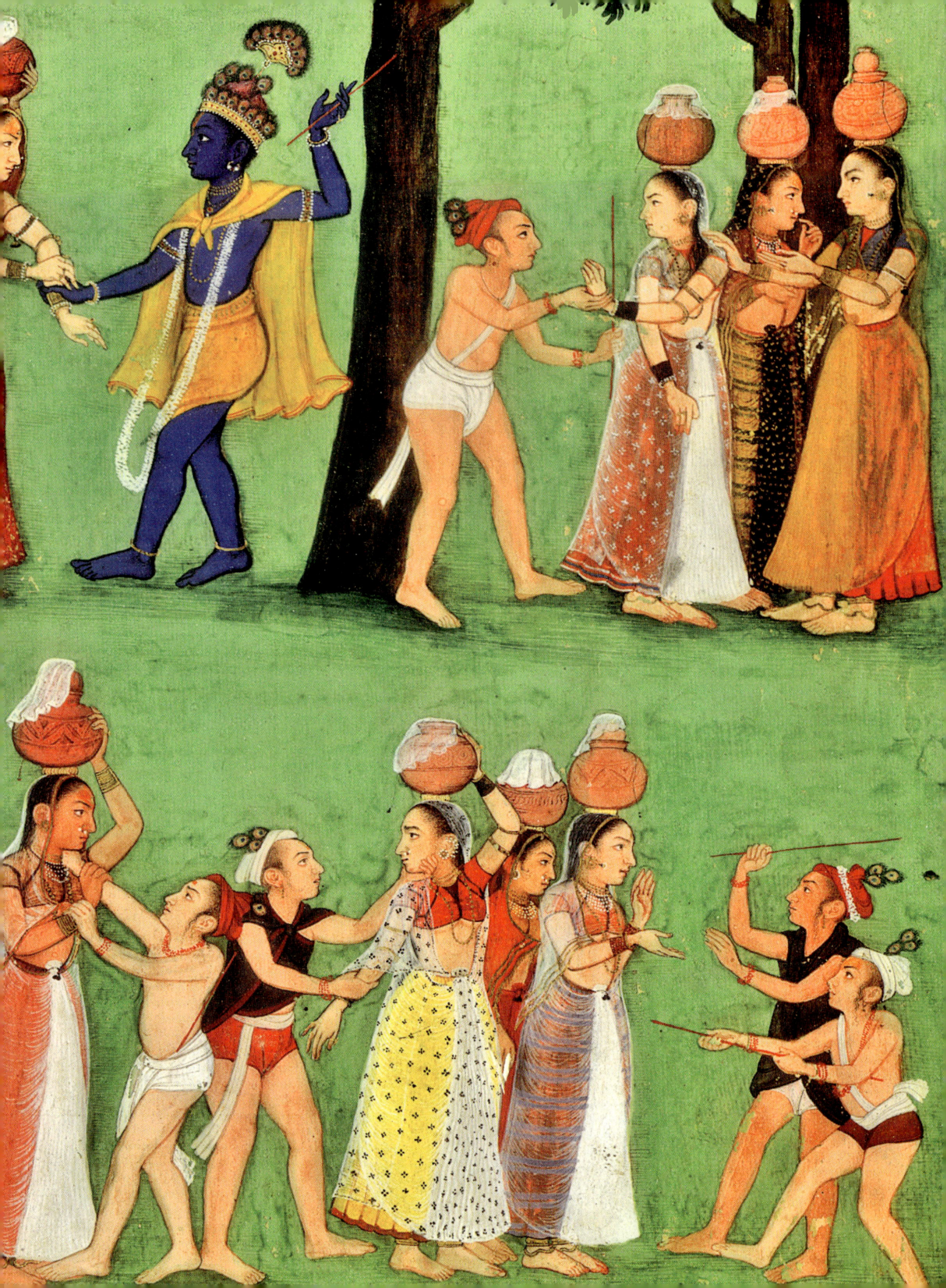

The secondary mode of ragas, known as raginis, was also expressed in the miniatures. The word ragini is actually homologous with the word *garbhini*, which refers to a pregnant woman. A ragini, therefore, is that which carries within itself the seeds of a future raga. Each raga and ragini is also supposed to manifest itself in two rupas or forms; the first is invisible and is called *nadamaya rupa*. Paintings and pictorial representations, however, fall into the second category, which is visible and is called the *devatmaya rupa*.

The Ragamala paintings demonstrate their potential to communicate by helping an observer experience the corresponding harmonies of a raga. This is believed to be the essential foundation of the mystical experience that leads to a feeling of openness, enabling participation in divinity and a state of yogic spirituality or realization.

Apart from the spiritual aspect, the Ragamala also served an aesthetic purpose, which was to synthesize poetry, music and painting in a manner that gave the viewer pleasure. Traditional miniature painters used poetic and religious symbols, scenes from royalty and architectural features, to visualize the text and poetry of the Ragamala paintings. Sometimes they even assumed divine proportions, depicting gods and goddesses.

Woman playing a veena, glass painting, Tamil Nadu, Crafts Museum, New Delhi

Celebrating Spring

Love between the nayak and nayika is represented in its myriad nuances, from shringara (sensual love) filled with desire and longing, to *vipralambha* (love and the sufferings of separation). Depiction of the local flora and fauna add a rich element of ornamentation, as well as enhance the mood. Some of the best examples of 18th century Ragamala paintings can be found in the depiction of Raga Vasanta or the melody of spring. This melody expresses the beauty and joy of spring and the glories of nature, using symbols that celebrate creation and fertility. In the paintings, one sees Krishna personified as a *devata* and symbolic of *purusha* (eternal male). The execution is sensuous and smooth with portrayals of musical instruments and images of dance. The human figures

Shringara—the many faces of Indian beauty

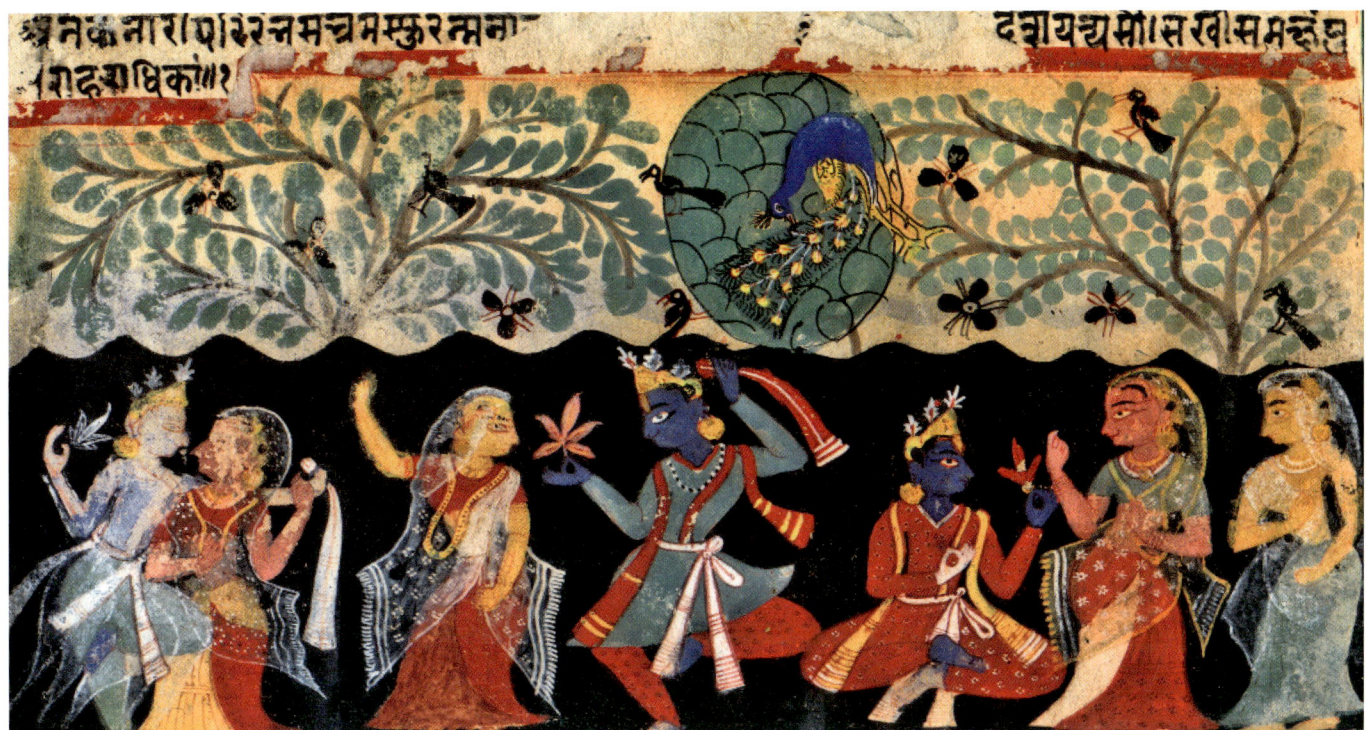

are delicately etched, and Lord Krishna is shown dancing to the strains of enchanting music with the gopis, symbolic of human souls craving for union with the Divine.

Early Gita Govinda, *Gujarat, 16th century, N.C. Mehta Collection, Ahmedabad*

Raga Vasanta paintings of the Kangra School depict the joyful dance of Krishna with the gopis holding musical instruments like the *dholak* (drum) and *khartal* (wooden cymbal with strings). Such paintings are treated with delicacy and do not use loud or vibrant colours; they are filled with images of the foliage and flowers typical of the Kangra valley during the month of March. The white plum and the pink peach blossom appear frequently, along with yellow blooms believed to be symbolic of youth, life and joy. While the yellow blossoms stand for physical and sensual beauty, the white blossom is believed to signify spiritual strength and beauty. Delicate streams, flowing tranquilly with floating flowers, indicate a gentle breeze.

In contrast to the Kangra style, the Ragamala from Bundi depict Lord Krishna as blue-skinned and dressed in yellow. He holds a vase full of blossoms and plays the *veena* while the gopis play drums, cymbals and the *ektara* (a single-stringed instrument). The paintings are filled with images of varied flora and fauna. A common feature in the Bundi paintings is the presence of the peacock, ducks and *hamsa* (swan), all of which are eternal symbols of love and passion, while the buds and blossoms symbolize new beginnings.

Chitra—lines of pleasure 95

The Ragamala painted by the Rajasthani artists are filled with bright, vibrant colours. Krishna and the gopis are shown dressed in the traditional Rajasthani style, wearing brilliantly embroidered clothes. The cowherd god appears often in a dark orange dhoti with golden frills and wearing wooden *khadau* (slippers) on his feet. The gopis are dressed in tight-fitting *cholis* and skirts fringed in bright red, yellow, orange, blue and green. The palette comes alive with an effusion of warm tones, with yellow and orange depicting the sunlit landscape of Rajasthan, green depicting the verdant splendour of its fields and forests, and blue denoting the infinity of the sky above and the waters below. These paintings make lavish use of primary colours to communicate the breathtaking beauty of the landscape as well as the romantic and erotic feelings inspired in men and women during this season of passion and desire.

The prince in his chamber with his lady, shooting an arrow of love, (the bow and arrow symbolize Manmatha's lotus bow) while the hand maiden cools the chamber with a fan of peacock feathers

A Complex Tapestry

The Ragamala paintings witness the coming together of several facets of painting. The nayak and nayika, for instance, are portrayed within the framework of certain aesthetic and traditional parameters. Lord Krishna is shown in the *avatar* of the Dakshina nayaka, one who loves all women; and the nayika are portrayed as Padmini or Chitrini. The first of these refers to a beautiful maiden, shy, soft-skinned, with a golden complexion and filled with fragrance, beauty, generosity and love. The Chitrini, on the other hand, is extremely beautiful, but in a more flamboyant manner. She is also accomplished in the arts, music, dance, poetry and all forms of love sport.

The manifestation of a state of mind through facial expressions and speech is called bhava. The stimulus of the bhava in painting is believed to evoke passion and the erotic flavour. The Ragamala paintings are examples of both kinds of bhava—*alambana*, that which sustains love, and *uddipama*, that which causes excitement. Both of these merge to create the *sthayi bhava* or underlying emotion, which is the basic element defining the intention behind the painting. It seeks to make the observer feel an emotion or experience, rather than merely see an image.

The Barahmasa series are similar to the Ragamala paintings. The word 'barahmasa' literally means twelve months, and the songs contain references to each month of the year. Here the changing seasons become symbolic of the varying moods of love and longing, with the melodies resonating the anticipation and desire of the lover and the beloved. In fact, shadrituvarnan, or the description of the six seasons—vasanta, grishma, varsha, hemanta, shravan and shishira—plays an important role in the Sanskrit kavya literature, which is also contextualized within the emotional gamut of shringara.

The Ancient Canons of Art

The best known of the kama literature, Vatsyayana's *Kamasutra*, mentions painting as *alekhya* (undefinable beauty) and includes it among the sixty-four fine arts. There is also an entire chapter on *shadanga*. The canons and ideals of Indian art dictated by texts such as *Vishnudharmottara Purana* describe the shadanga (six limbs) as inseparably connected with a *chitra* (painted image). No painting is perfect in its absence. The 'limbs' are akin to the legs, arms and torso of the human body and they represent the different aspects of a painting, which is complete only when all the parts are present.

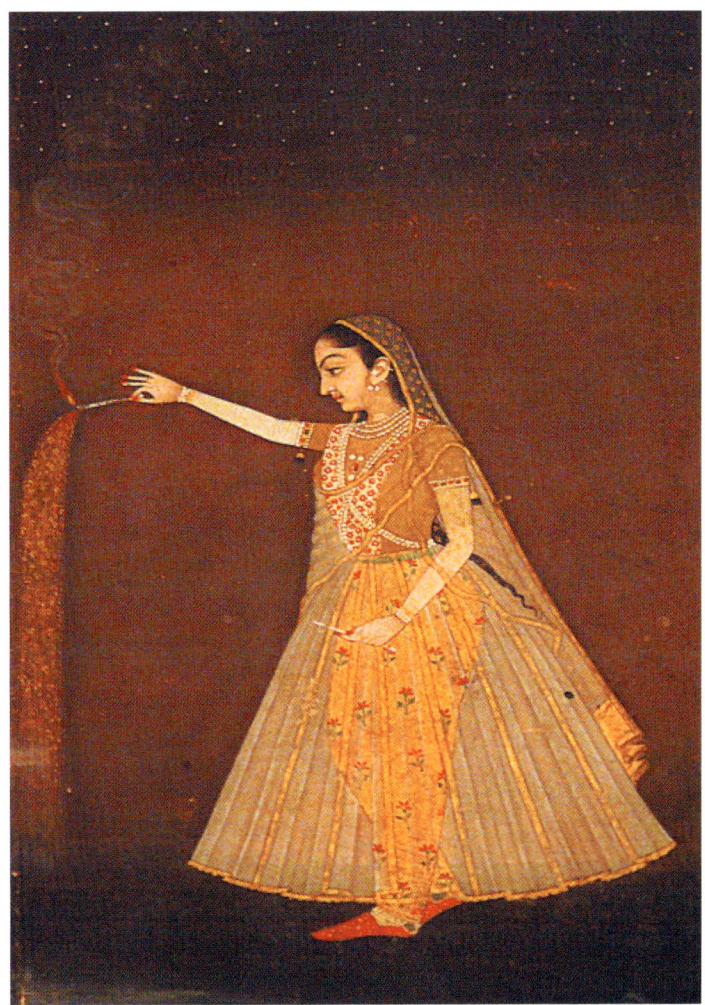

Lady holding a sparkler, Mughal period, National Museum, New Delhi

Five hundred years later, Yashodhara wrote *Jayamangalatika* on the lines of *Kamasutra* and enumerated the theory of 'shadanga' in the form of a *shloka*:

> *Rupabheda pramanani bhava lavanya yojana sadrishya varnika bhanga iti chitram shadangakam.*

The six limbs are enumerated as: rupabheda, pramanani, *bhava-yojana*, *lavanya-yojana*, sadrishyam and varnikabhanga, which translates into drawing, proportion, arrangement of line, mass, design, harmony and perspective.

Vishnudharmottara Purana presupposes accurate draughtsmanship. Once the shape and appearance of figures have been decided, it is necessary to

Chitra—lines of pleasure

differentiate them. The forms must be articulated according to the principles of pramanani and sadrishyam. Sadrishyam demands that the form must be faithful to nature, not lost in imagination. Pramanani is an essential principle of form, not only with regard to individual figuration but also for the composition of the picture. Another essential quality is varnika-bhanga, which, in painting, refers to tonality of colour and in sculpture to the depth of three-dimensional volume.

Painting traditions in India have centred on naturalism, limitless self-expression, liveliness, finesse and sophistication. The fundamental intention was always to create a particular mood and evoke a specific feeling. Nature was an integral part of the process to achieve this goal. The painters used pigments and colours made from minerals, vegetables, animal products and lampblack. Art was thus based on nature in its widest and deepest connotation, reflecting what *Kaushitaki Upanishad* states:

What one sees is but the reflection of the mind.

From Prudery to Plain-spoken

The Mughal School of miniature painting flourished in the late 16th century under Emperor Akbar's reign. These works often recorded the court scenes and courtly activities like hunting expeditions, and detailed images of flora and fauna. The style was aristocratic, individualistic and portraiture-based, with some of the main examples being the illustrations of texts like the *Hamzanama, Tutinama, Akbarnama* and *Tuzuk-i-Jahangiri*.

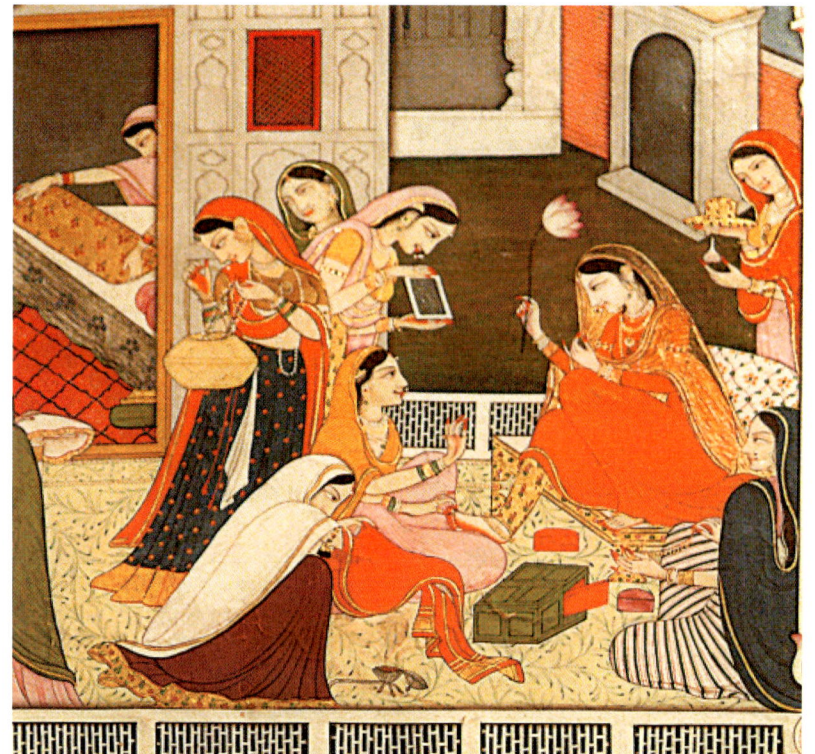

Rani enjoying her beauty, Pahari, National Museum, New Delhi

Due to lack of encouragement from Aurangzeb, and the collapse of the Mughal Empire thereafter, most court painters from the Mughal durbar shifted allegiance to generous patrons of the arts in Rajasthan and the Kangra valley. In Kangra they contributed to the Pahari School of art, typified by a refined delicacy and concentration on the nayak, nayika and religious themes. This was a total departure from the more ceremonial and

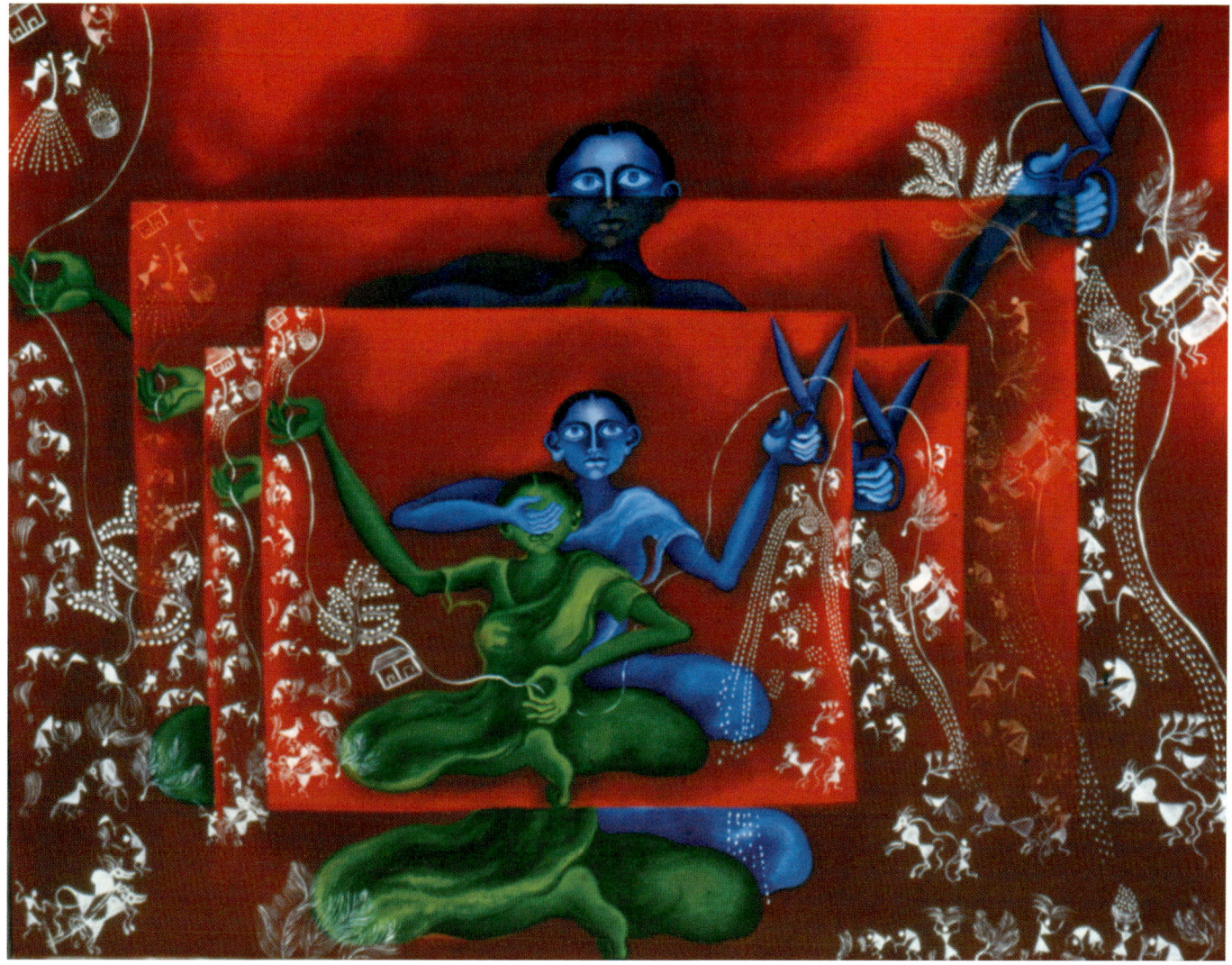

'Harvest', painitng by Arpana Kaur

lavish durbar art of the Mughals. The Rajput and Pahari schools of painting both emphasized the emotions of women, and their main theme was love, a primary source of inspiration with the Krishna legend at its centre. In fact, the Bhakti cult and the large corpus of shringara poetry such as Bhanudatta's *Rasamanjari* and Keshavadas's *Rasikapriya* and *Kavipriya*, did much to inspire painting in this tradition.

Indian erotica started losing its preeminence from the Mughal period onwards. Victorian prudery set the sun on the frank display of sensuality in Indian art, and with the increasing influence of the British on Indian society, sexuality became hidden and covert. Travelling through time, the erotic theme again found expression in the paintings of 20th century artists such as F.N. Souza, M.F. Husain, Bendre and Jatin Das, who blazed the trail for individual expression and liberated thought.

Chitra—lines of pleasure

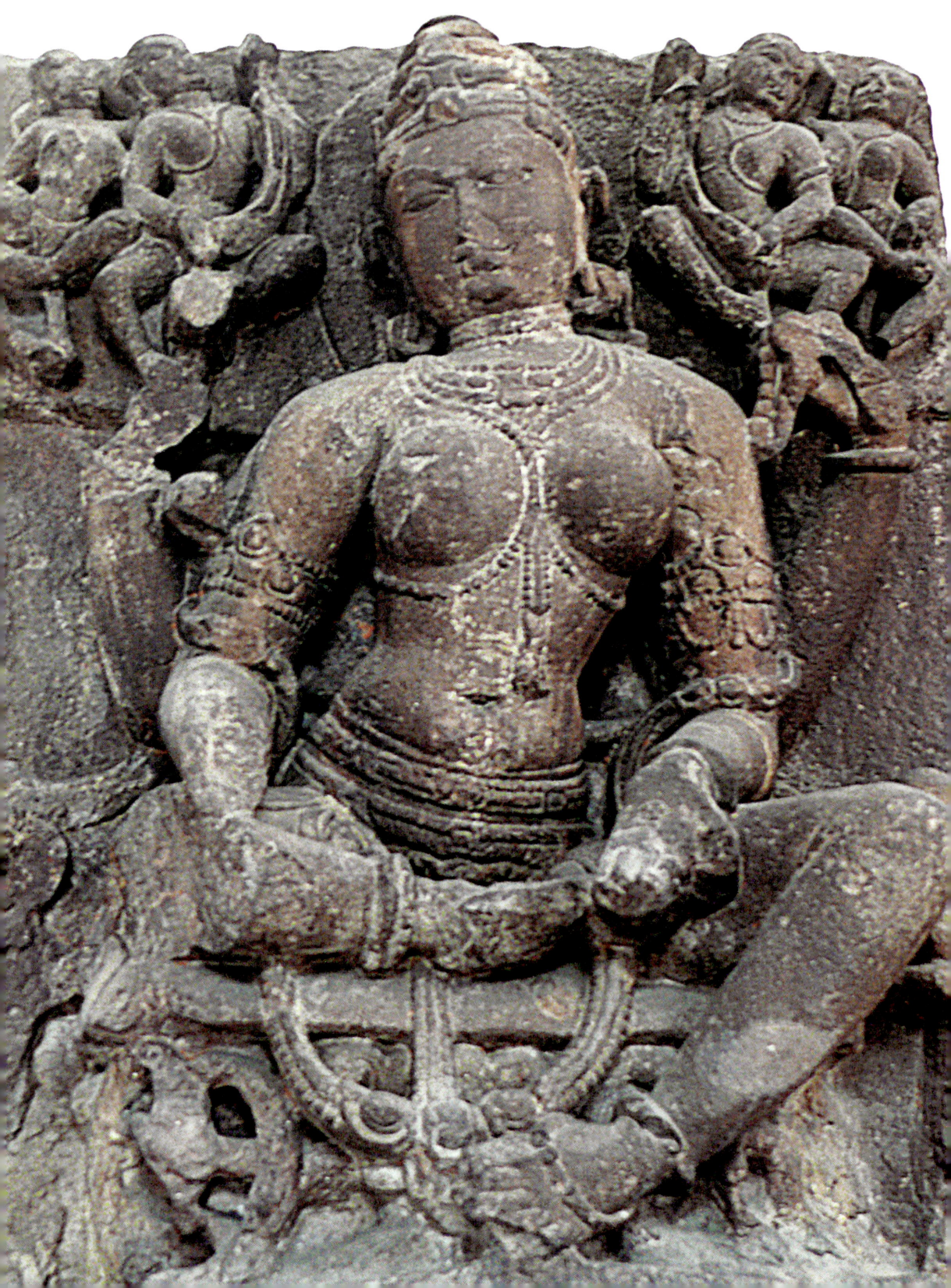

CHAPTER 7

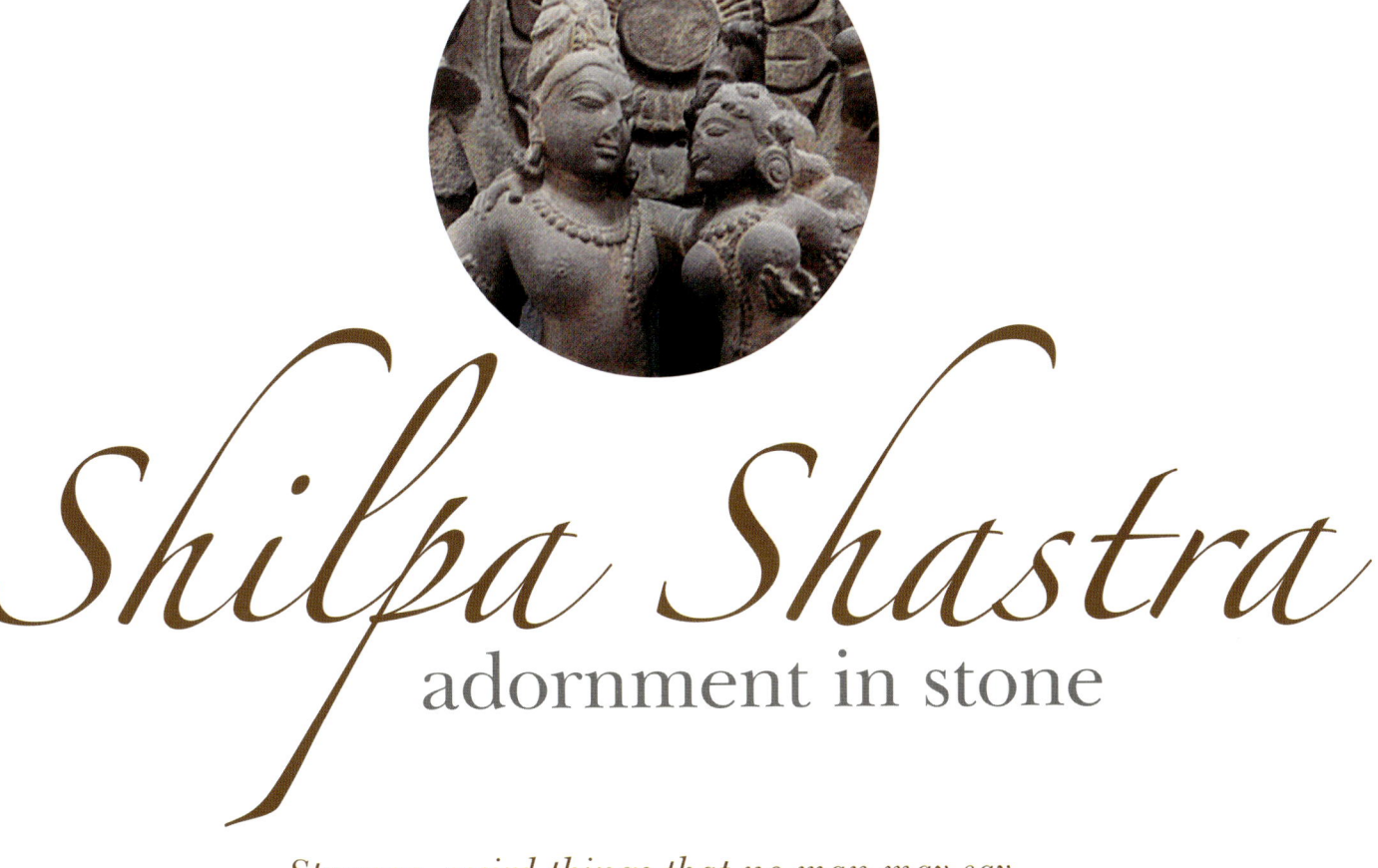

Shilpa Shastra
adornment in stone

Strange, weird things that no man may say,
Things humanity hides away—
Secretly done—
Catch the light of the living day,
Smile in the sun.
Cruel things that man may not name,
Naked here, without fear or shame,
Laugh in the carven stone.

THE GARDEN OF KAMA AND OTHER LYRICS FROM INDIA,
LAURENCE HOPE

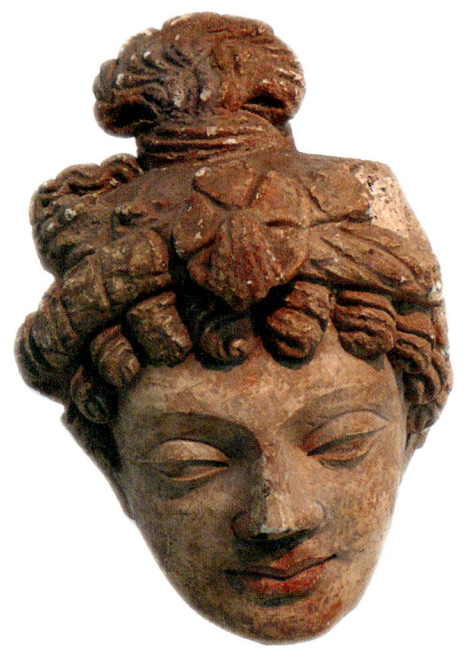

Female head, Gandhara, National Museum, New Delhi

(Page 100) Saraswati-Paramara, Madhya Pradesh, National Museum, New Delhi

The arena of Indian sculpture, particularly in the ancient and medieval times, abounds with sensual and erotic imagery, both explicit and subtle. It is important to have some knowledge of Sanskrit and Prakrit literature to recognize, interpret and appreciate the underlying themes in temple sculpture. Sanskrit texts on music, dance, architecture and sculpture, such as *Natyashastra*, *Mayamata*, *Kashyapashilpa* and *Vishnudharmottara Purana*, are essential reading to comprehend artistic iconography. The works of Bhavabhuti, Bana and Kalidasa, particularly the latter's *Meghadutam*, all enrich one's understanding of the tactile arts.

One can trace the history of Indian sculpture all the way back to the Indus Valley Civilization. One of the earliest sculpted images is a terracotta seal from that period depicting a male figure, enthroned in a particular yoga posture, with his feet crossed below an erect penis. He wears buffalo horns and is surrounded by four animals. The seated ithyphallic image of the primordial God has been identified as proto-Shiva. In its most obvious interpretation, it would be linked directly to sex and erotica. But on a deeper level, and according to many Indologists, the erect penis is symbolic of the life force, of creative energy and the harnessing of these energies. This erect penis, or the *urdhvalinga*, pressing against the abdomen, is also symbolic of the ascent of semen, characteristic of the Shiva image. Control of the seminal fluid is believed to culminate in complete 'control of all passions and the achievement of desirelessness'. (*The Tantric Tradition*, Agehananda Bharati)

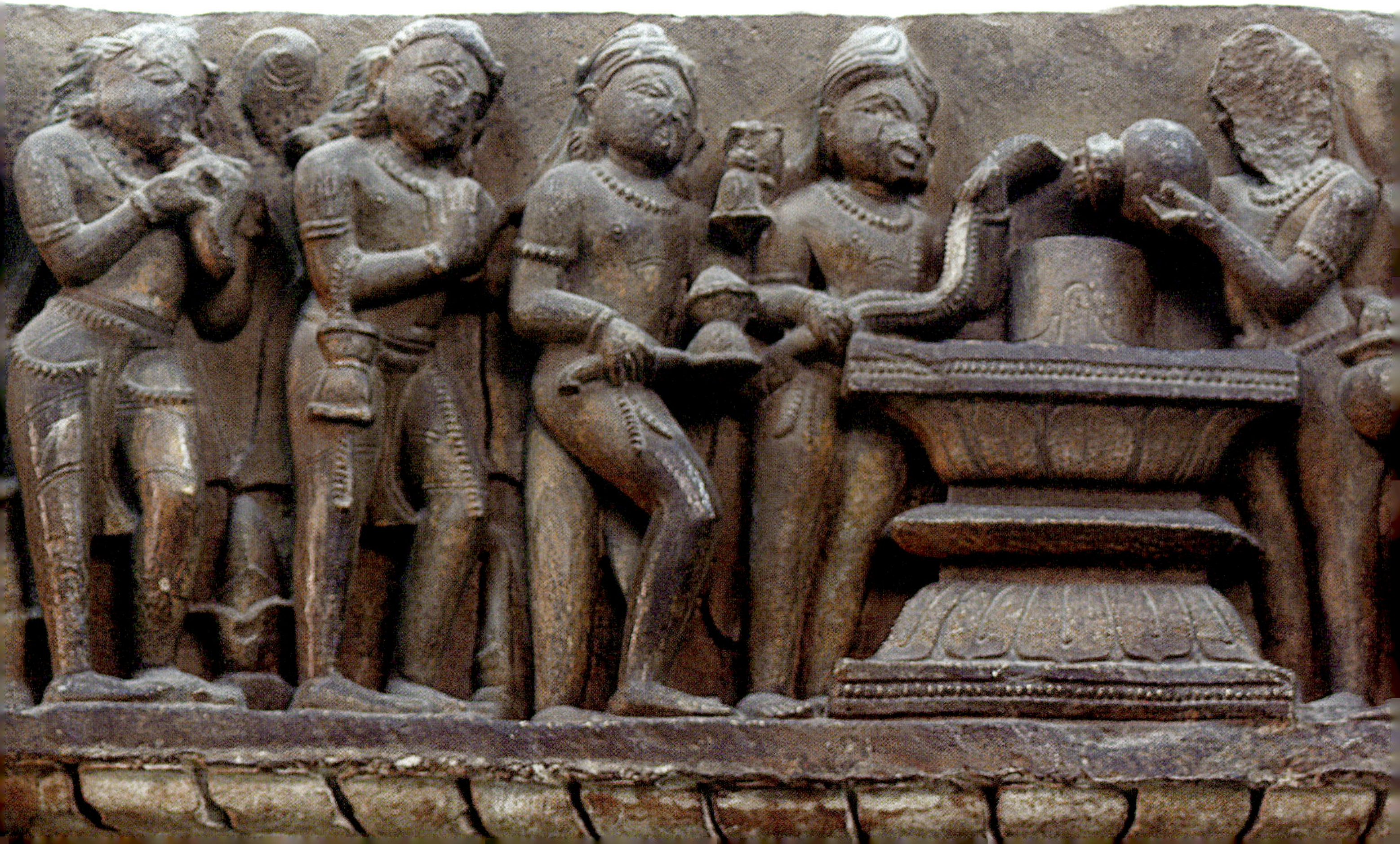

The Vedic Pantheon

Lord Shiva's erect phallus, or *shivalingam*, is one of the most widely worshipped icons by Hindu devotees even today. In Shiva temples throughout the country, the lingam rests on the yoni, symbolizing the union of Shiva and Parvati. In some temples, the shivalingam is represented as the separation between the pure male and female. These perfectly shaped white lingams are placed on a red cloth, white being the nucleus of 'being', while red is the active and passionate attachment projected into space and time.

Vedic deities were abstractions of natural phenomenon like rain, water, earth and wind. They displayed anthropomorphic characteristics: Rudra is the mighty god of storms; Indra is the god of rain and brandishes his thunderbolt; Surya, the sun god rides a golden chariot; Usha, goddess of dawn unveils herself and Agni, the god of fire approaches like a household priest, leading believers on the right path.

There is a human aspect in all these deities, originally derived from nature. The earliest representations of Surya and Indra at the Bhaja caves illustrate a simple and human conception. Indra appears like a terrestrial king, seated cross-legged on his elephant, Airavata. He moves through his celestial paradise just as a terrestrial king would ride on his state elephant through his domain.

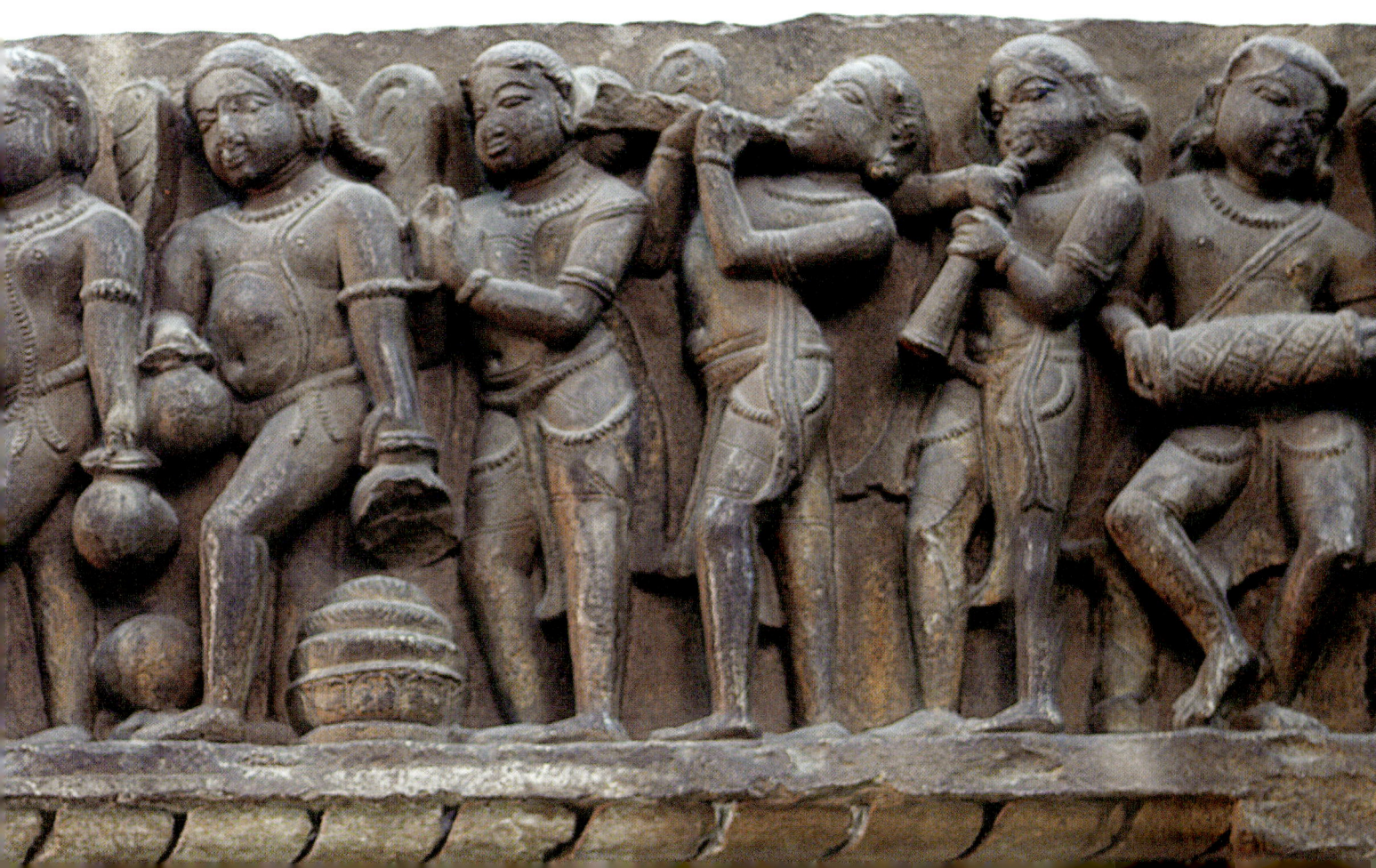

Devotees worshipping shivalinga, Chandela, National Museum, New Delhi

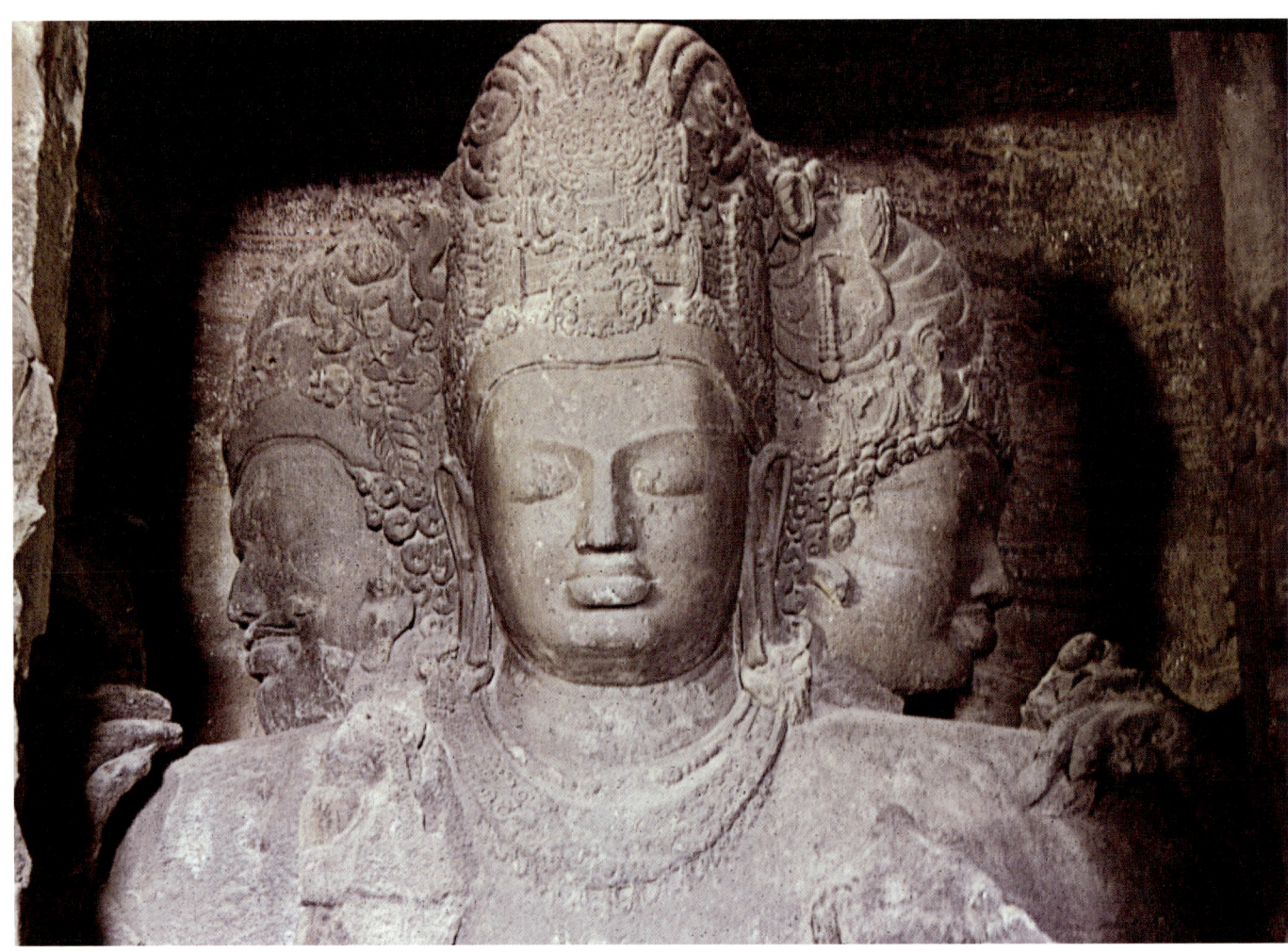

The Trimurti from the Elephanta Caves, Maharashtra

(Page 105) Uma-Maheshwara, Pala, 11th century, National Museum, New Delhi

Manifestations of the Holy Trinity

One of the central set of deities in Hinduism comprises Brahma, Vishnu and Maheshwara (Shiva), representing the forces of creation, preservation and destruction, respectively. Each god in the trinity has his consort—Brahma has Saraswati, the goddess of knowledge; Vishnu's consort is Lakshmi, the goddess of wealth and beauty; and Parvati (known variously as Durga, Kali, Amba among other names) is the goddess of power, destruction and transformation and the consort of Shiva. The gods may be worshipped either with or without their consorts.

The early representation of the holy trinity is a group of three images named Brahmeshvara-Vishnu-Laskshitayatanam that was made by the Pallavas and bears the Mandagapattu inscription. The temple is near Villupuram, Tamil Nadu and the inscription of King Mahendravarman I (610-30) declares that during the early medieval period, both in the Deccan and the far south, several temples were dedicated to the Hindu Trinity.

104 *Shringara*—the many faces of Indian beauty

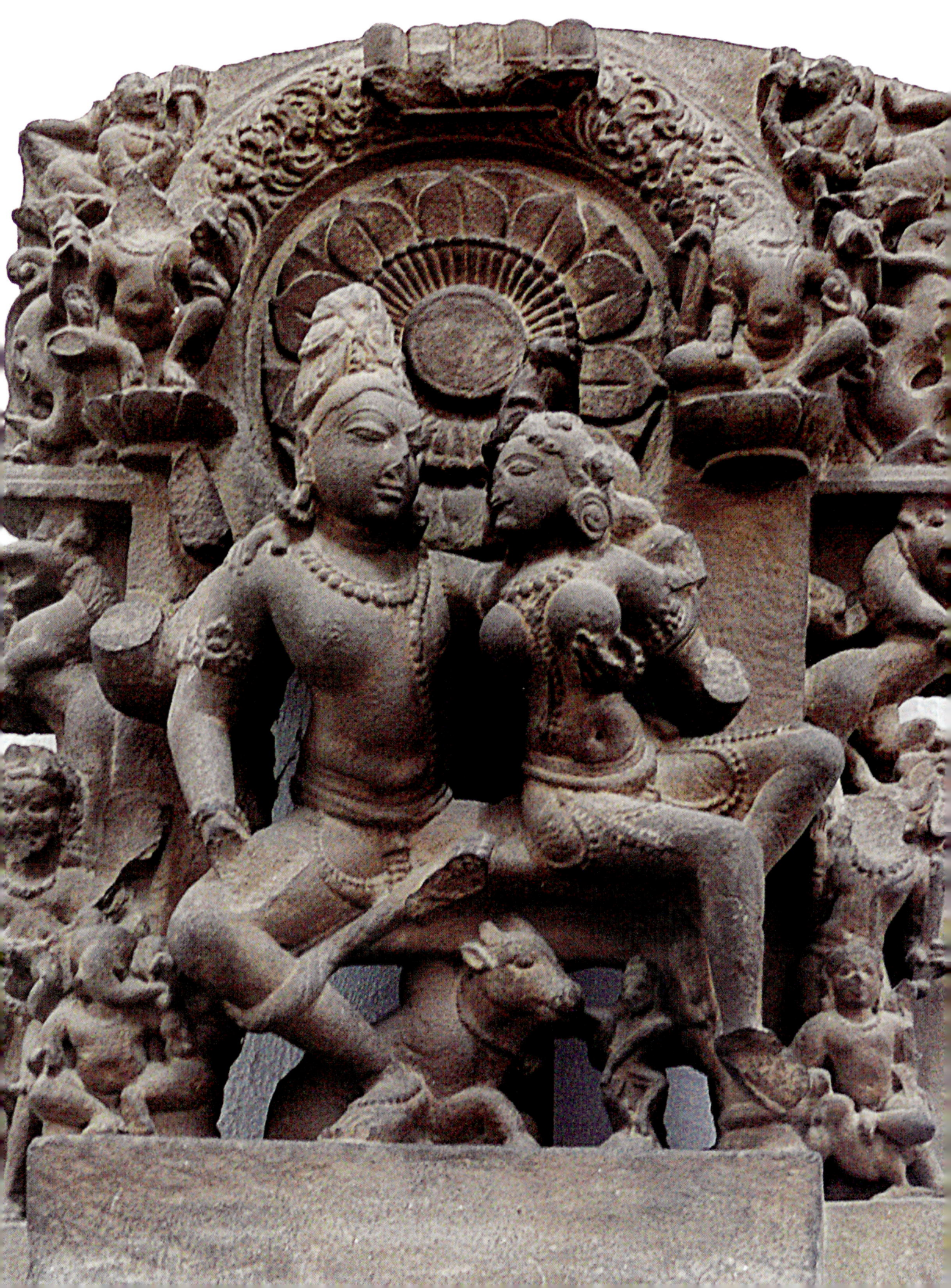

Lakshmi is often depicted as an aquatic deity. The theme of Lakshmi bathed by the elephants has been expressed in beautiful works throughout India. The avatars of Vishnu, suggested by the heads of the fish, tortoise, boar and man-lion. become objects of the beauty vested in the god. One of the finest depictions of Vishnu's first avatar, the fish or *matsya*, is housed in the Dhaka Museum. There is also a magnificent depiction of the marriage of Lakshmi and Vishnu, where Lakshmi rises from the milky ocean while Vishnu as Kurma, the tortoise or second incarnation, holds Mount Mandara aloft. Legend has it that Vishnu helped the gods and demons churn the sea for holy nectar and then married Lakshmi.

Also seen in temple sculpture are the Dityas, the twelve sons of Diti and sage Kashyapa. They make up a group of *devas* or celestial gods or angels. The Vasus are eight elemental gods representing aspects of nature and cosmic phenomena; they are the attendant deities of Indra and Vishnu. In Shiva temples one sees carvings of the eight Bhairavas, who surround Shiva (Mahabhairava). Some interesting stone representations are of the eleven Rudras, dreadful in form, who are supposed to have entered the minds of humans.

*(Page 107)
Ganga, Chandela,
11th century,
Madhya Pradesh,
National Museum,
New Delhi*

Marriage of Shiva and Parvati, Pratihara School, 10th century, Bharat Kala Bhavan Museum, Varanasi

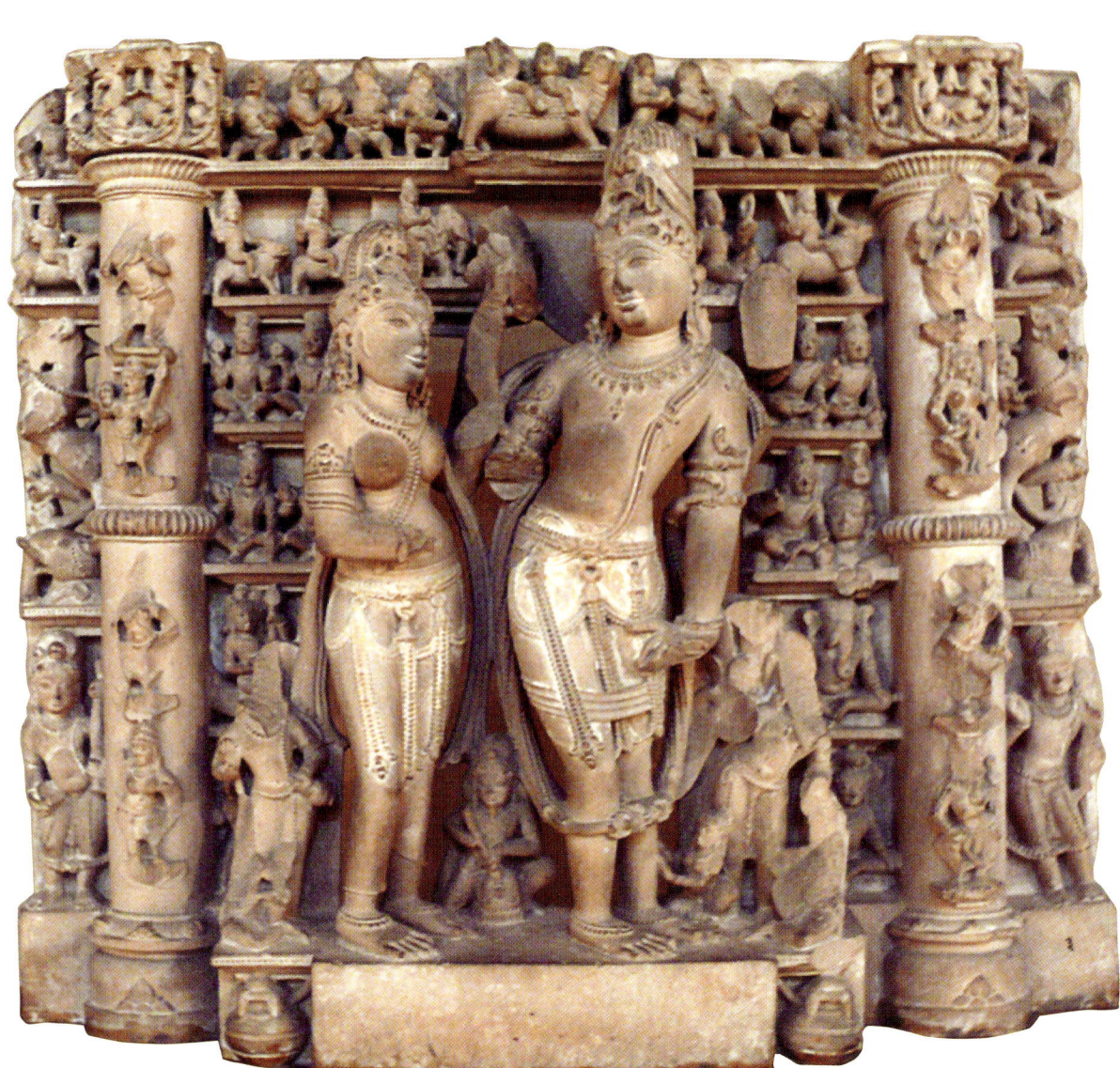

The Many Faces of Shiva

In Indian philosophy, gods are supra-human beings. Shiva in the three-headed form represents yet another notion of beauty: one head is the auspicious one, the second is Aghora, the terrible, and the third is Lalita, or the charming form of Devi. Kalyanasundara, Shiva as a bridegroom, appears in multiform iconography throughout India. Somaskanda, Shiva with Uma and their son Skanda or Kartikeya, and Umasahita, Shiva with Uma, are seen commonly in South India.

Images of Uma-Maheshwara, Uma and Shiva, are frequently seen in North India, but a prime example can be found in the Deccan, namely at the Ellora caves in Maharashtra. The theme of Shiva as Gangadhara, where a raging Ganga flows through his locks, has been expressed in rock and temple sculpture. Ardhanarishvara, Shiva as a hermaphrodite, has undergone many changes over the centuries. Nataraja, Shiva as lord of the dance, also brings out the notions of beauty attached to the image of Lord Shiva. The multi-armed Nataraja, in the Chatura or Lalita pose, is a recurring theme in many monuments throughout the country. The mother cult based around the seven or eight mothers and the sixty-four yoginis is also centred on Shiva.

Symbols of Significance

The rich tradition of philosophy, both rational and spiritual, found its way into Indian art and architecture. Both stupas as well as temples held within themselves a profound symbolic language based on visual representations of the important philosophical concepts. These included the *chakra*, the revolving wheel of time that symbolized the cyclical rhythms of the cosmos; the *padma*, or the lotus, representative of the universal creative force that springs from the bosom of the earth; the *ananta* (represented as a snake), symbolizing water and the infinite ocean from which all life emerged;

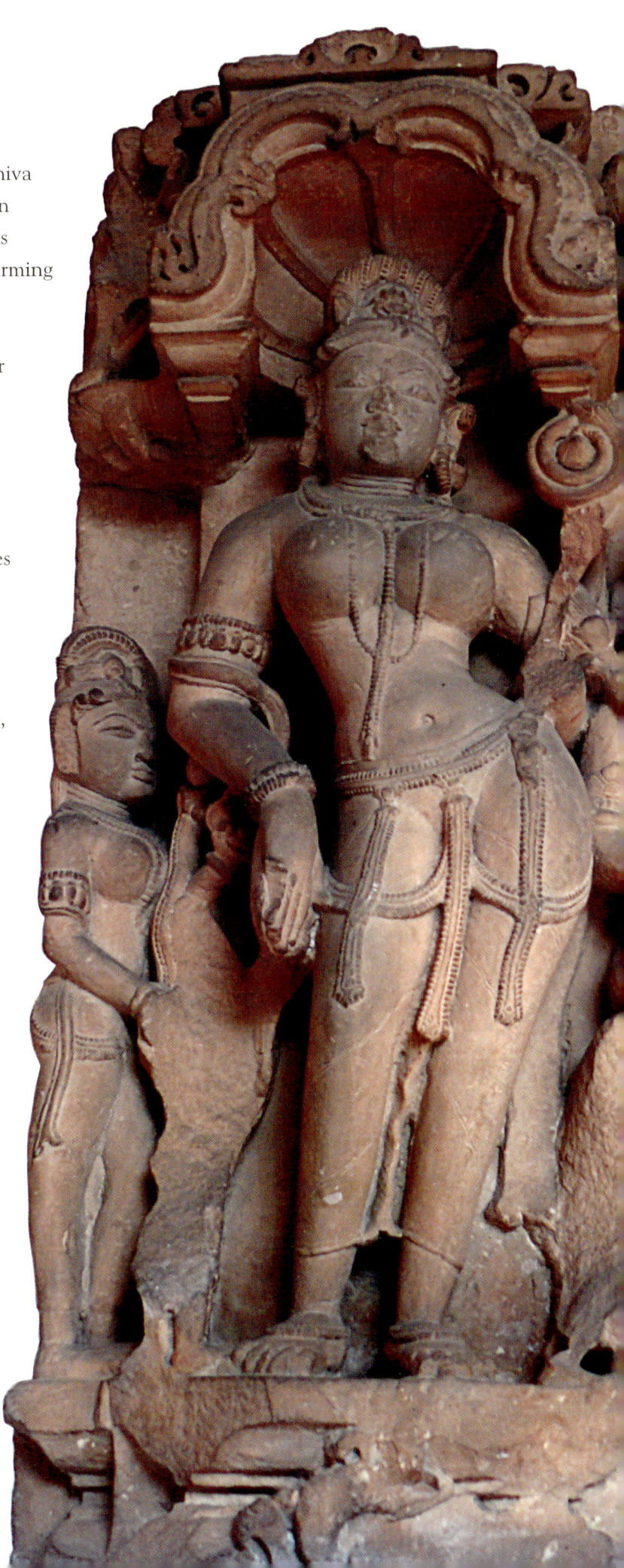

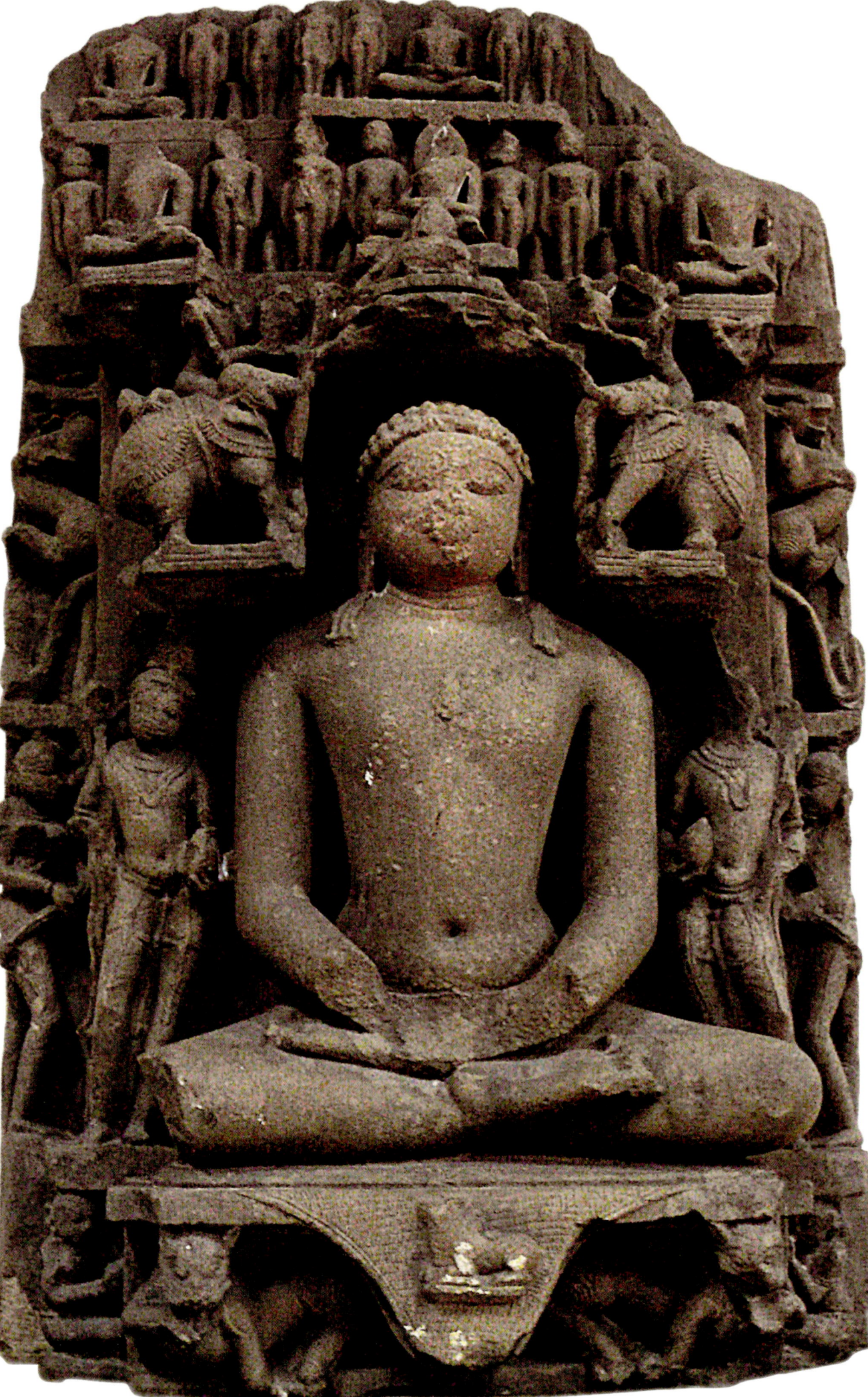

the *swastika*, representing the four-fold aspects of creation and motion; the *purnakalasha*, or the overflowing flower pot, a symbol of creativity and prosperity; the *kalpalata* and *kalpavriksha*, the wish-fulfilment creeper or tree that symbolized imagination and creativity. *Gavaska*, was a symbol sometimes understood to be the third eye; *mriga*, or deer, was symbolic of erotic desire and beauty; and the lingam and yoni, were the universal male and female fertility symbols.

Rules were also evolved to provide additional symbolic content through the hand gestures (*mudra*) of sculpted deities. Deities were sometimes given multiple arms to signify energy or power, or to suggest movement symbolic of the celestial dance. Different arm and hand positions embodied different virtues such as wisdom, strength, generosity, kindness and care. Multiple arms could thus be used to signify multiple virtues.

There are many in the Western world who have failed to comprehend the layered significance of Indian art and sculpture. For them it was a mere reflection of superstitions and archaic belief systems. But what eluded these observers was the fact that while a certain degree of superstition did no doubt exist, it was offset by the communication of philosophical and cultural constructs that inspired the people. The idea of shringara rasa elevated life and living to a level beyond the ordinary and mundane, to one that was sacred, beautiful and true to the essence of their traditional value-systems.

> *Strange, weird things that no man may say,*
> *Things humanity hides away—*
> *Secretly done—*
> *Catch the light of the living day,*
> *Smile in the sun.*
> *Cruel things that man may not name,*
> *Naked here, without fear or shame,*
> *Laugh in the carven stone.*
> —***The Garden of Kama and Other Lyrics from India,***
> **Laurence Hope**

The Buddha in Stone
Buddhist sculpture was divided into two styles: the Mathura and the Gandhara schools of art. The influence of the Greeks, especially in rock-cut art, led to the Gandhara School, while the Mathura School

(Page 108)
Adinatha,
11th-12th century AD,
Bharat Kala Bhavan
Museum, Varanasi

Standing Buddha,
Gandhara, 2nd-3rd century,
National Museum,
New Delhi

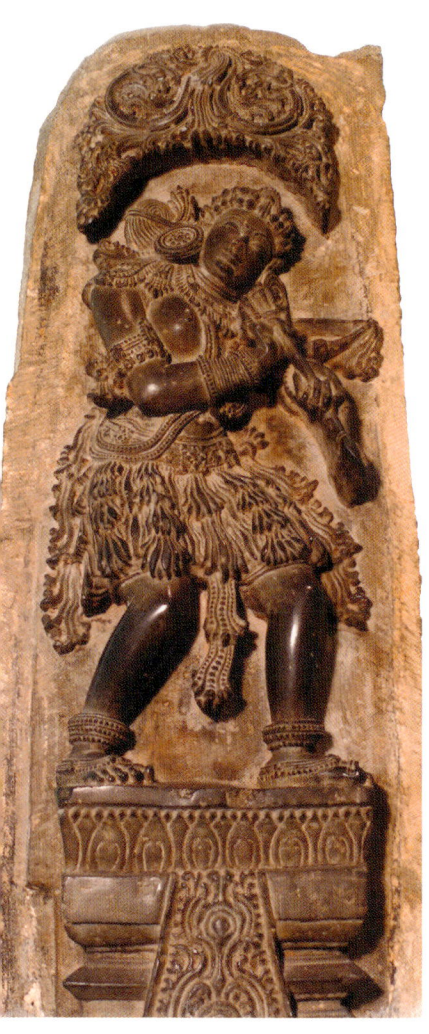

Huntress, Hoysala, Mysore, 12th century, National Museum, New Delhi

*(Page 111)
Buddha's life scene, Ikshavaku-3rd century AD, National Museum, New Delhi*

remained largely indigenous. The Hinayana and Mahayana phases of Buddhism also influenced the nature of rock-cut art. The Hinayana sect devoted itself to representing the artefacts used by the Buddha, while the Mahayana sect focussed on the creation of Buddha's images.

Till about the 8th century CE the Gandhara School of art, which was primarily Buddhist in its thematic content, was prevalent in the North and North-Western parts of India; the finest examples being the Bamiyan Buddhas in Afghanistan. Of Graeco-Roman influence, the Gandhara style was known for its sublime and classical beauty, the influences of which harked back to the idealized beauty of the Greek sculptures. The Bodhisattvas, scenes from the life of Buddha, and his nativity series, also exude a timeless beauty.

The Mathura School which flourished under the Kushan rulers in North India between the 1st and 2nd centuries had completely different aesthetics. The human body became less classical, more sensual, with transparent drapes adding an almost tactile quality to the sculptures which became larger than life. The feminine figures were exquisite in their representation, bearing an indelible hallmark of elegance, charm and sophistication. From yakshis to salabhanjika the women of the Mathura period draw their inspirations from the full-bodied Indian traditions of Bharut and Sanchi. The yakshis had nude upper bodies with globular breasts while the lower bodies were draped in transparent garments, suggestively parted, exuding robust vitality.

Buddha in his wisdom came to the conclusion that human life comprised pain, suffering, sorrow and emptiness, and was therefore not worth living. Existence is brought about and bound by desire, and yet it is desire that causes suffering, frustration and disillusionment. Kama (desire) is hence the root of all life and woman is its symbol. This explains the early Buddhist ideas of deprecation and denouncement of the female gender.

The attempt of Buddhism to banish women led to a powerful reaction. In *Cult of Desire*, Kanwar Lal talks of this reaction, stating that at one stage, temple after temple depicted the entire range of sexual acts – 'vulgar as vulgar can be, unnatural as unnatural can be, obscene as obscene can be, and indecent and shocking, disgusting and repulsive!... a new religion of love and passion was born.'

Monasteries and Stupas

With Mahayana Buddhism came the golden moments in Buddhist sculptural traditions. When the Mauryan ruler Ashoka converted to Buddhism and

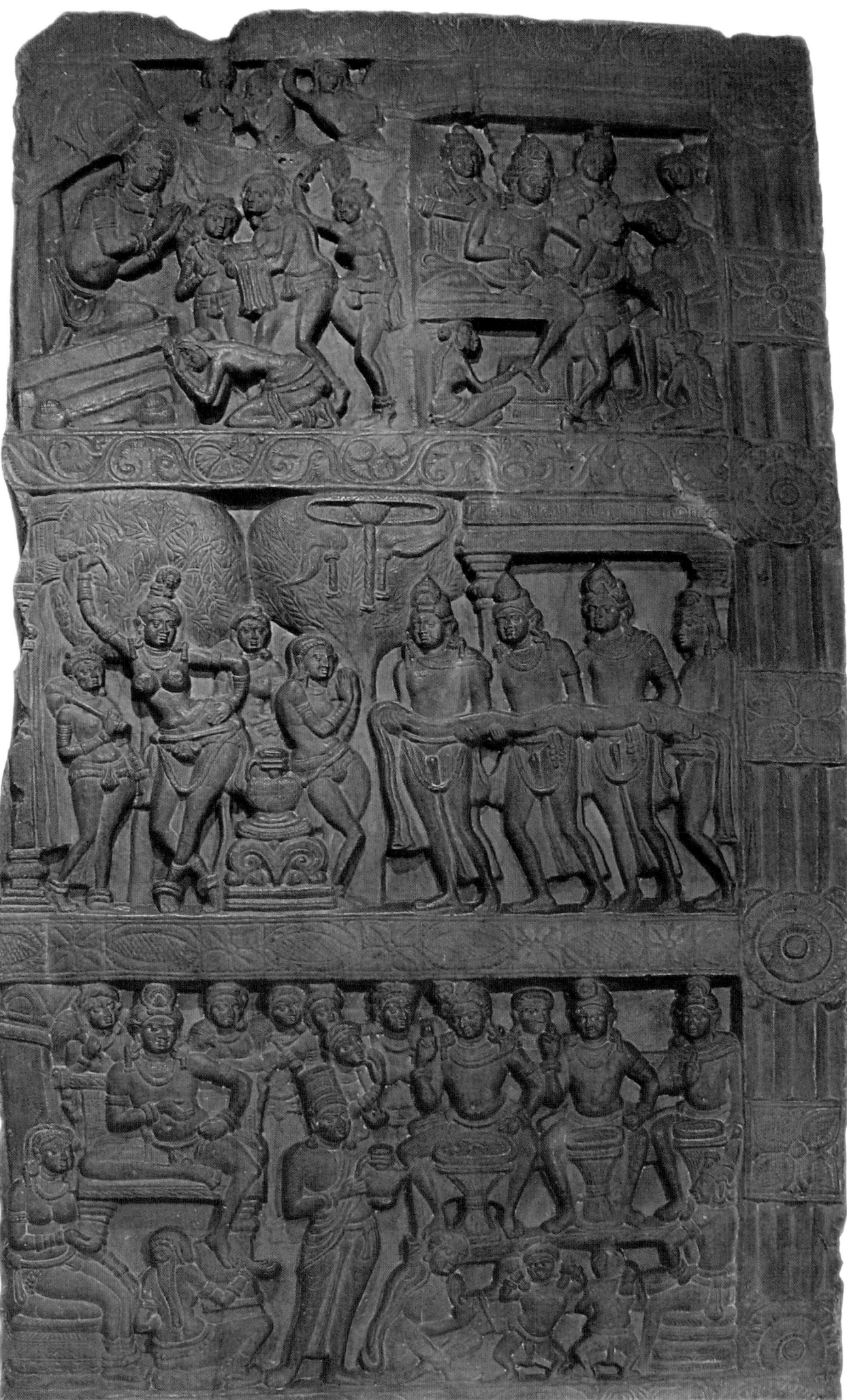

declared the drum of war be replaced with the drum of *dhamma* after the tragic battle of Kalinga, he built 85,000 stupas. Each of the stupas were engraved on rocks and pillars with the teachings of the Buddha. The famous pillar at Sarnath in Madhya Pradesh in polished sandstone is known as the Ashokan Pillar with inscriptions which served as edicts of Buddhist teachings. The sacred wheel of the pillar is the Dharmachakra which is symbolic of the first sermon which Buddha delivered at Sarnath.

The ancient cave monasteries of India are another magnificent testimony to the tradition of sculpture. Decorated with carvings and adorned with paintings, these remarkable caves were intended as religious centres. For a millennium, rock cutting was to remain a favoured mode of artistic expression. The pantheon of Hindu gods and goddesses is found all over such centres of art, especially in western and southern India.

One of the earliest Buddhist architectural forms that deserves mention is the stupa. Buddhism gained prominence during the reign of Emperor Ashoka and the religious architecture was typified by three main elements—the *chaitya* hall (place of worship), the *vihara* (monastery) and the stupa (hemispherical mound for worship/memory). Some of the best examples of this can be found in Sanchi and the Ajanta and Ellora caves.

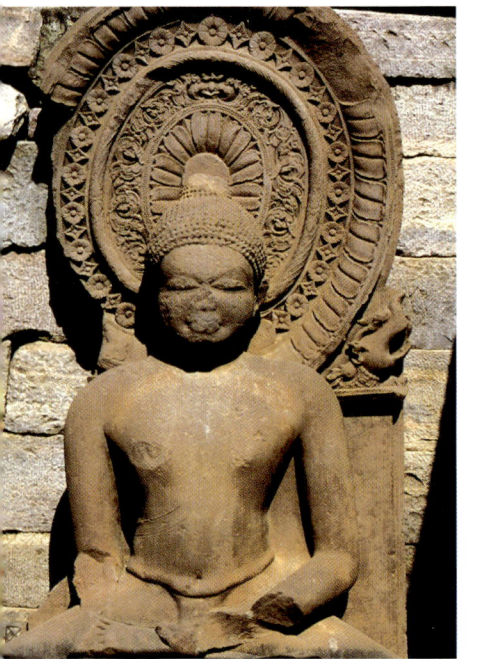

Buddha, Sanchi, 273-236 BC

Conversion of Jatilas, Kushana, 2nd century, Gandhara, National Museum, New Delhi

Few Indian stupas are as well-known as the Sanchi stupa in Madhya Pradesh. However, in Sri Lanka, the stupa reached tremendous proportions. The Abhayagiriya Dagaba at Anuradhapura, the capital of the early kings of Ceylon, was 327 feet in diameter, and larger than some Egyptian pyramids. In India, stupa architecture became more and more ornate. The Amaravati stupa, for example, was larger than the one at Sanchi; it was adorned with carved panels telling the story of the life of the Buddha. Sarnath and Nalanda are the most famous of the later stupas. The Sarnath stupa was an imposing structure of beautifully patterned brickwork, with the high, cylindrical upper dome rising from a lower one.

The chaitya hall of the rock-cut monastery also developed in size and splendour. As the accommodation needs of each monastery fell short for its

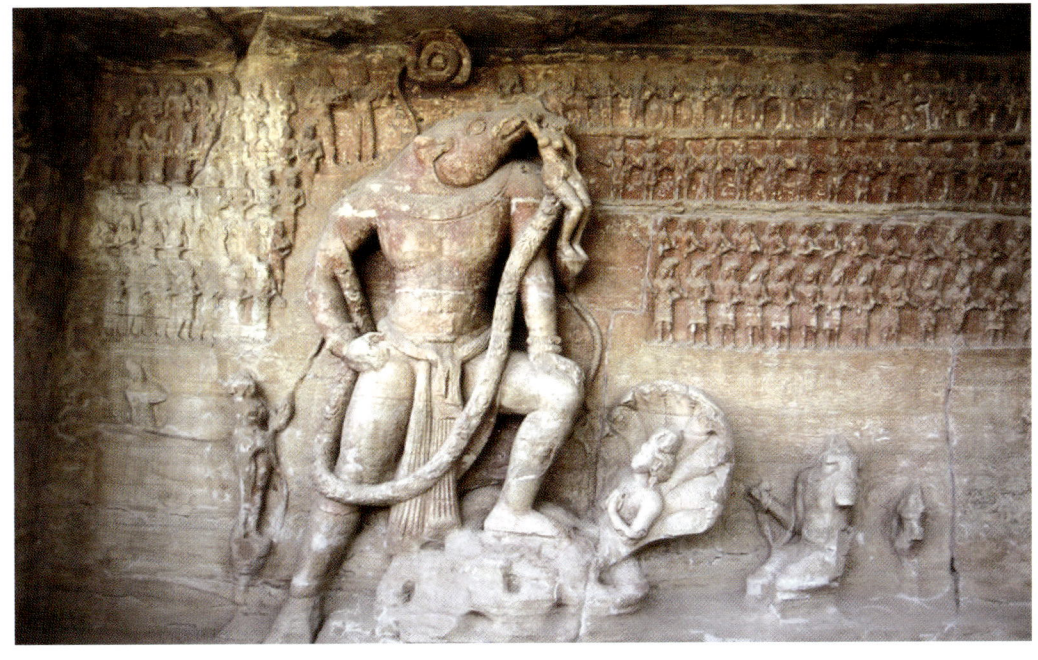

Vishnu as a boar, Vidisha Cave 5, Udaygiri, Orissa

Manjushri, Pala, 8th century, Nalanda, National Museum, New Delhi

inhabitants, a new cave was carved. The most famous of these cave groups is in Ajanta, with no less than twenty-seven caves, some carved a hundred feet deep into the rock. The splendid sculpture found in these caves make them among the most glorious monuments of India's past.

The magnificent Kailashanath temple at Ellora, the first rock-cut temple in the history of Indian architecture, was started by King Krishna I of the Rashtrakuta dynasty (717-775). As his architectural ambitions grew, he was not satisfied with the mere hollowing of rock to create caves. He ordered the entire rockface to be cut and a splendid temple carved, like a statue from the hillside, complete with a shrine room, hall, gateway, votive pillars, smaller shrines and cloisters, entirely adorned with divine figures and scenes, large and small, of a grace and strength rarely seen.

Temple Art

Indian temples have been traditionally classified into three types: the Nagara or 'northern' style, the Dravida or 'southern ' style, and the Vesara or 'hybrid' style seen in the Deccan area. Regions such as Bengal, Kerala and the Himalayan states have their own unique styles. In each case, the distinctive architecture was shaped by the broad geographical, climatic and cultural variations that existed in the region.

Naturally, the geographical conditions dictated the nature of raw materials used, which in turn, significantly affected the carving styles and construction techniques. In the Hoysala temples of the 12th and 13th centuries a soft

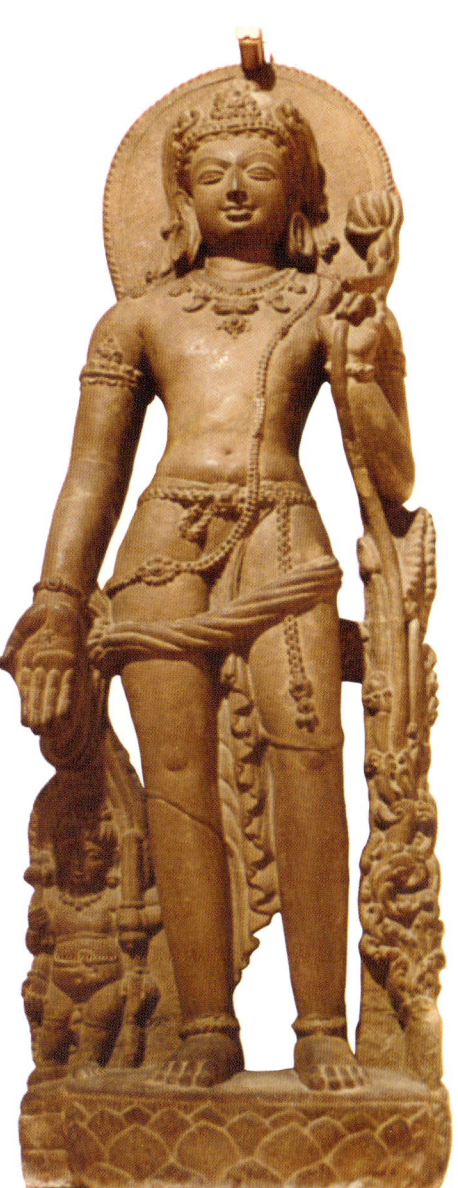

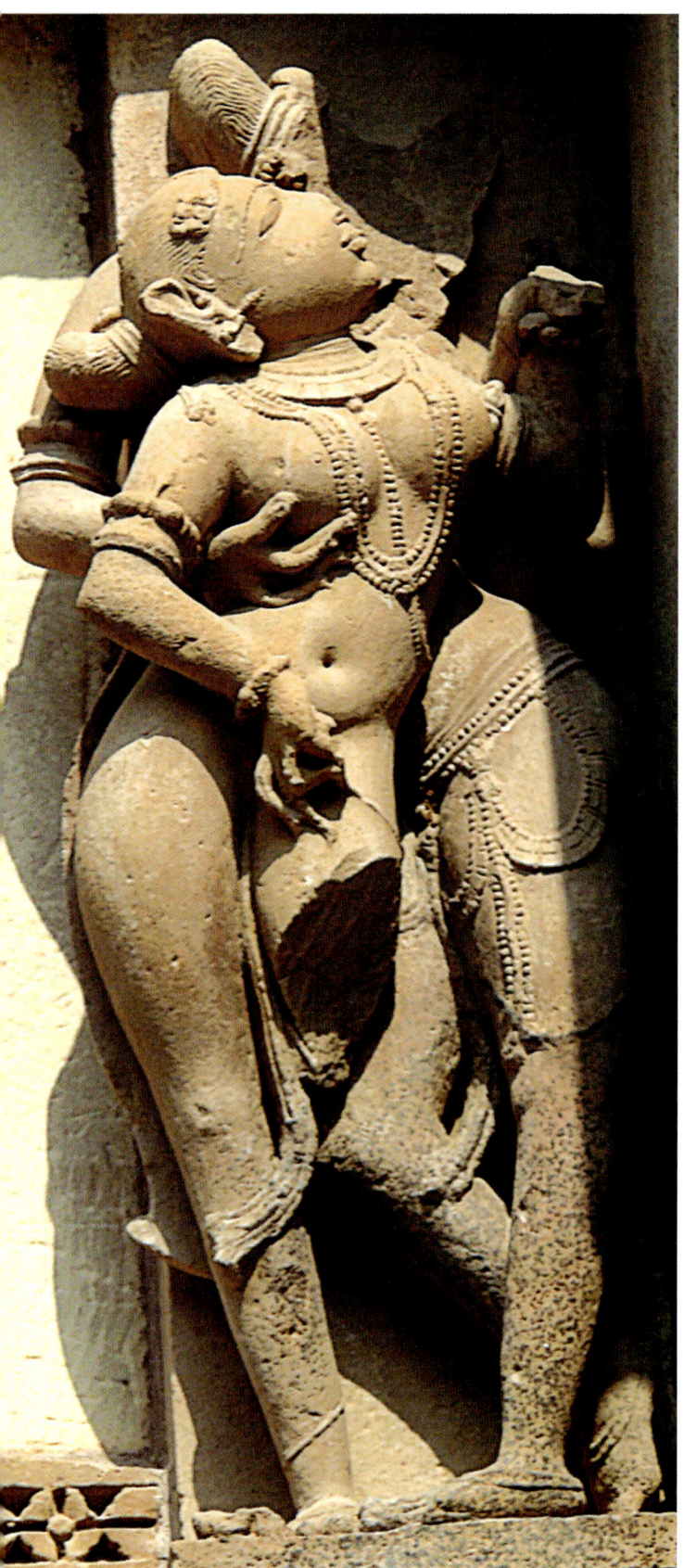

soapstone was used and this led to the evolution of later creations in ivory and sandalwood. These materials allowed for detailed and filigree work. In contrast, the hard crystalline granite-like rocks typical of the area around Mamallapuram did not allow such fine work. Granite was limited to the carving of shallow reliefs, as can be seen in the Pallava temples of the 7th century.

Sex as Sacred

According to *Kamasutra*, sexual enjoyment is complementary to the moral, material and spiritual well-being of a person. The sex act was regarded as natural as sight and scent, not something to be hidden in shame and then brooded on with guilt. One of the main intentions behind the creation of the Khajuraho temples and *Kamasutra* was to educate the people and make them more aware of sex as an integral and sacred part of life, an element they must master rather than be subservient to. Indian artists sculpted temple walls with representations of sexual activity covering all aspects of life. Sexual orgies, of both the natural and unnatural kinds, were immortalized by the graphic stone carvings of different periods.

In fact, the architecture of the temple itself symbolized human coital union. The sanctum sanctorum was the bridegroom, the main hall or the *mandapa* the bride, and the *antarala* or the passage between the two was the *milana-sthala* or meeting place. The joys and pleasures of life were celebrated on the façades in carved panels of entwined or conjoined couples.

Temple architecture in India has been an important vehicle for the expression of erotica and is unsurpassed for the sheer celebration of the feminine form. From the beautiful, scantily-clad women of the Ajanta caves and the temples of Khajuraho, to the gorgeous alasya kanyas or women at their toilette, the female form has been represented in its full and abundant glory. A stock erotic image is the maithuna couple showing voluptuous figures of a man and woman fondly grasping each other around

114   *Shringara*—the many faces of Indian beauty

the waist and shoulders, symbolic of wealth, prosperity and love. These sculptured couples also had a protective function, and depicted the strong link between sexuality, fertility and the auspicious in Indian society.

Thus the temple, once reserved for temple patrons, was opened to the common man in modern day life. It has become a public arena where erotic images meet a wider gaze. Whether in Ramgarh (Rajasthan); Aihole, Badami, Pattadakal, Srirangam, Kanchipuram, Nagarjunkonda (South India); Konark and Bhubaneswar (Orissa); Ajanta and Ellora (Maharashtra) or Khajuraho (Madhya Pradesh), passion breathes upon the walls of temples.

The Pinnacle of Adornment

Known all over the world as the highpoint of erotic art in India, the architectural style of the Khajuraho temples stands apart. Divided into the western, eastern and southern groups, the temples are built from east to west. They have three main sections: the entrance or *ardha mandapa*, assembly hall or mandapa, and an inner sanctum or the *garbhagriha*. The western group is the largest, with its Kandariya Mahadev temple dedicated to Lord Shiva, containing 900 sculptures carved in sandstone and built without any mortar. The exquisitely carved exterior offers a contrast to the plain interior space that houses a shivalingam in the womb of the temple that is located beneath the main spire (*shikhara*).

The Jagdambi Temple is finely decorated with numerous erotic carvings. In the temple *griha* is an enormous image of the goddess Devi. Built in the Nagara style, it bears a beehive shaped tower (shikhara). Over time, the central shaft of the temple was surrounded by many smaller reproductions of itself that resulted in a spectacular visual effect. (The Nagara style travelled east to the Parasurameshvara temple at Bhubaneswar and the Surya temple at Modhera.)

The Vishvanath temple is one of the finest of the Khajuraho temples and was built by the Chandela ruler, Dhanga, in 1002. The temple's sculptures are particularly striking in the quality of their carving and subject matter. Dedicated to Shiva, the temple enshrines a shivalingam, his vehicle, the Nandi bull, as well as an image of his consort Durga. In another shrine at a farflung corner, is a shivalingam with four faces carved on its surface.

(Page 114)
Lovers, Chitragupta Temple, Khajuraho

Lakshmana Temple, Khajuraho

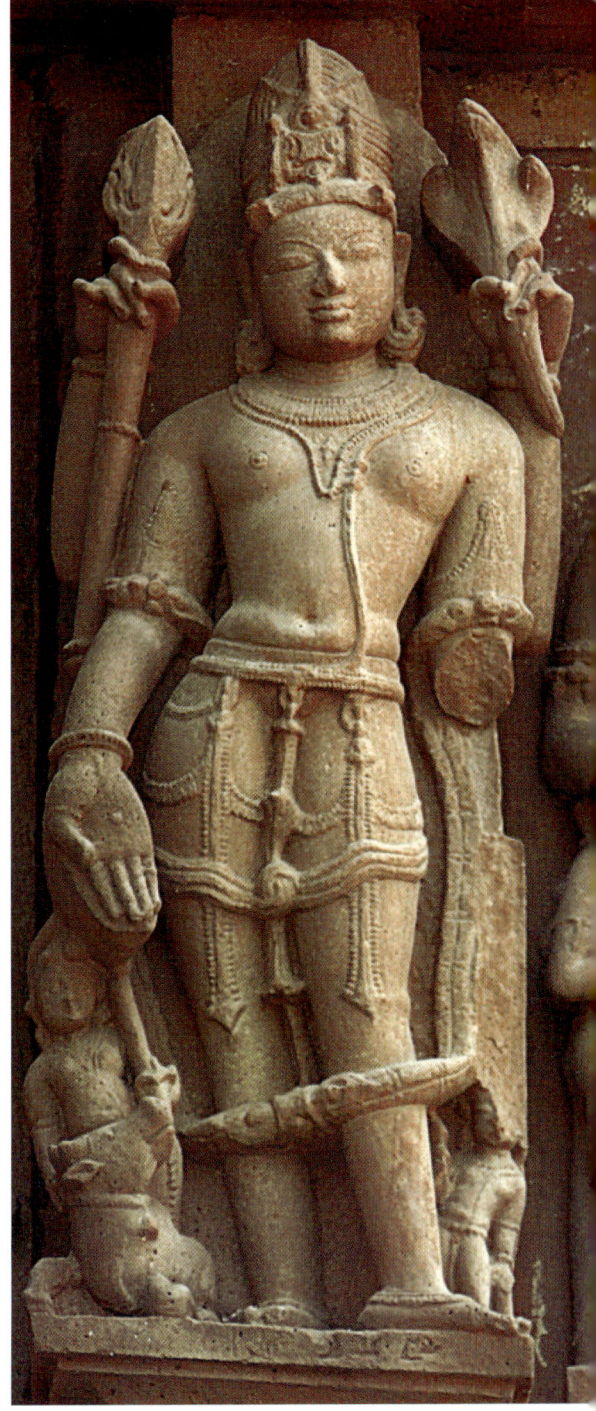

Shilpa Shastra—adornment in stone

Tantric Rites

The sexual activities and positions displayed on the façades of many temple groups all over India are linked to tantric beliefs.

> *This thread is the idea that tantra is a cult of ecstasy focused on a vision of cosmic sexuality.*
>
> —***The Art of Tantra**, Rawson Phillip*

(Page 117)
King and queen, Chitragupta Temple, Khajuraho

Vamana, 12th Century, Central India, National Museum, New Delhi

The Tantric iconography of sexual union has travelled through time. The union of man-woman as a metaphor for Shiva-Shakti is the foundation on which Tantric thought rests, and all its imagery spreads from this basic idea. The repertoire through which the artist created images includes *mandala* designs, *yantras*, snakes, triangular female emblems, lingams, explicit copulating couples, symbolism of fire, and colour and form. However, in Tantric art, creativity has not been the hallmark; rather it is the transferring of text into image.

The Eternal Image

Ideas and imagery pass on from generation to generation in India and there is a continuum in the imagery. From the ovoid lingam adorned with a five-hooded serpent symbolic of cosmic energy, executed by ancient artists, to the serpent heads painted by the contemporary Indian painter Manu Parekh, to the explicit depiction of male and female genitalia by Ranbir Kaleka, the theme is eternal.

Erotica was not just a matter of pleasure but had a deeper scientific rationale. It was elaborated not only in texts relating to the visual and performing arts, but also those on religion and literature. The shivalingam is perhaps the high point of Indian erotica. Minimal at one level, it achieves the final abstraction of its concept and form in the *svayambhu* or self-originated. Subtly rounded on the surface, and curved on the top and bottom, it is representative of the transcendent cosmic energy where male and female can be seen as distinct. It is this separation and union of the male and female which makes Indian erotica so holistic, giving equal importance to both the sexes and their shared energies.

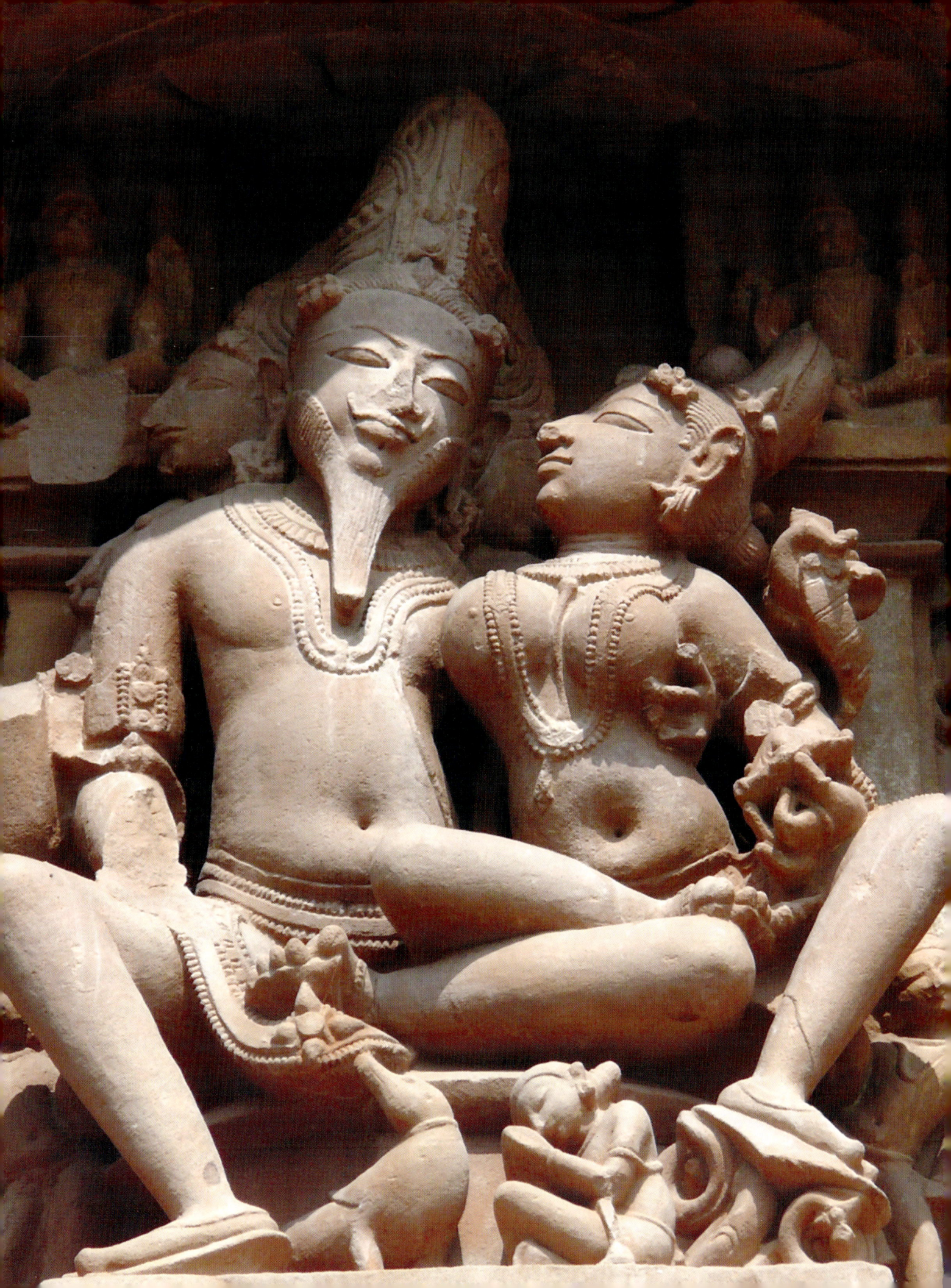

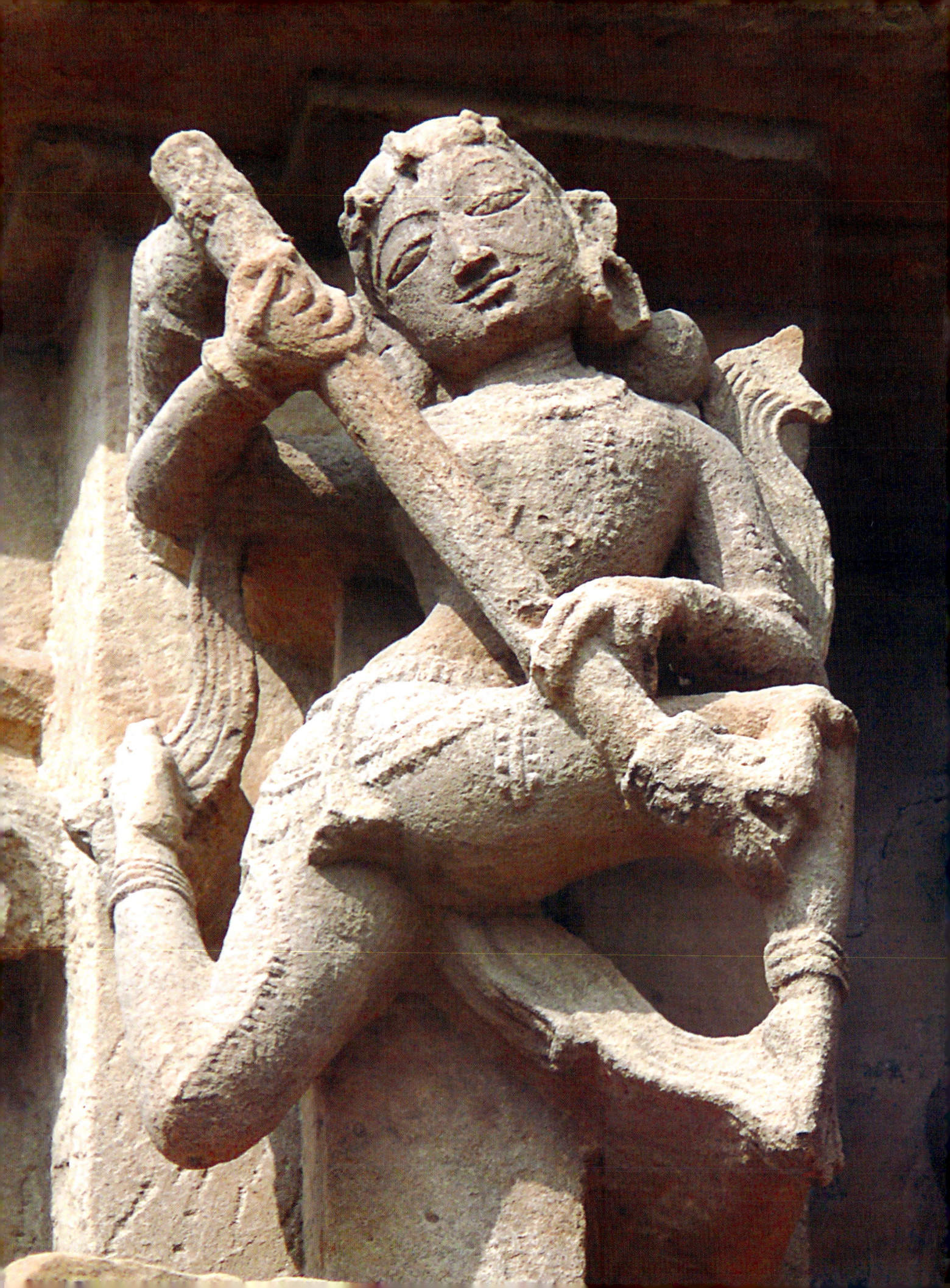

CHAPTER 8

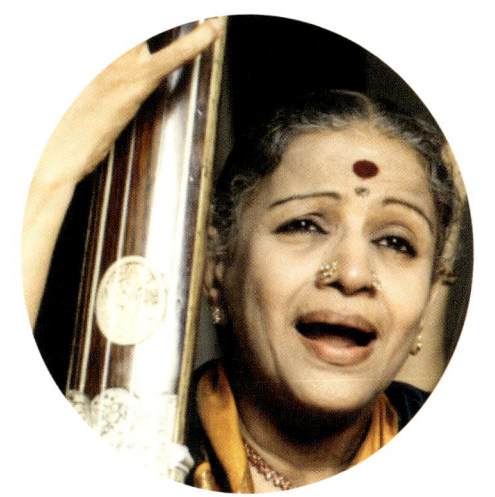

Sangeet
food for the soul

It is cruel you know, that music should be so beautiful. It has the beauty of loneliness and of pain, of strength and freedom. The beauty of disappointment and never satisfied love. The cruel beauty of nature, and the everlasting beauty of monotony.

BENJAMIN BRITTEN

The Indian aesthetic tradition is based on the fundamental premise that music, dance and drama are artistic pursuits that have the potential to influence people deeply. *Natyashastra* with its rasa theory exemplifies this belief system and divides the constituents of all emotional expression into the following categories:

i. *Vibhavas* or the cause/catalyst of emotion
ii. *Anubhavas* or the external expression of the emotion aroused
iii. *Sattvabhavas* or physical and involuntary responses to emotion
iv. Bhavas or emotions and moods.

In the final analysis, the emotional state comprises two states of mind that are called *sthayi* and *sanchari*. The former refers to the more concrete and lasting emotions and the latter to the fleeting or transitory. While sthayi is applicable to all human beings, sanchari is much more individualistic and person-specific. Bhava, therefore, can be elicited through music, or a synthesis of certain musical progressions and configurations that are based on harmonic, rhythmic and melodic detailing.

(Page 118)
Musician, Duladeo Temple, Khajuraho. The temple has several carvings of dancing apsaras and flying vidyadharas

(Page 121)
Venugopala, brass, Crafts Museum, New Delhi

Nayika, Basholi Kalam Pahari, 1685-1690, N.C. Mehta Collection, Ahmedabad

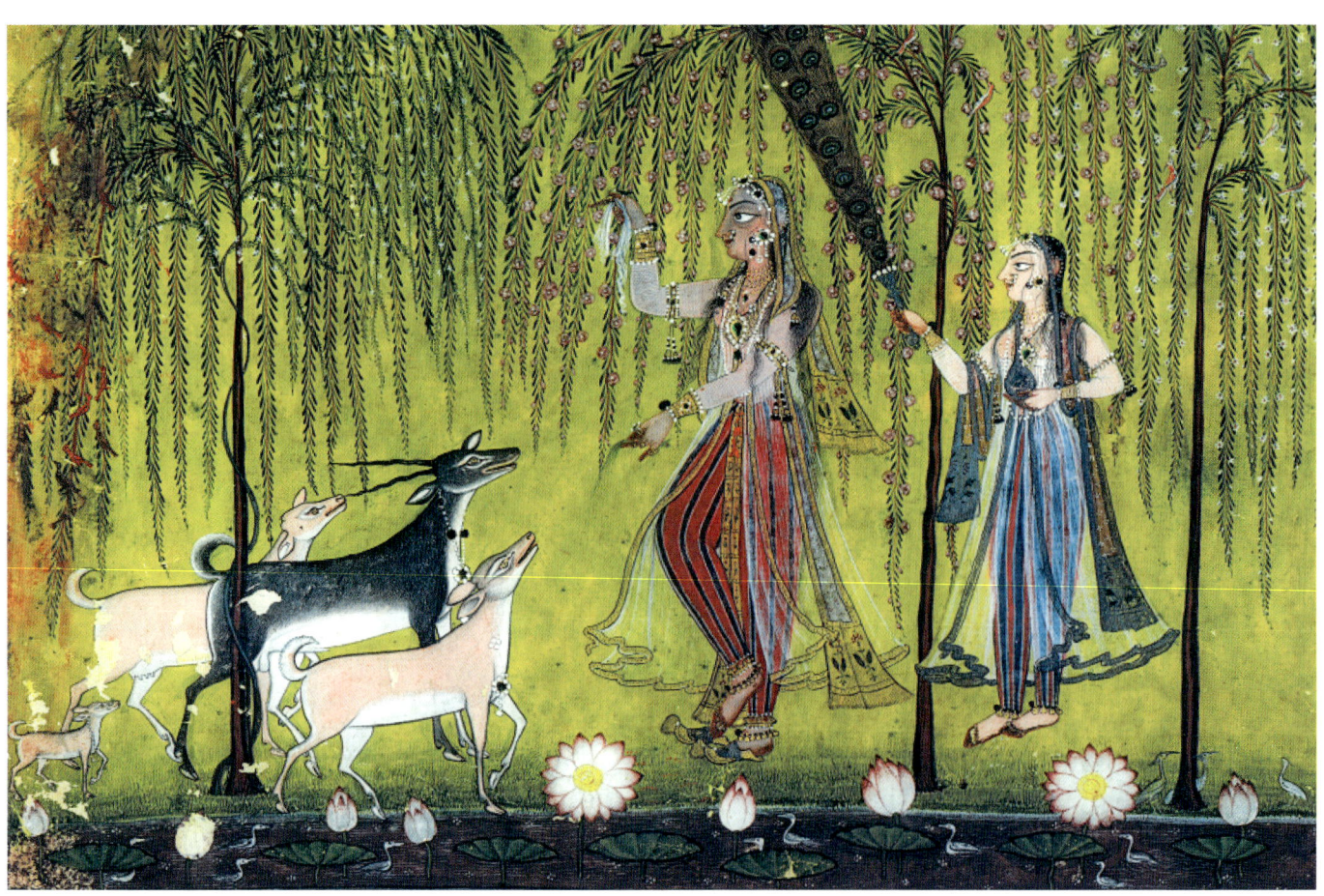

120   *Shringara*—the many faces of Indian beauty

The Divine Art Form

Within the aesthetic tradition itself, music occupies pride of place. So elevated is this particular form of artistic expression, that the gods themselves have played an active and vibrant role in the making of music: Goddess Saraswati plays the veena, Lord Krishna the flute, and Lord Shiva his *damroo*. From the earliest times music was used to calm the disturbances of the mind, making it more susceptible to receiving the vibhavas embedded in a situation or composition, helping the listener to identify with the different rasas evoked and the various bhavas generated. It is here that we can find the rasaraja shringara, or that which elevates one to a peak of pleasure. It is this particular emotional component, distinct from all the other rasas that is seen as the basis of an aesthetic experience, and through it, metaphorically, of a mystical experience.

Shringara in music is essentially an experience, moving between the performance and the transference of the rasa. The concept of rasa in music, in an extension of the same logic, is inextricably linked to raga. Derived from the Sanskrit root *ranja*, the word 'raga' literally means 'colouring'. In the context of music it refers to a medium through which the listener's mind can be coloured with a specific emotional response and arouse in it certain passions.

Musical Stepping Stones

Broadly defined as that which allows a musical composition to create a certain mood in both listener and practitioner by using specific notes in a specific manner, the raga was actually brought into mainstream musical terminology by sage Matanga (AD 500–700). Matanga wrote *Brihaddeshi*, a canonical text in which he initiated the 'raga' tradition, defining it as something that is essentially and purely musical—something that produces different emotional effects by using

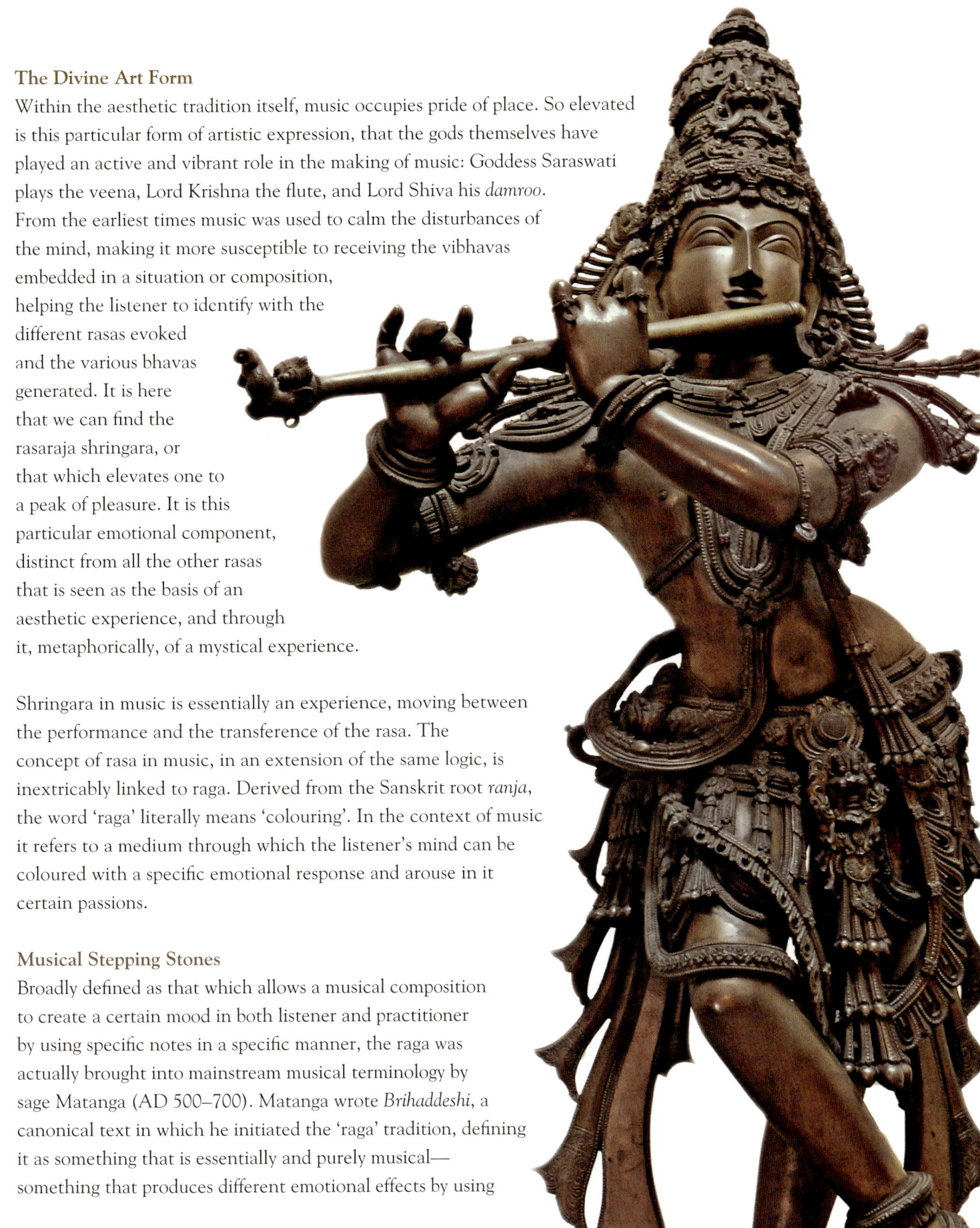

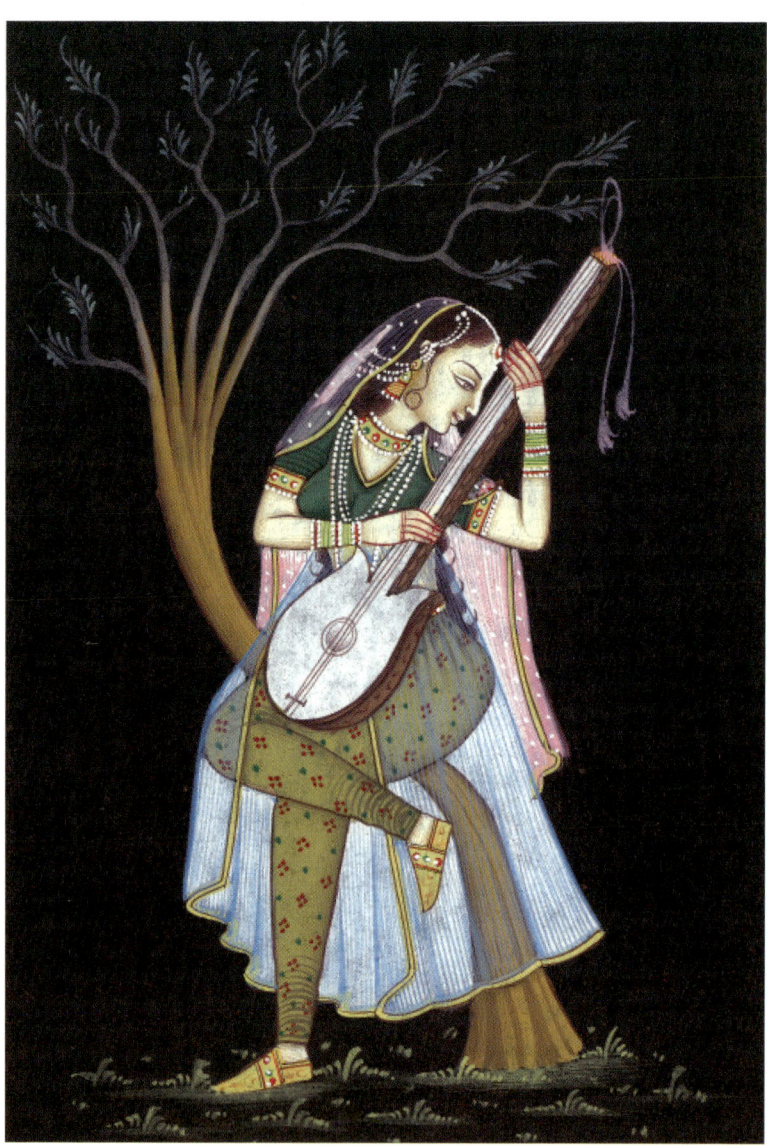

The 'ashta nayikas' or the eight nayikas are often a popular theme with Rajasthani artists. Here, one of the nayikas, the Abhisarika, is seen waiting for her beloved at the appointed place

different *dhvanis*—even when the notes on the scale remain the same.

For Matanga therefore, raga is connected to dhvani, which, in turn, is derived from poetics and refers to the creation of an impact beyond that which is directly expressed. What distinguishes any one raga from another is the presence of a dominant note called the *vadi swara*, and the avoidance of certain other notes called the *vivadi swara*. It is in the combination of these notes that the entire gamut of human emotions can be experienced. The emotive note of each raga or ragini is also called its *swaradevata*; it is through this note that the overall essence of the raga or ragini is established, a pattern most beautifully expressed in the Ragamala paintings that are believed to be the pictorial representations of musical expressions.

Fundamentally, the experience of music brings into play the interaction between three main elements—tone (svara), rhythm (*laya*) and form (rupa). One is drawn into states of varying emotionality as these elements merge in different combinations. These are then further enhanced by the addition of lyrics and other musical embellishments. *Natyashastra* looks at music within the context of theatre and dramatics, or natya, and as a medium through which emotions evoked by performance can be accentuated. And that is how music is linked with the different rasas, since all these different aspects of traditional aesthetic convention merge in the creation of specific sensations.

Evoking the Mood

Every musical composition is governed by a specific moment in time that is closely associated with it, or evoke, a specific emotion. The morning, for instance, is the time for bhakti rasa and shanta rasa that ragas like Bhairav are linked with; ragas such as Kafi, Asawari, Todi and Bhairavi are best played in the morning and afternoon; and ragas such as Bilawal, Kalyan and Khamaj, with suitable lyrics,

122 *Shringara*—the many faces of Indian beauty

create an atmosphere of shringara rasa when played in the late evening and the early part of the night, a time for romantic dalliance.

According to Bharata, there are eight categories of bhavas and these are distributed across the seven notes of the octave—sa, re, ga, ma, pa, dha, ni—with specific rasas attached to specific notes. The fourth note—ma—is connected with the shringara rasa. All musical compositions and ragas have their own melodic embellishments and ornamentations. Unlike Western classical music, where each note is written and the musician and performer follow the dictates of the composer, in India the performer is himself the composer—improvising and innovating melody and rhythm with complete technical mastery over the five key notes—vadi, samvadi, niyas, anuvadi and vivadi—which form the basis of each raga.

Emotion is evoked through volume, breath control and intonation, all of which combine to determine a specific rasa. Along with the *alaap*, essentially a dialogue between the musician and the raga itself, the *taan* or quick movement of notes which displays technical virtuosity, have their own impact. The subtle shades of the various bhavas emerge and re-emerge and, one being more prominent, surge forward towards the formation of a rasa, or predominant emotive tone of the song.

The decoration of a composition occurs through various musical devices like the *kan, meend, murki, gamak, khatka, behalava, ghaseet, krintan* and *jamjama*, all different nuances of vocal embellishments and virtuosity. A wide variety of taans, all of which accentuate the rasa, intensify the passion.

One of the fundamental elements required to evoke a particular rasa is the *bandish* or composition, which is also the central pillar of the raga in *khayal sangeet*. Khayal, the medieval form of vocal classical in northern India, was popularized by the Muslim rulers. While in certain forms like *dhrupad*, khayal and *tarana*, the bandish helps in the development of the raga, other forms like *thumri* and *dadra* need to be composed, keeping in mind that these are *shabdapradhan* (text-dependant) genres—the beauty of the words is very important for the creation of the desired melodic effect.

The Romantic Forms

The thumri, in particular, marks a significant development in the evolution of Hindustani music. Originating in the court of Wajid Ali Shah in the 19th century, thumri is based on the expressive aspects of music and was initially the song of the *tawaif* or courtesan, accompanied by dance. The songs deal with romantic love that

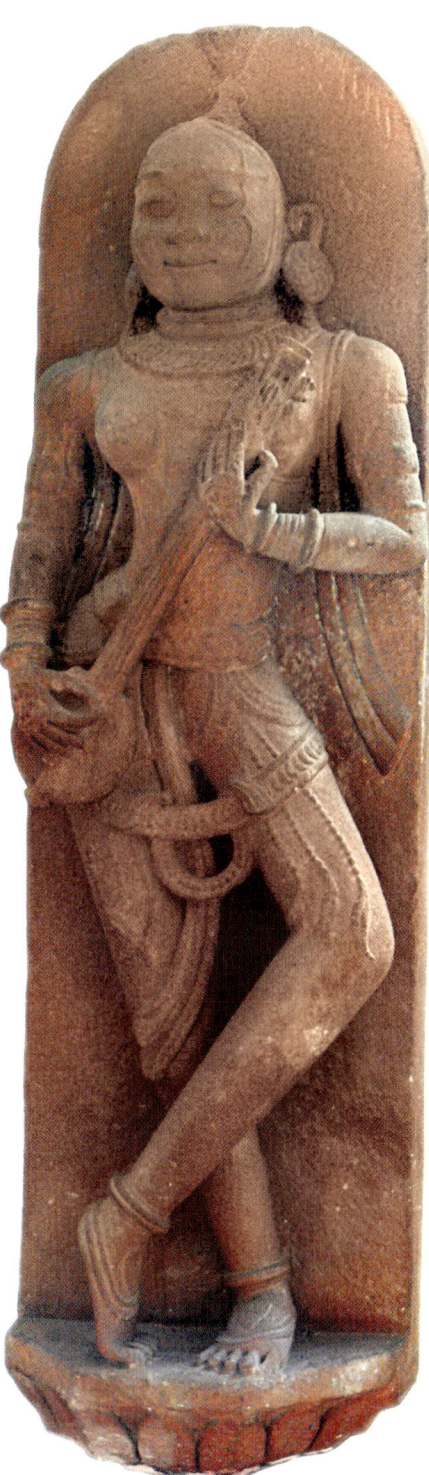

A lady playing an instrument, 19th-20th century, National Museum, New Delhi

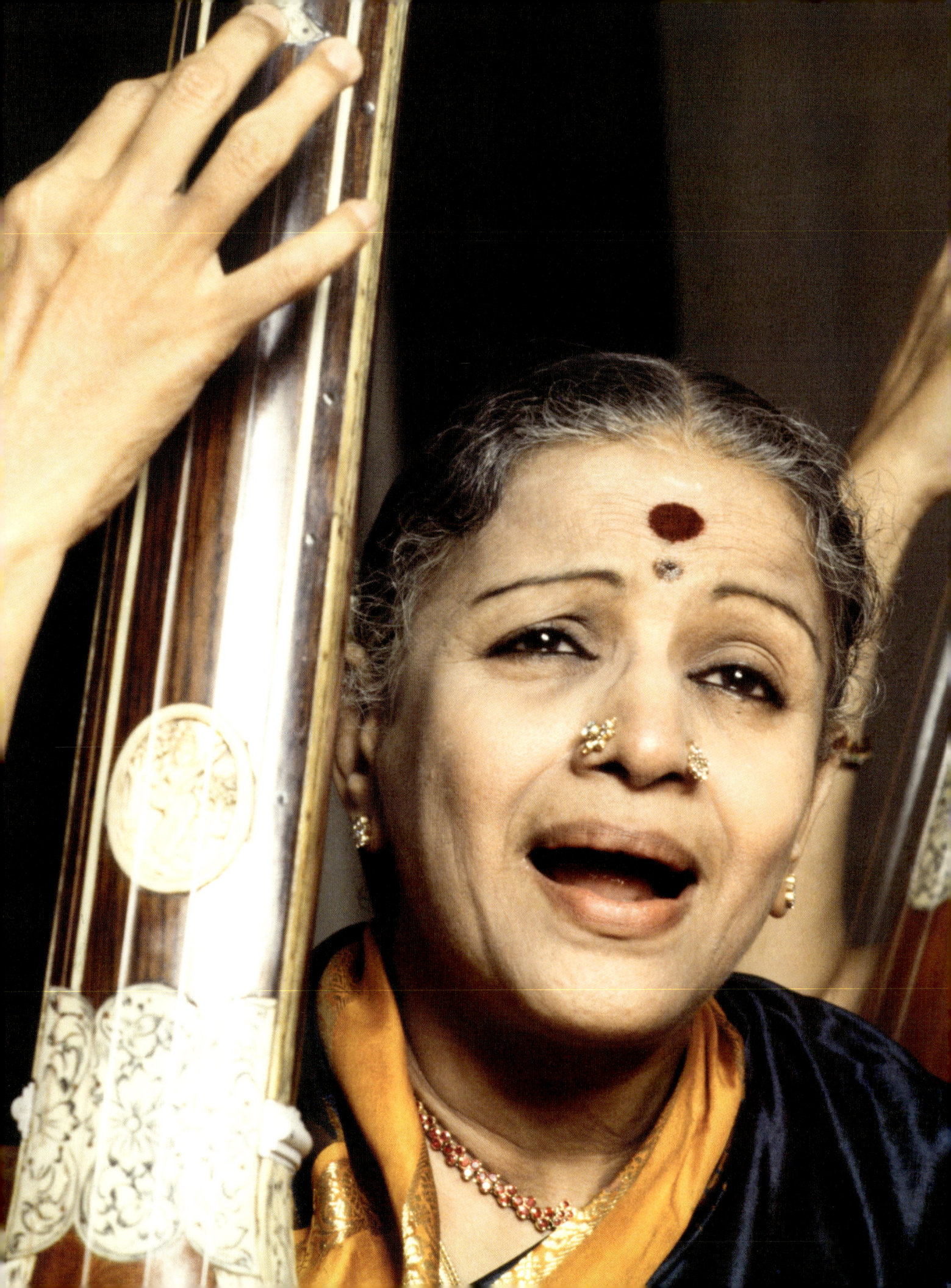

is, in fact, symbolic of spiritual love. They are usually written in Braj bhasha, a dialect prevalent in Uttar Pradesh and associated with the legends of Krishna.

Other popular themes include the pangs of separation, jealousy and an overwhelming passion for the beloved. The music in thumri and its variations like *barsati*, *chaiti*, and *kajri* are infused with folk influences, but the structure remains essentially classical. First written by Amir Khusro, ghazal *gayaki* appeared on the musical scene in the 13th century.

Like the thumri, the ghazal focusses on emotional and romantic themes rendered lyrically through couplets in Persian or Urdu. Yet another genre that deserves mention are the songs of the nautch girls or courtesans who practised their art in India till the end of the 19th century. The word 'nautch' is actually an anglicized version of the Hindi or Urdu word *nach*, which in turn, is derived from the Sanskrit *nritya* and the Prakrit *nachcha* and means dance. The professional exponents of a refined variety of cultural entertainment, the courtesans were known for their beauty, training in classical dance and music and the sophisticated art of seduction. So evocative and imbued with rasa was their performance that officers of the East India Company are known to have described it as 'superior to all the operas in the world'.

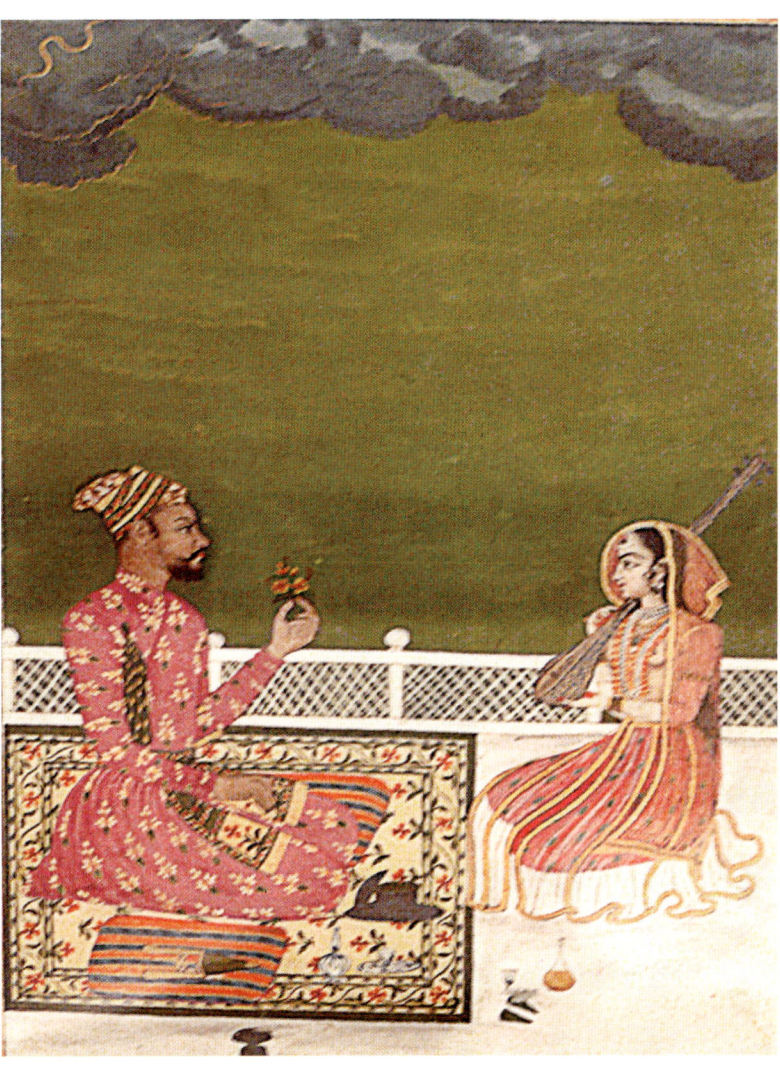

A prince enjoying music, Golconda, Deccan, National Museum, New Delhi

(Page 124) M.S. Subbulakshmi

The courtesans sang of love, wine, and the amorous escapades in the lives of the gods. They based their songs on traditional romantic folklore and legends that spoke of the lover's yearning for the beloved. The musical renditions, accompanied by facial expressions and body gestures all combined to arouse feelings of love, passion and yearning in the audience. While the songs usually spoke of the gods, the words became more nuanced and took on different levels of meaning when a courtesan had a special liaison with a patron, or wanted to oblige someone.

Sangeet—food for the soul

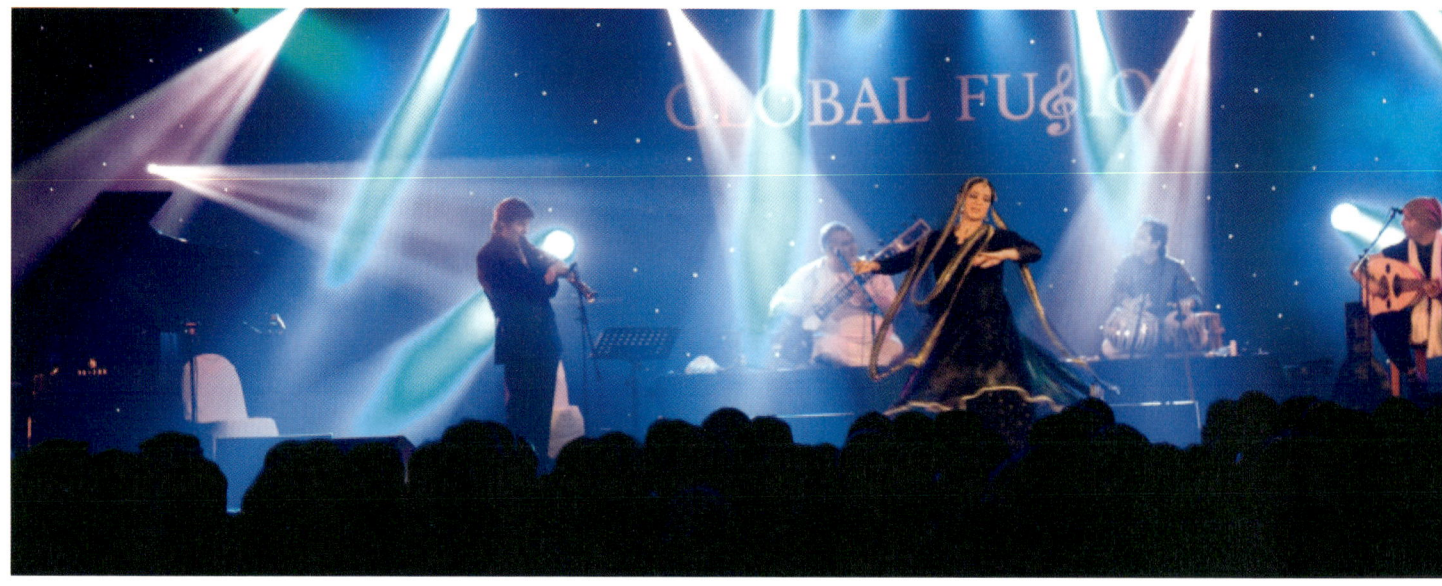

Sufi Kathak by Manjari Chaturvedi along with (L-R) Tim Ries (Rolling Stones), Ustaad Shujat H Khan, Yogesh Samsi, Dhafer Youssef, Nguyen Le at Global Fusion Concert, Dubai

The Other Face of Joy

Since the nature of shringara is spontaneous, unrehearsed and unpredictable, its evocation becomes more elaborate and subtle. So much so, that the same emotion can be created vicariously within the soul of the audience or *rasikas*. It is therefore, only the skilled poet, musician or artist who can capture its spirit and convert it into a bhava, leading to a moment of emotional release.

For many practitioners of music, the search for beauty does not exclude sadness or unhappiness. The darker aspects of life are recognized and transformed into other avatars when they are touched with art and music. Joy and sorrow, in such conditions, are inextricably linked and have to be experienced together to be true. The shringara rasa is tinged with viraha, or the longing of the beloved, and until the moment of union finally arrives the karuna rasa is enriched by despair. However, it ultimately culminates in shanta rasa, that is 'ultimate bliss'.

Seasonal Songs

The barahmasa or the seasonal songs that are sung around the year, form a distinctive genre of romantic poetry. The changing seasons become symbolic of the varying moods of love and longing, with the melodies resonating the external ambience, the feeling of anticipation and the desire of the lover and the beloved. In fact, Shadrituvarnan or the description of the six Indian seasons play an important role in Sanskrit kavya literature. Kalidasa's poem, *Ritusamhara*, for example, is devoted to the beauty of the six seasons, almost like a garland of seasons. Contextualized within the emotional gamut of shringara, the barahmasa poems form a rich repertoire of romantic songs.

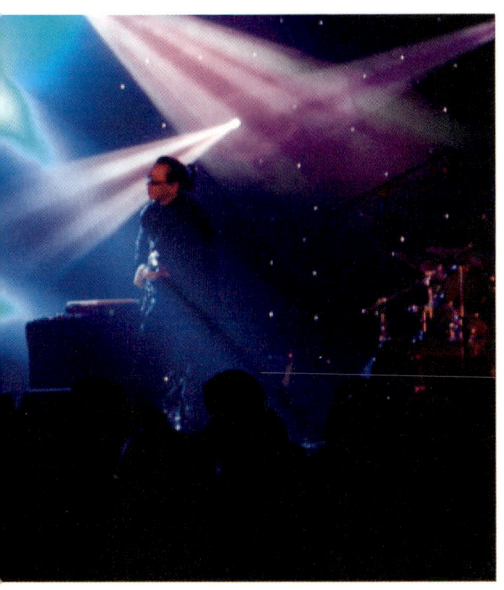

Some of the finest barahmasa was written by Guru Nanak Dev, the first of the ten gurus, who laid the foundations of the Sikh religion. He developed the Raga Tukhari to be sung in the early hours of a winter morning. A number of *shabads* or devotional compositions were sung in this raga, revealing new levels of diction, imagery and thought:

Pari-a baajh duhaylee ko-ay na baylee gurmukh amrit peevaa.

(Without my Beloved, I am miserable; I have no friend at all.
As Gurmukh, I drink in the Ambrosial Nectar.)
—***Tukhari Chant, First Mehl, Barah Maaha***

The Guru takes his imagery from nature and the lives of the common people around him, thereby making philosophical ideas and concepts intelligible. A certain song speaks of a married woman who awaits the return of her husband, her longing aggravated by the arrival of the monsoon that makes separation unbearable. Another barahmasa, popular in the rural areas in Punjab, is found in the *Adi Granth* written by Guru Arjan Dev in Majh Raga.

*Gur Poorai har naam dirhaa-i-aa
Har nichal har dhan palai jee-o.*

(The Perfect Guru has implanted the lord's name within me.
I have the imperishable Treasure of the Lord in my Lap.)
—***Raag Majh, Chau Padas, First House, Fourth Mehl***

Such an expression of intense feelings overwhelms the human heart. Its appeal lies in the universality of all human emotion. Amongst the Sufi poets of Punjab, the barahmasa of Ali Haider and Bulleh Shah won much admiration and popularity as they spoke of the divine, mystic and spiritual aspects of existence. In the more contemporary times, Amrita Pritam, the well-known Punjabi writer and poet, also wrote an artistic barahmasa, though her work broke away from the traditional format and dealt with subjects that were revolutionary and modern.

Sufi Kathak at Global Fusion Concert, Dubai by Manjari Chaturvedi

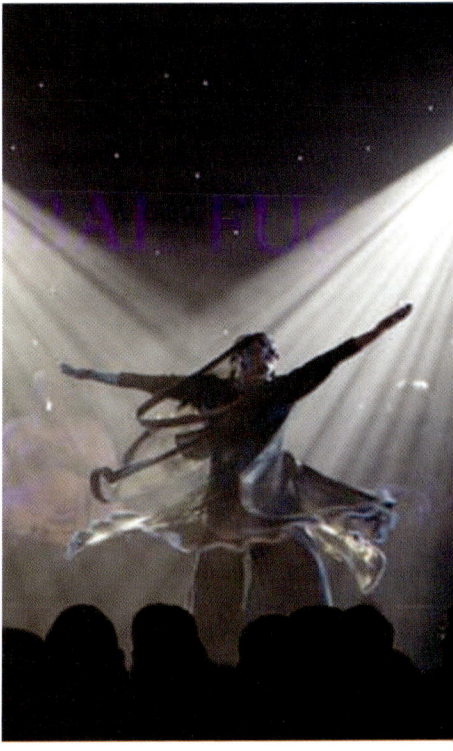

Sangeet—food for the soul

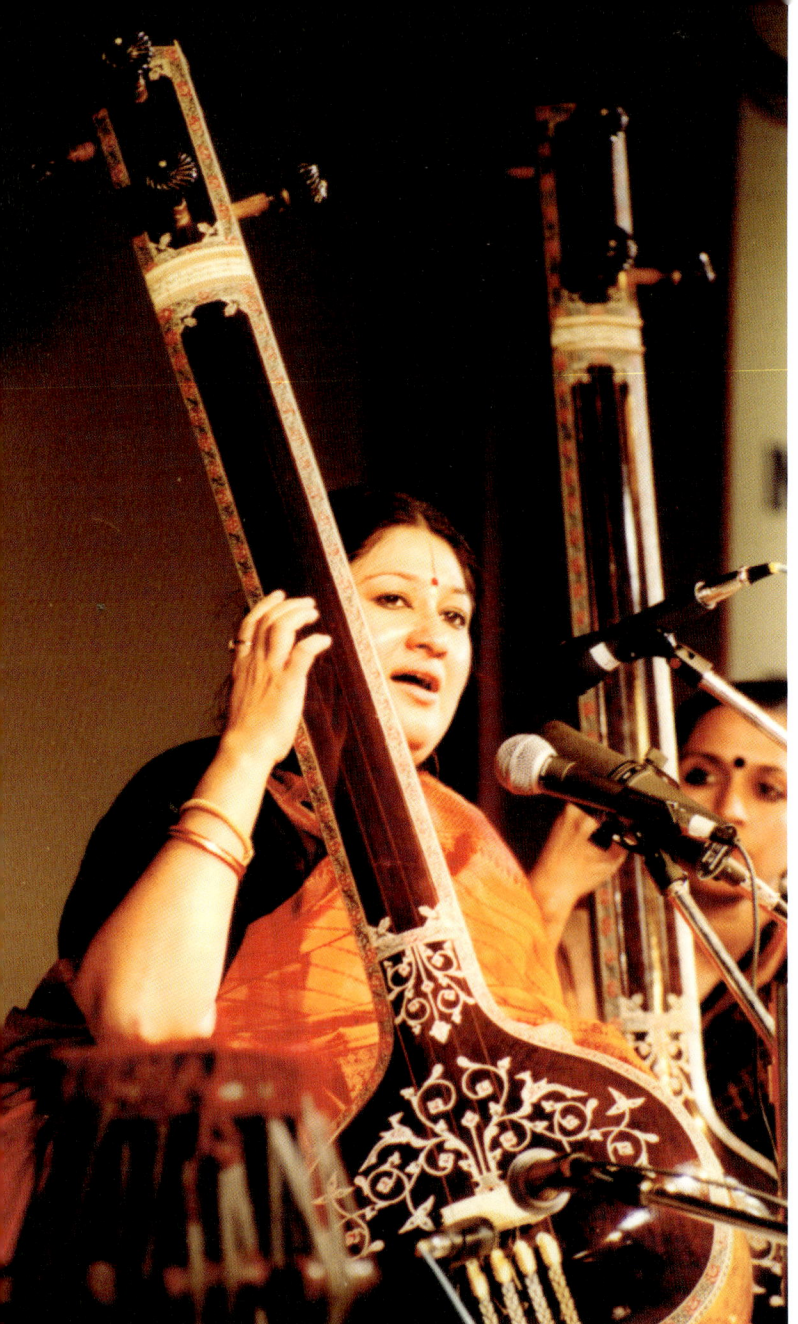

Hindustani classical vocalist, Shubha Mudgal

The Pathos of Separation

Mulla Daud was the first poet to write a barahmasa in Hindi in the 14th century. His narrative poem, *Chandayan*, contains two barahmasas and focusses on separation, using the twelve months of the year as figurative mediums for its expression. In the Hindi barahmasa, the central theme is generally of separation, detailing the pangs suffered by the nayika as she pines for her beloved. In some cases the songs end with the return of the beloved, filling the nayika's heart with ecstasy. However, in the case of others, the woman remains in a state of viraha, describing the beauty of nature, which makes her separation even more painful. A second narrative voice tries to persuade her to meet another man and find pleasure with him so that the joys of the season are not wasted. But the nayika refuses, preferring her anguish to a betrayal of her love.

This particular format of the barahmasa serves three purposes—first, the song is infused with all the throbbing beauty that surrounds the nayika, arousing her passions; second, it conveys the depth of emotion that the nayika experiences in terms of virah and loneliness; and third, by resisting the temptation to fulfil her cravings with another man, the poet depicts the triumph of righteousness.

Across the villages of North India, the folk versions of the barahmasa are sung by women, usually through the months of Ashadha to Ashvin (the monsoon). They express the longings of wives as they either wait for the return of an absent husband, or, in a context of impending departure, urge him not to go away leaving them alone surrounded by the beauty of nature that should be enjoyed together.

There were many variations to this basic thematic framework. Sanskrit shadritu poetry, for instance, describe the erotic joys of the lover and the beloved in union, while the chaumasa deals with the nayika's longing and fear of separation. Not only do the barahmasa songs comprise the very core of the shringara rasa, they also symbolize the consonance between the psyche of the heroine and the moods of the seasons.

In expressing the anguish in her heart and associating it with the nature that she sees around her, the nayika or *premika* draws several parallels—the throbbing of her heart is compared with the pulsating sap of the trees, the trembling of her body is reflected in the plaintive cry of the *chakravaka* bird calling for its mate, and her sighs are like the gusts of breeze that brush against the clouds. The natural world shares her romantic urges that are no different from the lifeforce that moves the trees and the birds around her.

Unravelling Layers

Much of the eroticism and beauty of such portrayals has been passed down over the generations through an oral tradition where song, melody and verse come together to communicate stories, mythological tales, chants and hymns. The written word was converted into a musical composition (bandish) composed in a particular raga—the combination of which intensified its emotional appeal. The ragas could become chitra or visual expressions like the Ragamala paintings; the songs could merge with gesture, movement and expression to become natya (drama). When the same poem or song was given expression in concrete form, it became shilpa or sculpture and architecture.

It is, therefore, not accidental that the Sanskrit word shringara has within it a similar fluidity that defies narrow definition. It refers to romantic love, and at the same time, to layers of emotion and nuances—ranging from the adornment of the nayika to the sensuality of moments of togetherness; from the pathos of separation to the passion of union; and from the bhakti of the divine to the eroticism of the mortal.

In the Indian tradition all these emotions merge into one another, defying the rigid structuralism of any hierarchy; they go beyond distinctions of the profane and the sacred, the divine and the mortal, the spiritual and the physical, merging imperceptibly into the larger ambit of love. The premise here is that adorning or decorating the body is linked to the anticipation of meeting with the beloved. To love the beloved is to elevate the self to a peak of ecstasy until it becomes a manifestation of the cosmic leela, which then intertwines the emotions of love and devotion completely and imperceptibly. This synthesis of the bhakta and the rasika, of the beloved and the divine, is the essence of shringara.

The Eternal Couple

It is interesting to note that the model of the romantic couple is generally represented as *parakiya shringara* or illicit love. However, in a tradition where love and eroticism are celebrated in all their myriad forms, in no way does this

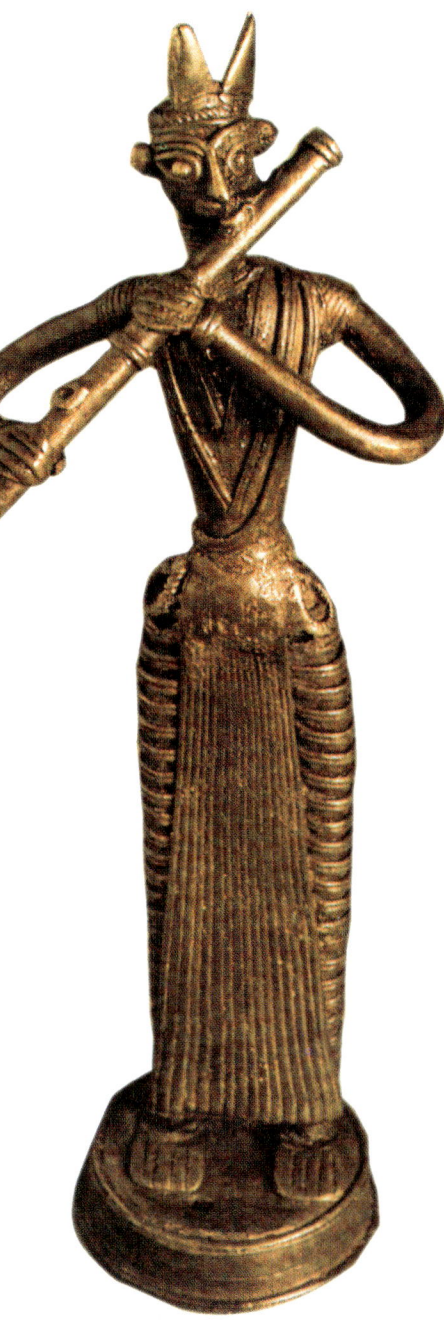

Krishna playing the flute, bronze, 18th century, National Handicrafts and Handlooms Museum, New Delhi

Sangeet—food for the soul 129

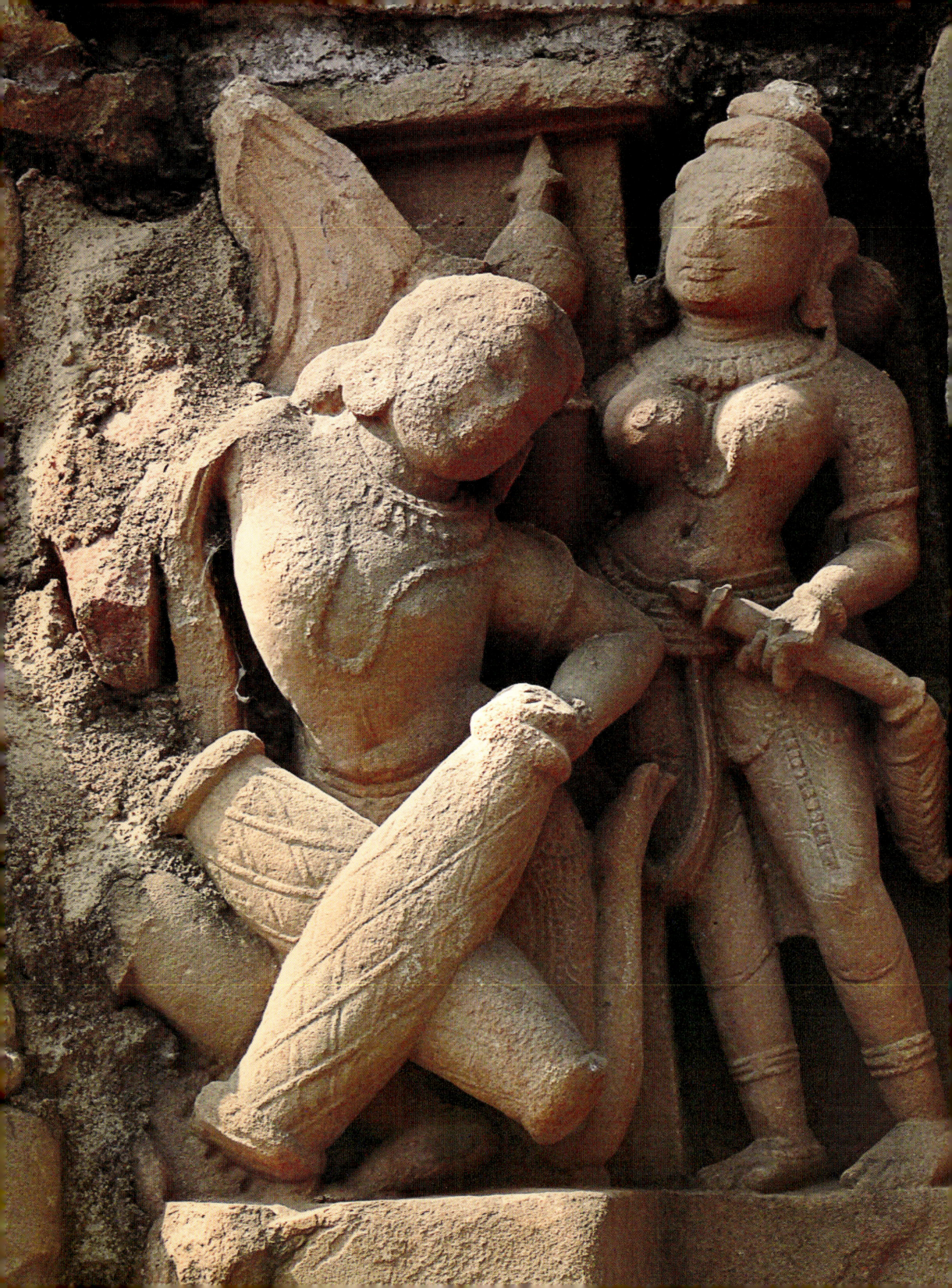

take away from the aesthetic beauty or depth of the emotion; in fact, love or *prem* become pivotal to the artist's composition and also to the re-creation of that emotion in the rasika. In broader terms, much of the shringara rasa in music is based on different nuances of *rati*, or love between a man and a woman, that has its own aesthetic dynamics and artistic expression.

One of the prime examples in this tradition is the eternally celebrated romantic couple, Radha and Krishna. In their love, sensuality blends imperceptibly into spirituality, shringara merges with bhakti, and mortal love goes beyond the conventional norms of adoring and desiring the divine, expressing itself instead in a state of emotional fervour no different from the human quest for bliss and ecstasy. And this desire has found representation in music, dance and painting.

In Jayadeva's poetical work, *Gita Govinda*, written in the 12th century, the physical love between Krishna and Radha is celebrated without reservation or apology. Kalidasa's *Kumarasambhava*, written in the 5th century, contains explicit descriptions of Lord Shiva and his consort Goddess Parvati making love over a thousand years. Other examples of poets and proponents of this genre are Vidyapati, Chaitanya, Kabir, Chandidas, Bhakta Narsimha and Meerabai.

Antar Bhakti—Bahir Shringara

During the 14th and 15th centuries, the Bhakti cult branched into the Rama and Krishna cults with poet-saints like Kabir and Tulsidas, who were devotees of Rama, and others, like Vallabhacharya and Chaitanya, who worshipped Krishna. The followers of Vallabh laid emphasis on music and contributed to both theory and practice, especially through styles like Ashtachap, Haveli sangeet and Pushti. The Ashtachap, established in the early 1600s, was based on the revival of earlier musical streams. It derives its name from the eight musical genres established by the poets belonging to Pushti Marga, or the Path of Grace, a sect of Hinduism founded by Shri Vallabhacharya. The Ashtachap poets composed the principles and methodologies of the musical renditions that typified the cult.

The Pushti Sangeet style saw the gradual dissociation of dance and music, the shift in classical instruments from the *pakhawaj* to the *tabla*, and the birth of styles like dhrupad, khayal and tappa, each with their own characteristic embellishments. Haveli Sangeet was one of the forms of Pushti Sangeet popular in Rajasthan where god Vishnu was venerated. The music is temple-based, and the temple itself is perceived as the *haveli* or palace where the god chooses to live.

(Page 130)
Musicians, Chitragupta Temple, Khajuraho

Venugopala, late Chola, 12th century, National Museum, New Delhi

In the 16th century, the Bhakti movement gave the shringara rasa a further impetus in music. The *Bhagavata* had already established Krishna as the prototypical romantic hero, but with Surdas' *Sur Sagar*, bhakti took on a new manifestation giving equal importance to the romantic, human and divine aspects of Krishna, investing the entire concept of devotion with a greater intimate dimension.

In weaving the shringara rasa into the fabric of bhakti through his evocative devotional songs, Surdas paved the way for the evolution of the Pushti marga tradition. This in turn merged different shades of philosophy, worship, romance, longing and passion in the imagery of the gopis, the archetypical confluence of Krishna's lovers and devotees. Much of the music and songs of the Bhakti movement bring out the subtle nuances of *bheda-abheda* (different-and-yet-not-different) found in Vaishnava philosophy. While the devotee is in trance with the lover/god, the latter is equally drawn to the former's devotion and love, and takes on numerous forms to dance with the devotees (gopis), thus fulfilling the longings of each one. The core characteristic here is the surrender of all ego and complete submission to the divine beloved and as Surdas says:

I reside in the hearts of those
who have abandoned pride and sing my praise
in a voice that is choked with emotion
drowned in love for me.

Ideally, the bhakti rasa is necessary to the shringara rasa to correctly express 'antar bhakti—bahir shringar', i.e. a state of internal devotion expressed through external manifestations of love and desire. This continuum is best found in the traditions of dance and music, which is considered a form of worship, an offering to the divine and where the shringar and bhakti rasa are found in syncretic union.

The Bhakti cult is similar, to the cult of Sufism where desire for union with the Divine is akin to the passions and longings of a mortal lover. The musical form of the *qawwali* also replicates this same pattern where love for the divine leads to a pitched, often frenzied state, where union and complete surrender are the only emotions that exist. Once again, one sees the shringara rasa in all its glory as the devotee gives himself up to a level of bliss where the self is annihilated in love for the divine.

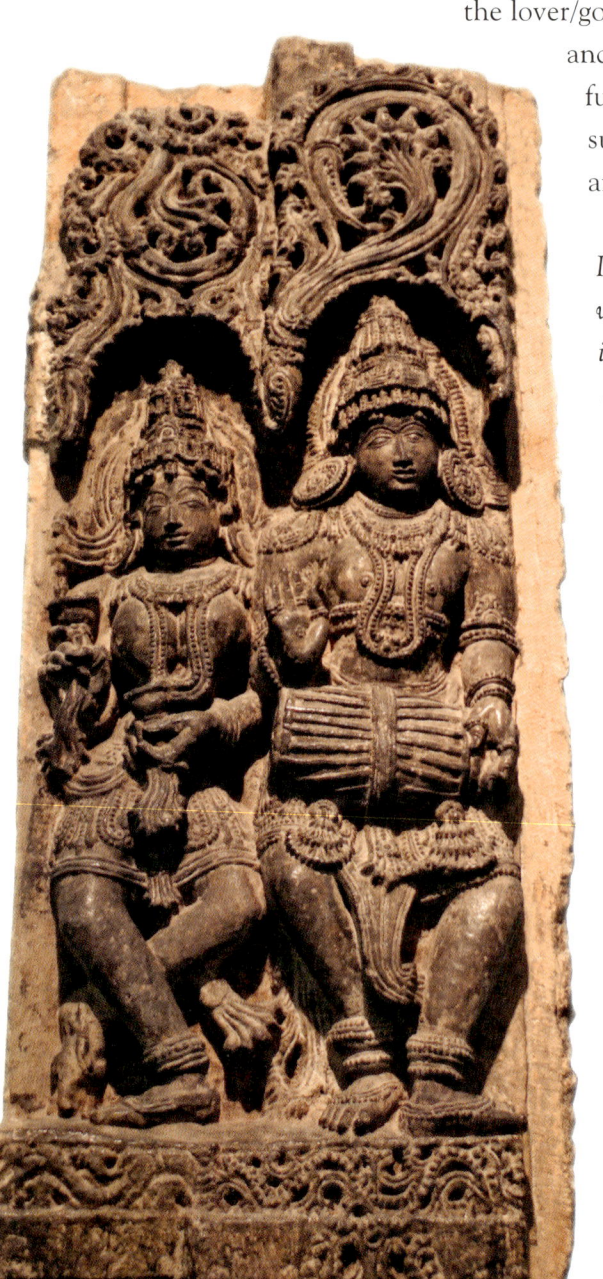

(Page 133)
The elegantly attired musician is seated on an ornate carpet playing the rudra veena

Musicians, Hoysala-Halebid, 12th century, Mysore

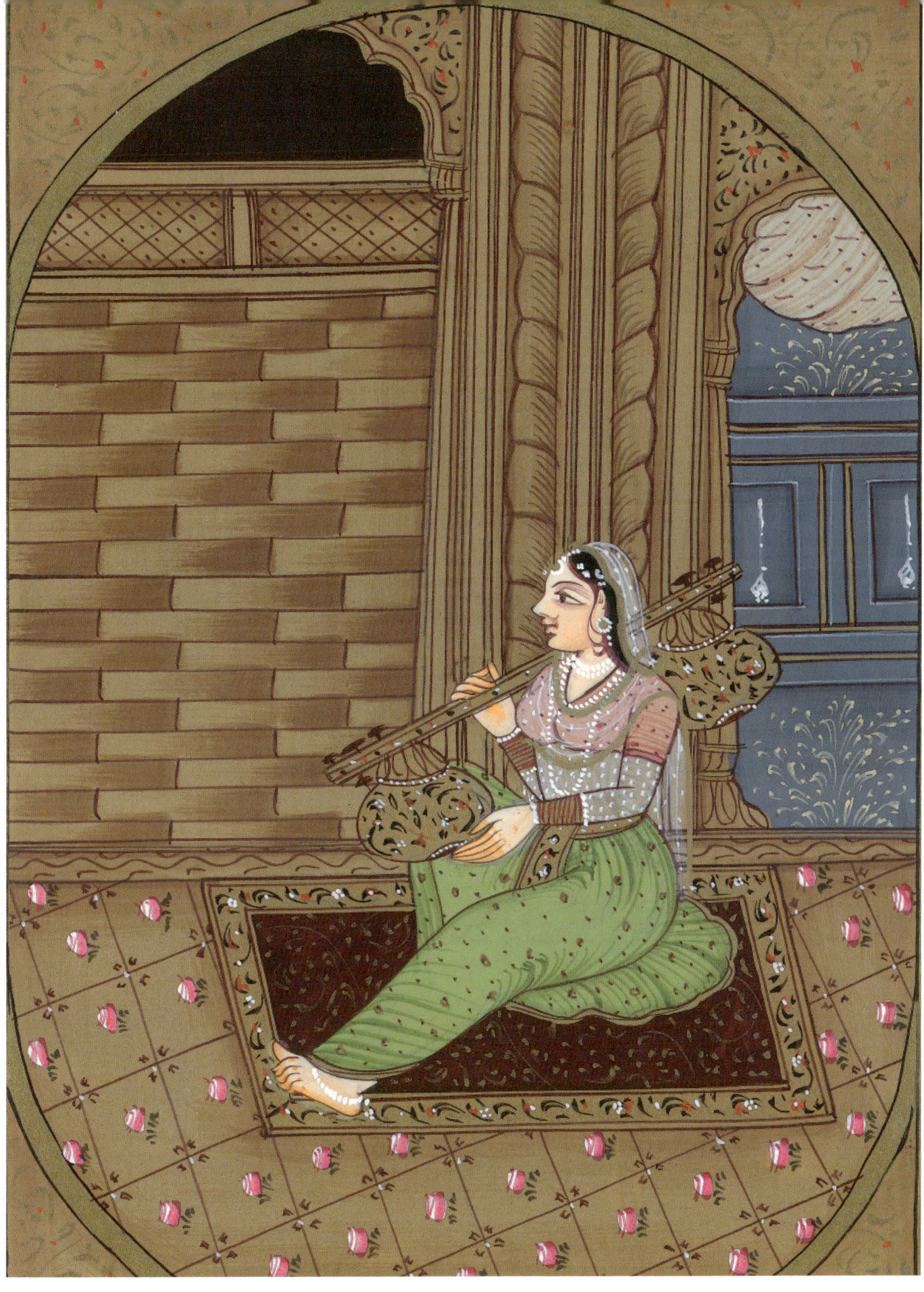

Sangeet—food for the soul

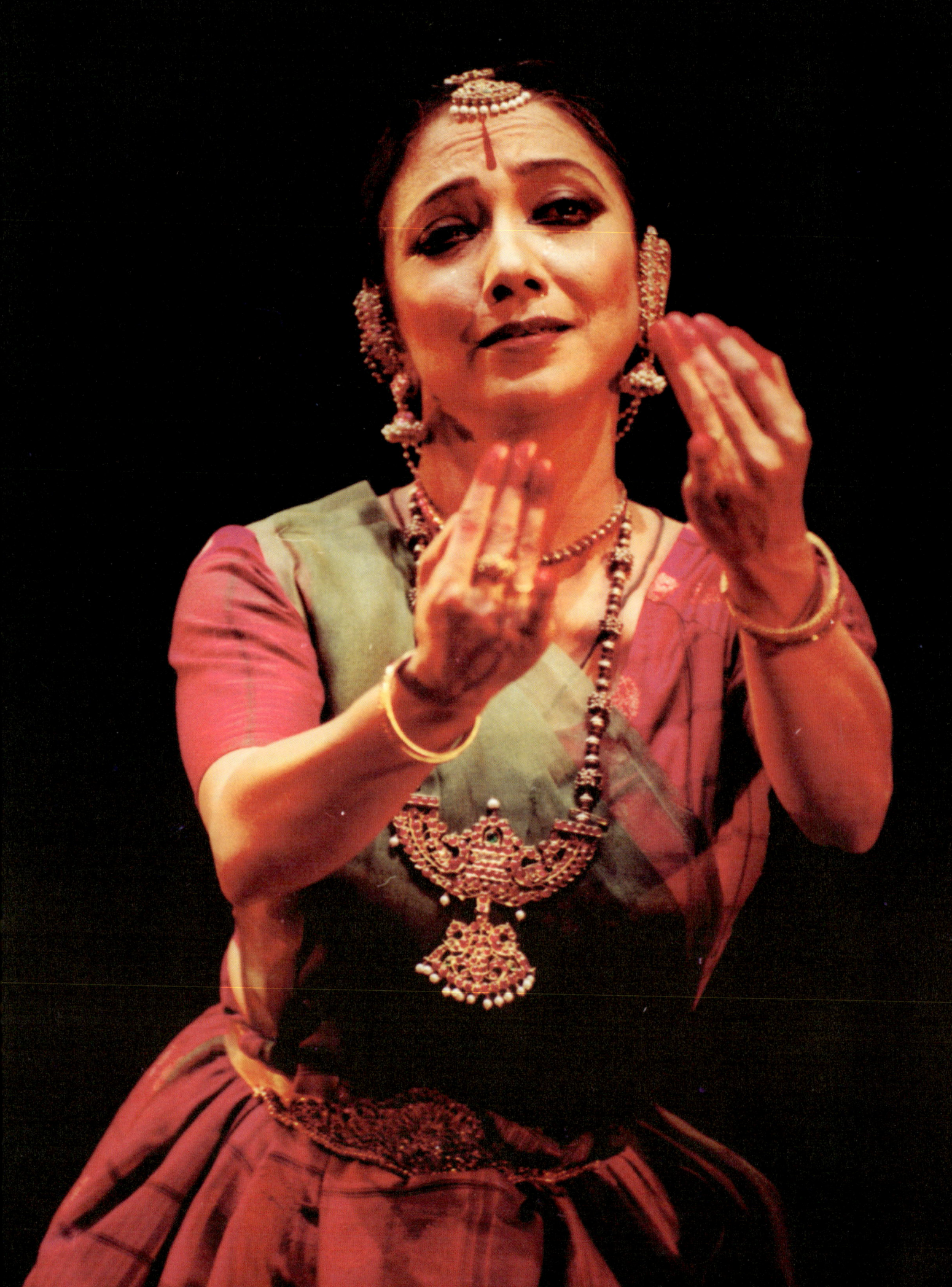

CHAPTER 9

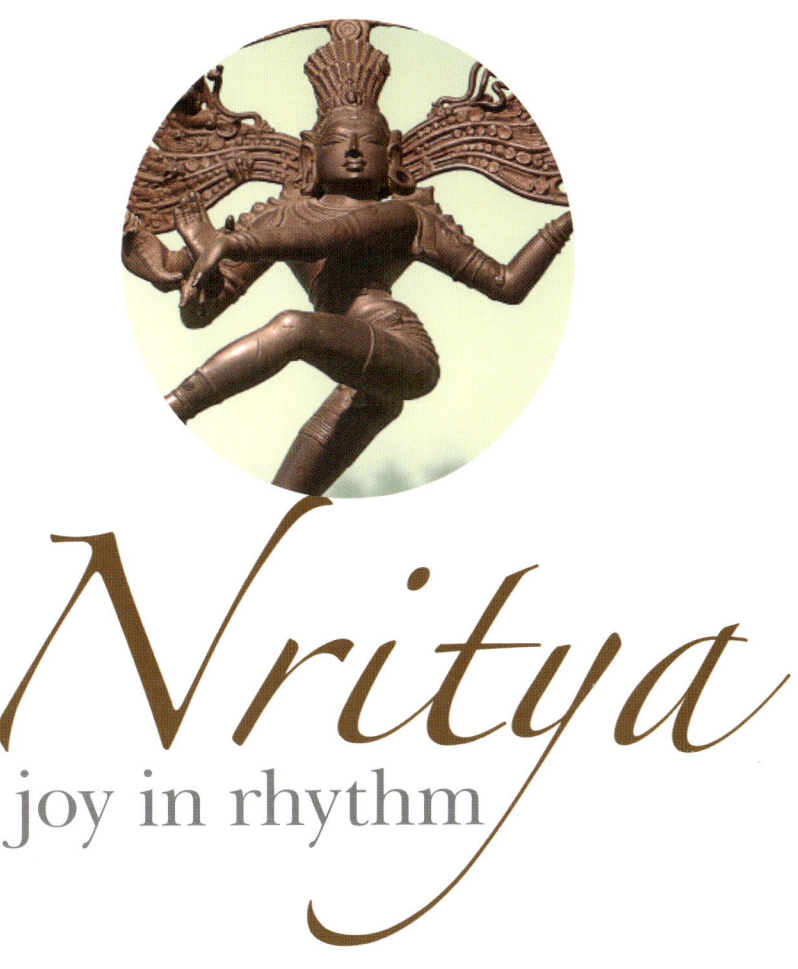

Nritya
joy in rhythm

Where your hands go your eyes follow;
Where your eyes go your heart follows;
Where your heart goes your expression follows;
Where your expression goes, there is your gift to the audience.

NATYASHASTRA, BHARATA MUNI

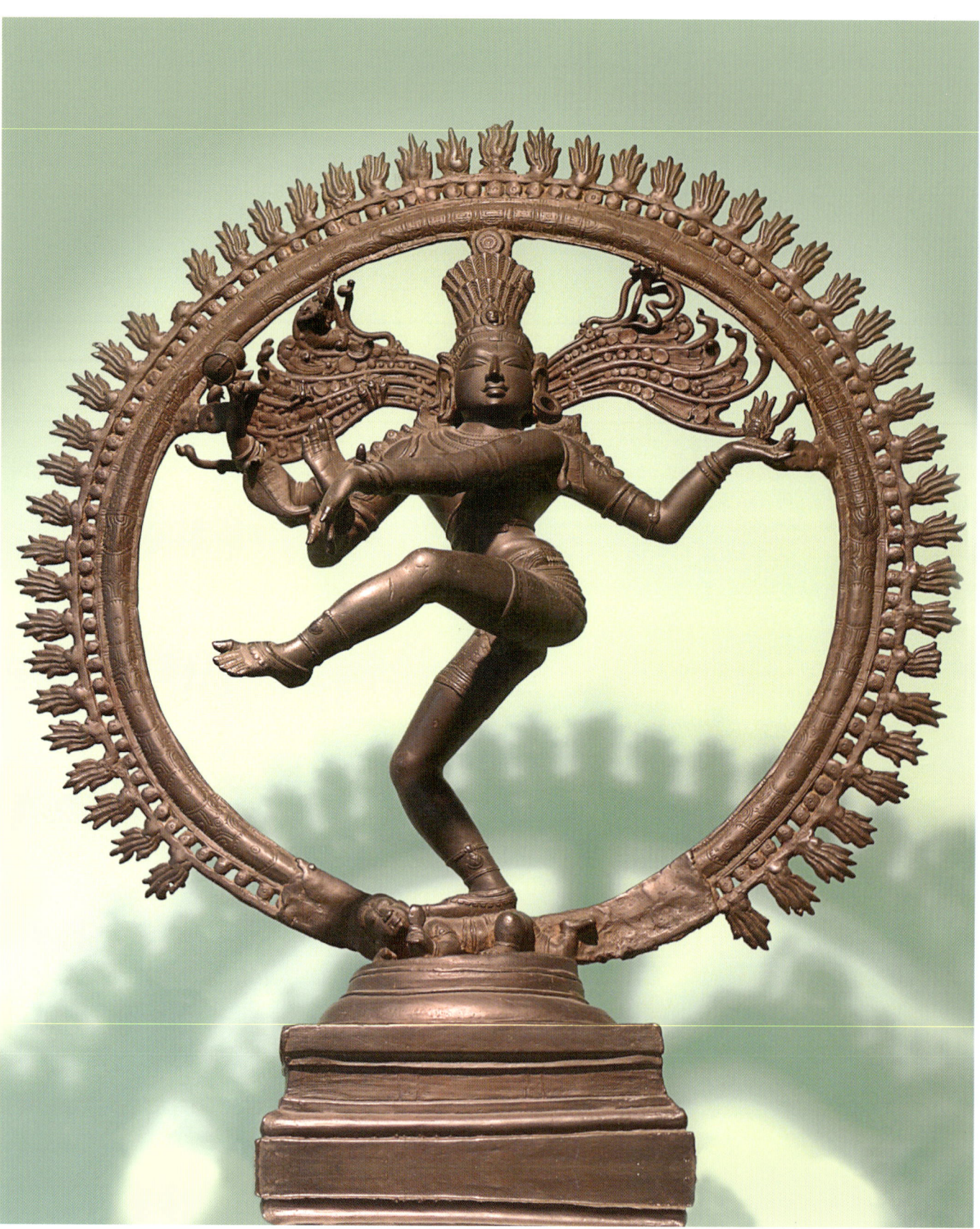

It is in dance that the shringara rasa is represented in all its manifestations. The emotion of love depicted in Indian dance has a deeper philosophical and metaphysical intent because it has always been a medium of worship (bhakti) or an offering to the gods. The search of the human soul (atman) for the Supreme and its desire to unite with the Ultimate (Brahma) is best depicted in the movements of dance, the perfect basis for antar bhakti—bahir shingara (internal devotion in the external manifestation of love) where love goes beyond the earthly to the sublime.

Tandava, the First Dance

More than a beautiful form of cultural expression, Hindu temple dance (which is the root of classical dance forms) is a spiritual experience for both the dancer and the audience. According to traditional beliefs, all dance forms have their genesis in the Tandava Nrityam or Lord Shiva's Dance of Eternity, which was said to have created order out of chaos. It is customary today at any classical dance performance to display a Nataraja statue—Shiva in his form as the divine dancer—on the stage. Nataraja stands, dressed in a headdress of moon and stars, his sacred snake hung like a garland around his neck, crushing the dwarfed demon of ignorance under his feet. His pose suggests a combination of dynamic and static forces.

In its best expression, Tandava is believed to be the ultimate coming together of the male and female energies—of Shiva, the male principal, and Lasya, the female principle. For any dance form to be true, it must, therefore, combine within itself explosive energy, vigour and strength, as well as elegance, grace and seduction. The masculine and the feminine, the god and the goddess come together, and in doing so, become the ultimate expression of the shringara rasa.

The Origins of Dance

Dance in India is extremely layered in its expression, and cannot be seen as a monolithic whole. Bharatanatyam form, for instance, is believed to contain eight distinct, idealized unions of heroes and heroines in different manifestations of shringara. These are categorized by Anne-Marie Gaston in her work *Bharata Natyam*:

> *Vasakasajjika, the one who arranges everything to receive her beloved;*
> *virahotkanthita, the one who pines for him;*
> *proshitapatika, a more extreme state of the latter who waits for her beloved;*
> *vipralabdha, the maiden upset with her lover who has not been true to his word;*
> *khandita, the angry mistress;*
> *kalahantarita, the one who is estranged because of jealousy;*
> *abhisarika, the one who ventures forth because she cannot wait for her beloved to arrive;*
> *and svadhinapatika, joyous after their union.*

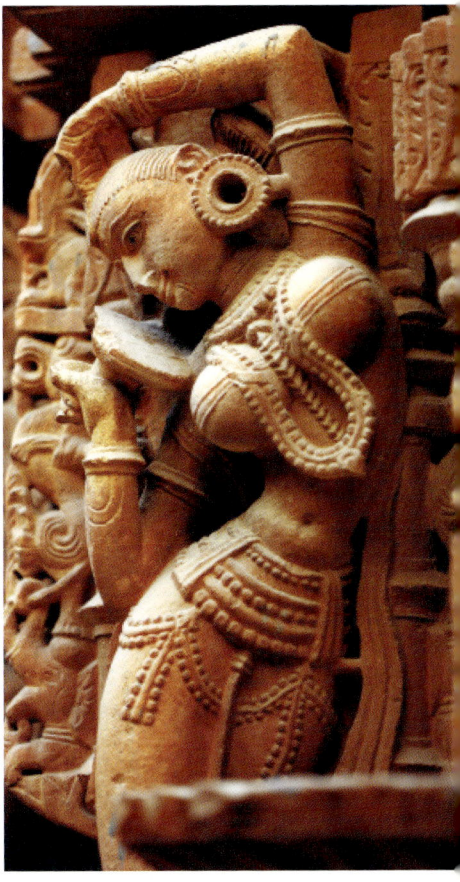

Lady with the looking glass, Khajuraho

(Page 134)
Bharatanatyam dancer
Leela Samson

(Page 136)
Nataraja, bronze,
Late Chola, 12th century,
National Museum,
New Delhi

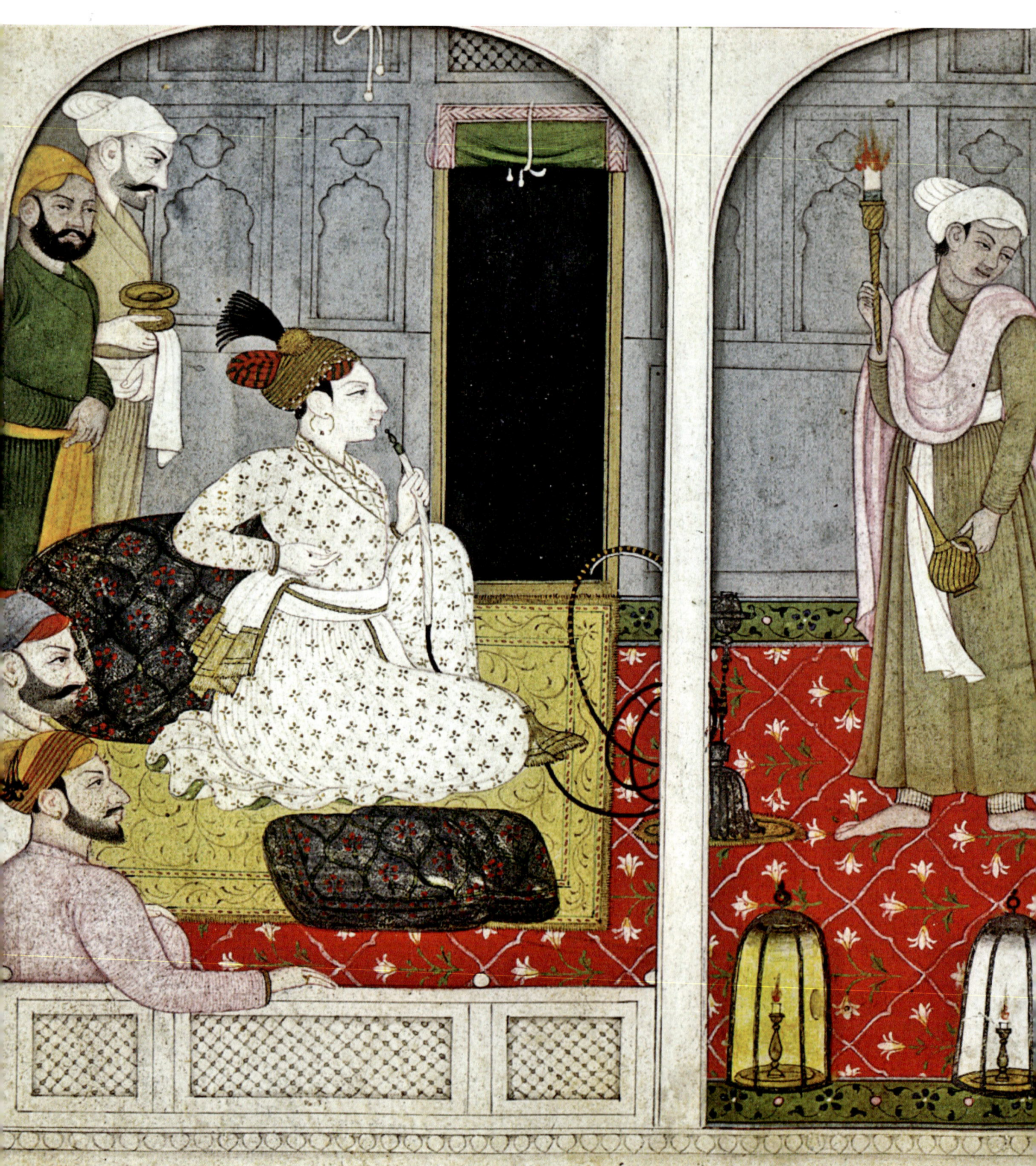

Raja Raj Singh of Chamba. Artist Ram Sahai, dated AD 1772, N.C. Mehta Collection, Ahmedabad

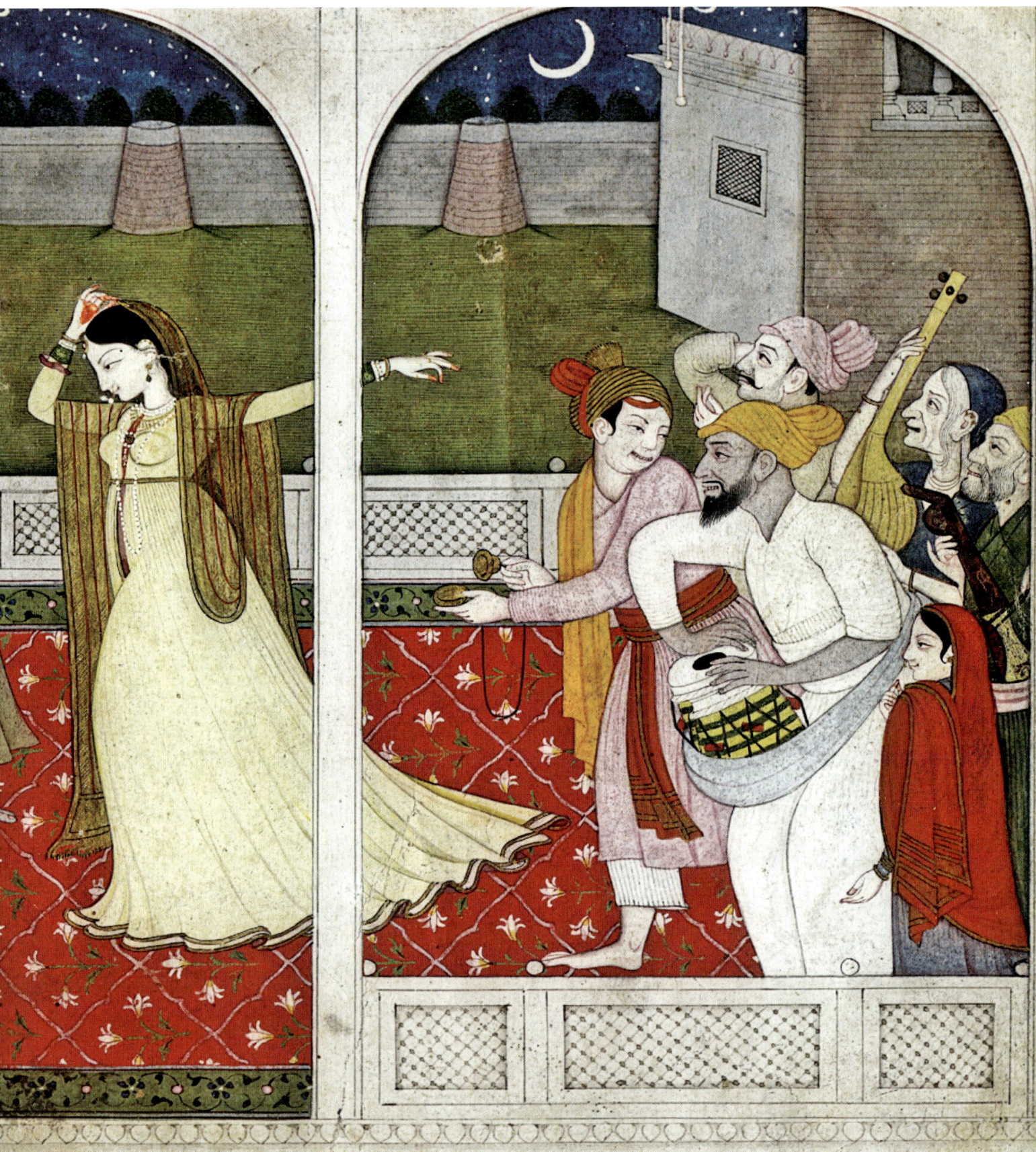

(Page 141 and below) The nayikas are attired in the traditional Rajasthani ensemble of ghagra, choli and chunni

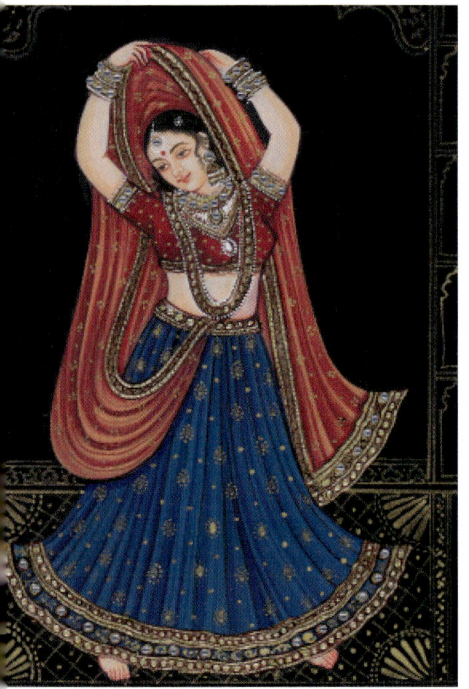

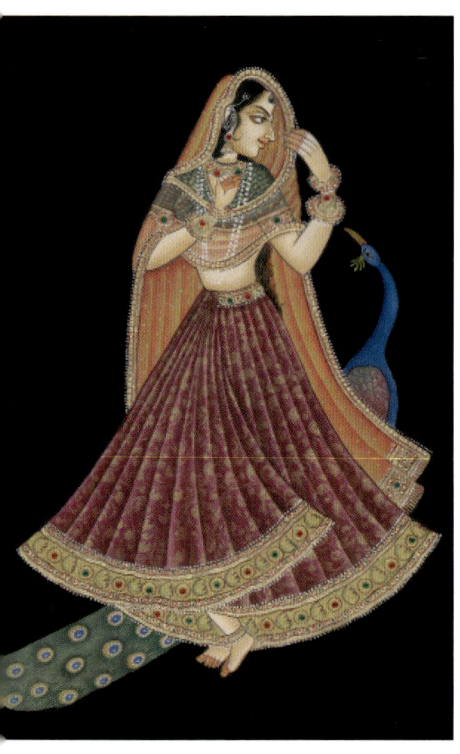

All the above deal with one form of separation or another, because the longing borne of distance is believed to enhance the sentiment of shringara. At another level, they also refer to the fact that the erotic love shared by human beings is but an echo of the desire of the mortal soul to merge with the divine love that is the aim of all existence.

Bharata Muni's *Natyashastra*, written between 200 BC and 200 AD, is the most iconic text for aesthetic theory and is often referred to as the 'Fifth Veda'. Literally meaning 'theory of dance', *Natyashastra* lays the foundations and codified rules of the rasa theory; these in turn became the theoretical basis for all art forms in India, primarily dance and drama. The dance form, Bharatanatyam, meaning natya or dance as seen by Bharata, takes its name directly from this work.

Among the other major classical disciplines of Indian dance is Kuchipudi, a dance-drama form that originated in the Kuchipudi village of Andhra Pradesh, as a part of the vernacular theatre. Mohiniattam from Kerala is a simplified form of Bharatanatyam, while Kathakali, from the same state, is a purely masculine style of dance-drama with elaborate facial makeup, expressions, hand gestures and techniques. Kathak is a north Indian style that developed during the period of Mughal rule in India. From the eastern part of the country comes Manipuri, a simple and graceful form, largely evolved from the local folk traditions in the Northeast, and Odissi from Orissa, with its distinctly regional stylistic techniques.

A dance performance of any classical style is divided into two parts: the shloka and the *nritta*. The shloka, meaning prayer or hymn, is a combination of dance and chant without a set rhythm. It is usually brief and rendered by a single singer with no accompaniment. The music is timed according to the movements of the dancer. While the shloka is being recited, the dancer conveys its meaning through hand gestures, body movements and facial expressions, helping the audience to move into a receptive and spiritual frame of mind.

The nritta, on the other hand, is fast, rhythmic and energetic. It could be a simple or complex narrative, based on stories from Hindu mythology, with gestures taken from the iconography of temple sculpture which the audience is familiar with. The nritta section involves more than one classical musician and vocalist who help keep the rhythm and beat (tala) of the music. The beats are evenly spaced and there is no emphasis of one over the other. Sometimes the rhythm changes slightly, or even completely, within a particular piece and the dancer adjusts his/her movements to the change. The dancer wears ankle bells or *ghungroos* that sound the rhythm as she strikes her feet against the ground in time to the music.

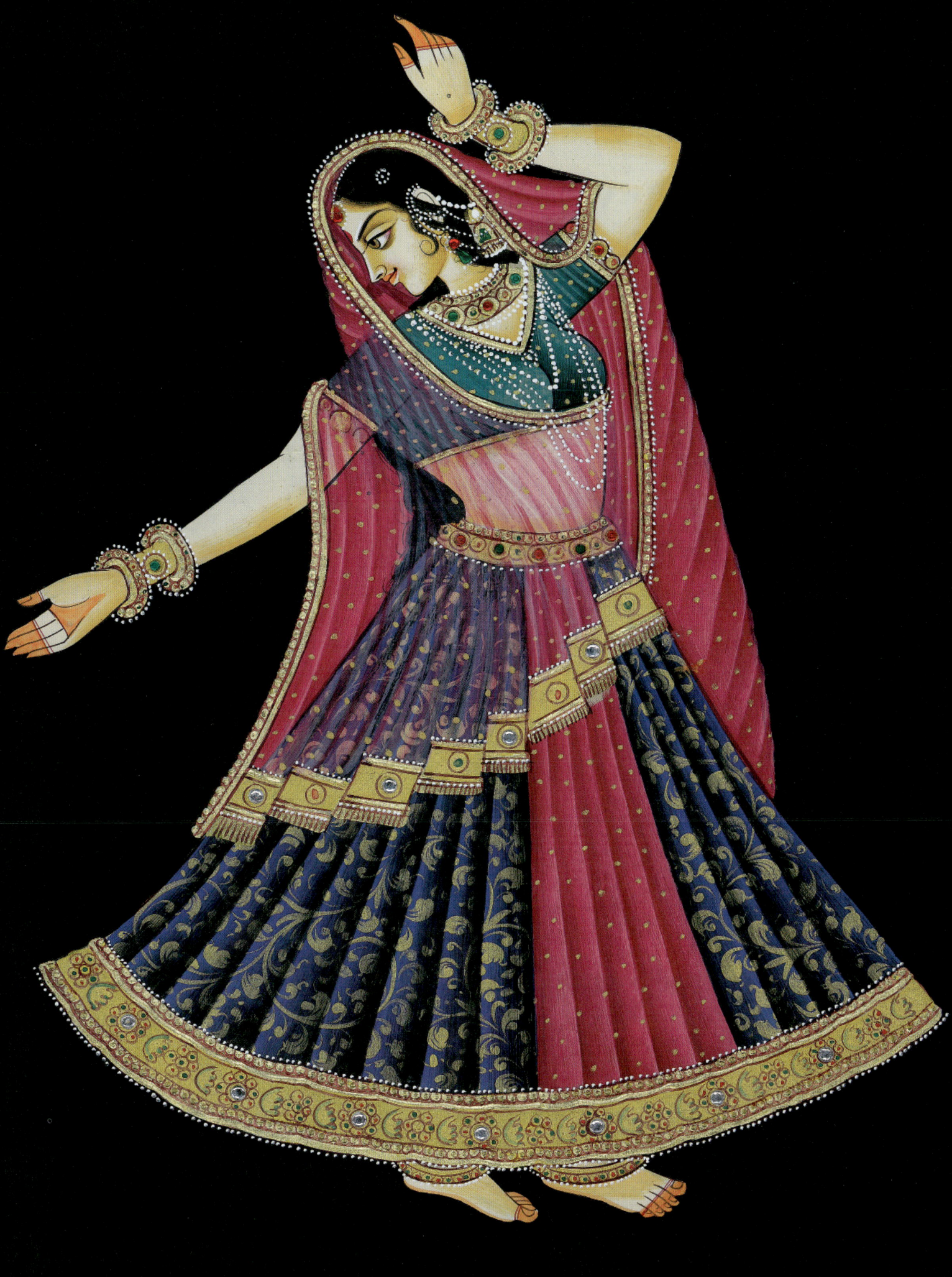

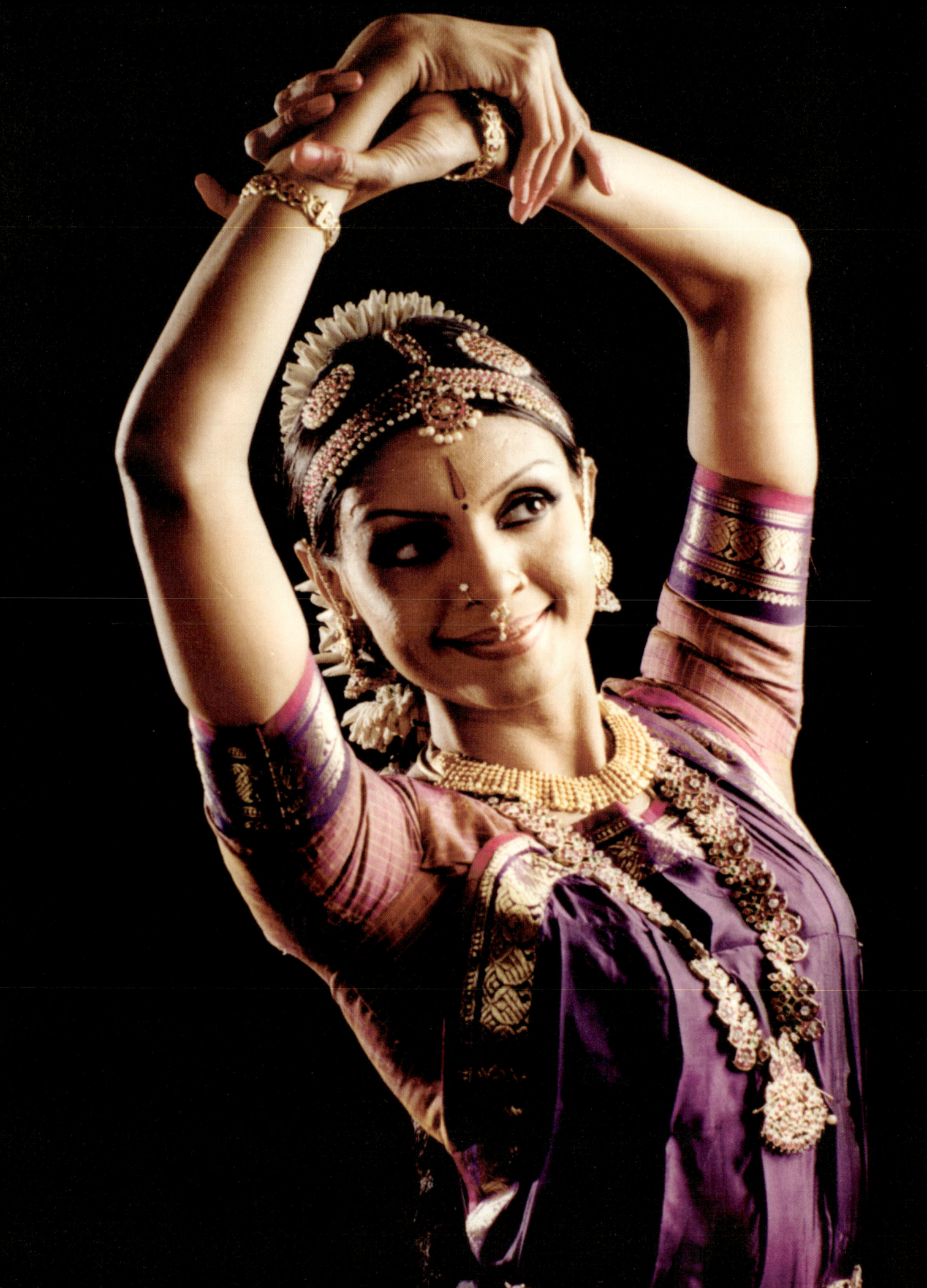

The ghungroos are so sophisticated that different angles, or ways of striking the ground, produce a variety of sounds that add to the overall dance experience.

The beginning and end of a dance performance consist of common elements, but also differ from one dancer to another. Dancers generally touch the ground upon which they are to perform in a gesture of reverence. The palms are then raised to the eyes and held folded in prayer and veneration in front of the torso. This is a sign of respect towards the art form, the teacher (guru) and the accompanying musicians.

By the end of the 16th century, dances and their movements had been codified to create a synergy across the forms. The common elements were—the body (*aangikam*), the costumes of the dancers (*aaharyam*), the music and poetry (*vachikam*), and the audience and the surrounding space (*bhuvanum*). This synergy communicates itself in a combination of poses and gestures accompanied by hand movements (*mudras*) and footwork (*goti*).

Each mudra conveys a meaning, specific or general. For instance, dancers have a definite gesture for the shivalinga. The gesture known as *alapu* stands for a flower, that could represent either a particular flower, flowers in general or even an abstract expression of joy. The meaning of each mudra, therefore, has to be understood in the context within which it is presented, rather than just as a physical gesture. Different regions and schools sometimes have separate names for the same gestures that become increasingly nuanced. In order to help the audience see and interpret gestures, some dancers paint the tips of their fingers red so that they can be interpreted from a greater distance.

The footwork or goti is based on three kinds of postures—standing, squatting, and sitting. Of these the squatting, or *aramunda* pose is the most common, largely because it allows for a greater variation in the kind of ways that the feet can be raised and stamped, each resulting in a different sound. The pose also facilitates the execution of several leaps and spins, all of which contribute to different centres of focus in the dance.

The standing posture, *samamundi*, is mainly used as an introductory position. In it the dancer stands with the feet together and legs straight. Although limited in the variety of poses it makes possible, the samamundi position makes for a graceful walk. The dancer uses it to make entrances, exits, and quick changes in location. The final position, sitting or puramundi, takes the aramunda position to the ultimate extreme and is physically the most challenging. It involves sitting on one's heels with the knees outward, and allows for hops and similar movements accompanied by mudras and arm movements.

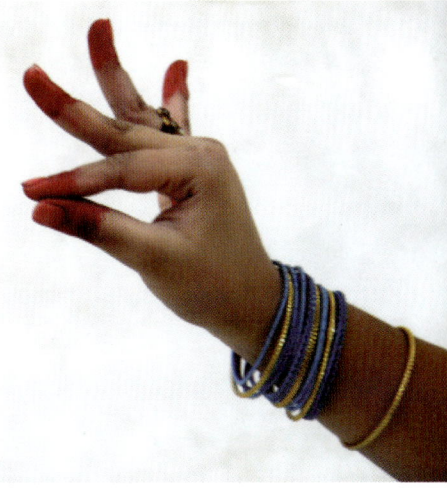
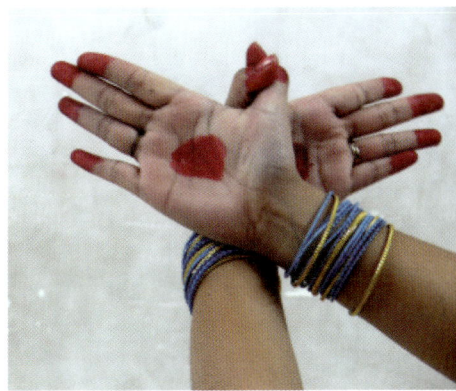

Mudra: Swan (top), Bird (bottom)

(Page 142) Bharatanatyam dancer, Priyadarshini

Traditional training in Indian dance includes intense practice of the squatting and sitting positions. This helps in the development of muscle structure and fast and smooth movement. In order to train the memory and provide a core set of movements, dancers learn formalized sets of practice movements, called adavu, which can be easily incorporated into the main dances.

In addition to these elements are facial gestures called rasadrishtis. By the early 1900s, most people, especially those belonging to the higher Brahmin castes, considered Hindu temple dance obscene. Consequently, it had to move into the domain of a formalized dance culture, patronized and practised by the educated and wealthy elite. The transition occurred gradually, but at the cost of the erotic aspects of the performances; dancers and teachers alike eliminated these expressions. The refinement achieved in terms of facial expressions was, as a result, devoid of the sensuality and shringara-infused eroticism that had been integral parts of the dance portrayed in temple sculpture.

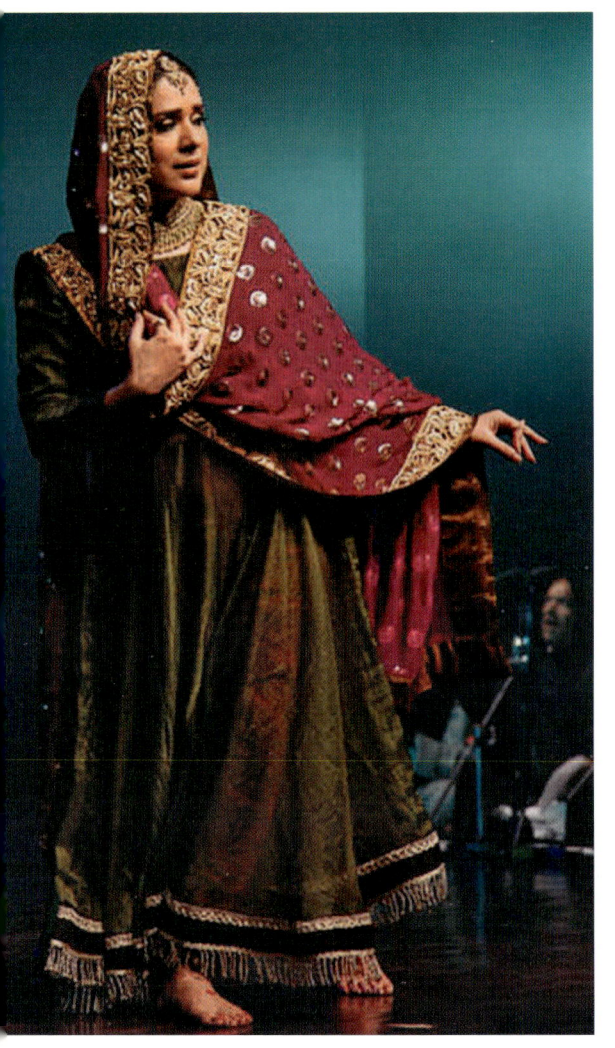

Sufi Kathak dancer, Manjari Chaturvedi

Even now, forms like the Bharatanatyam make very little use of the mouth. The reason for this, according to Anne-Marie Gaston, is that 'the mouth movements were considered the most obscene and, therefore, were omitted when proper ladies performed the dance'. Eye and head movements are very important in Bharatanatyam. There are eight distinct movements for the head: *utvahitum* (uplifted), *adhomukum* (lowered), *arlolitum* (rotated in a circle), *dutum* (shake of the head), *kapitumsha* (nod), *varahitum* (looking forty-five degrees to the side), *upshiptum* (forty-five degrees to the side, raised slightly) and *parivahitum* (slow head pivot side to side). These movements are then combined with those of the eyebrows and eyes to emphasize and communicate the meaning of hand gestures. Sometimes the head and eyes follow the hand as it creates a mudra; sometimes they follow the feet drawing attention to complex footwork; at other moments they simply shift and move from side to side in independent moves.

No discussion on classical dance can be complete without the mention of the original temple dancers called *devadasis*. Believed to be brides of the temple god, these women were usually at the mercy of the Brahmin priests who controlled the temple. By about 1900s, most of them had been forced to prostitute themselves for lack of patronage by the wealthy. The devadasi tradition was eventually outlawed in India by the British and dance was separated from temple ritual.

However, much before such laws were enacted, the ancient scriptures like Dharmasutras, or law codes concerned with the life and rituals of an ascetic and his student, also discouraged religious-minded students from associating with dancers, often going so far as to declare the teaching of dance a sin punishable by loss of caste. This was possibly because the dancers' profession made them impure; or because the distractions and temptations of music and dance were not conducive to the concentration required for serious study. It is easy to see that a set of texts focussing on enlightenment through sacrifice and privation might discourage the pursuit of a different, more worldly path. Bana, who wrote between 600-650, also noted that courtesans in the royal court performed erotic dance as part of court ritual.

While these views can be contested in the modern-day context, it should be kept in mind that Dharmasutras were aimed specifically at ascetics and their students, and therefore were not meant to be applicable to all and sundry. An alternative worldview included vocal and instrumental music, and dance, as a part of the sixty-four arts associated with cultural accomplishment.

The prejudiced perception of the devadasi was not the only one to exist. There were many who saw her as lucky, and above all misfortune since she would never be a widow or fall upon misfortune by virtue of being married to the god of a temple. Gaston mentions the ritual of *arati*, whereby luck could be transferred by a devadasi circling a lit lamp over an individual's head.

The knowledge of *abhinaya* or acting was an integral part of dance and included a mastery of the stylized gestures and postures that evoked rasa and saundarya in combination with other movements. Dancers have an advantage over painters, for instance, as they can imitate motion, which is the essential expression of life and its defining events, whether it is inward or suspended at particular points of motion.

It is motion that constitutes beauty in dance and the literature of dance in the Sanskrit tradition, unmatched both in its volume and its comprehensiveness, records the movements of the body in great detail. Sarangadeva's *Sangita Ratnakar* (1210–1247) is the most important treatise on music after Bharata's *Natyashastra*, and also a reference point for both the Carnatic and Hindustani classical music traditions. Sarangadeva conveys this enigmatic idea of beauty in the concepts of *rekha* (line) and *saunstha* (where line is said to be a pleasing composition of the body when there is a harmonious combination of the movements of the head, eyes, hands and body).

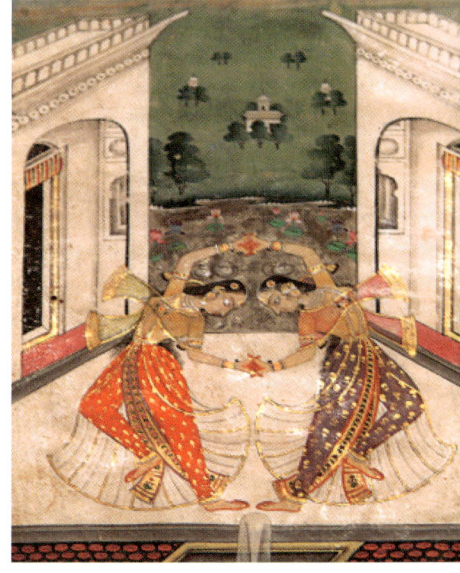

Dancers, Hyderabad-Deccan, National Museum, New Delhi

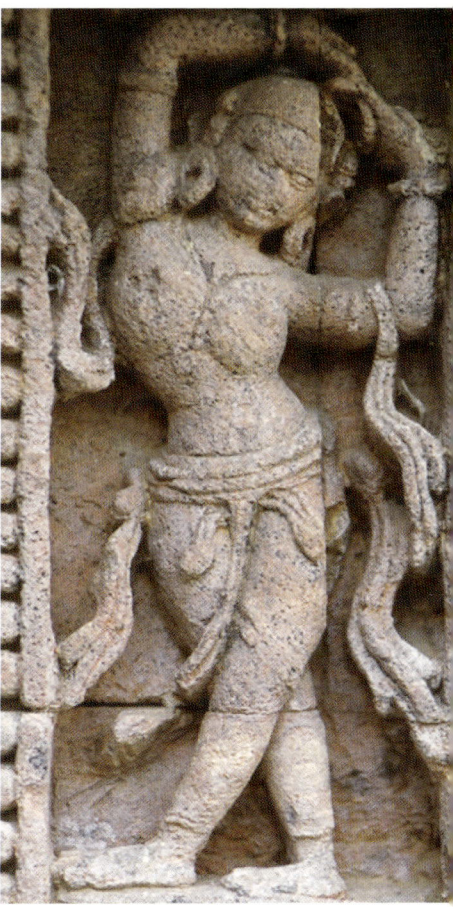

Dancer, AD 1238-64, Konark Sun Temple, Orissa

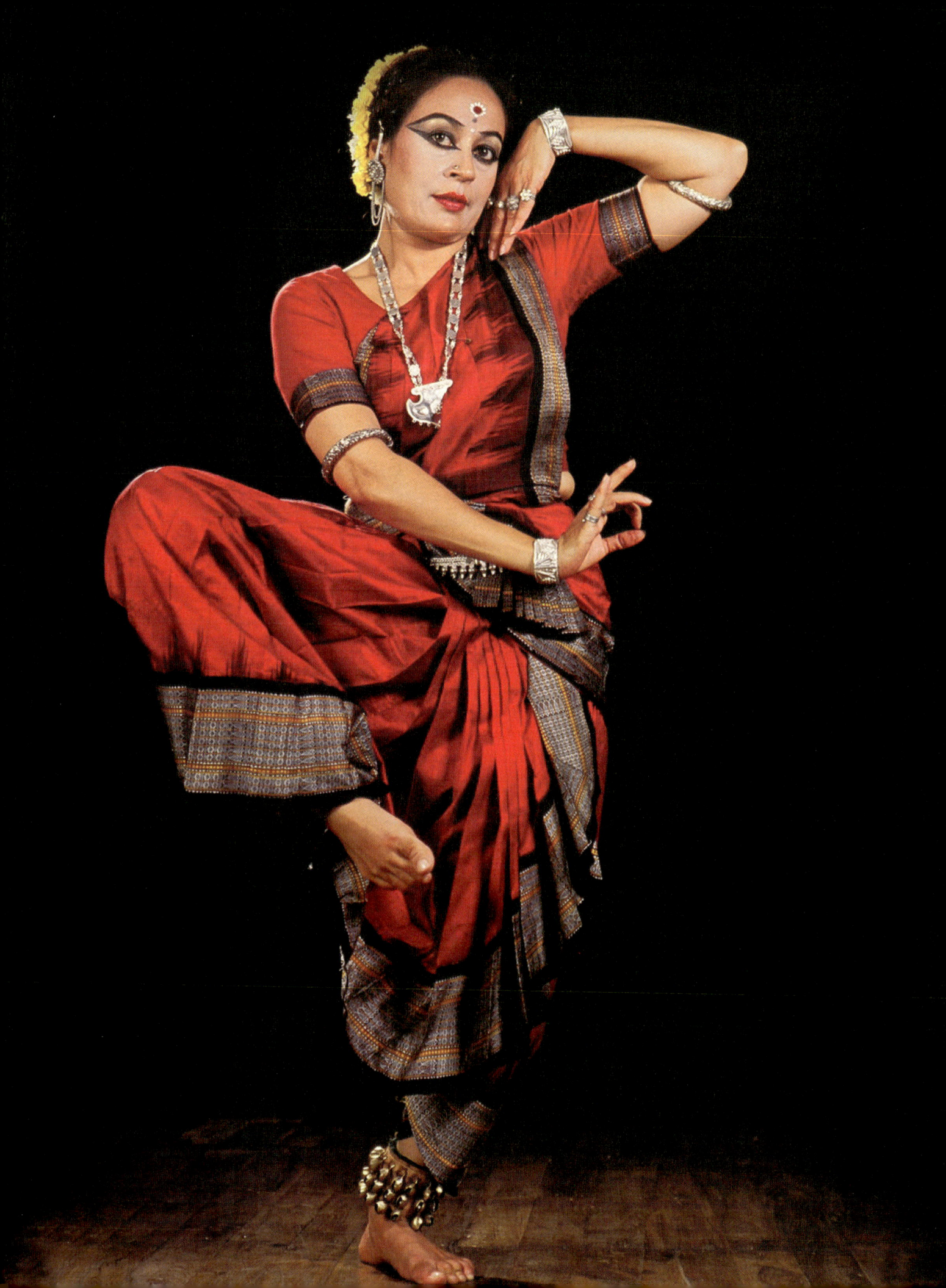

Movements for each part of the body, no matter how small, are prescribed as a means to represent objects, processes, ideas and mental states. The simplest imitation is that of natural objects, such as flowers. For instance, *Vishnudharmottara Purana* describes a simple hand gesture:

All five fingers gently curving upward and meeting at their tips form the figure called mukula. The object it represents is a budding lotus or water lily, whose natural form the hand imitates. The figure also signifies the gesture of worship or the act of eating. Another gesture is called alapadma: beginning with the little finger, the fingers are curved and separated from one another. This indicates a fullblown lotus, wood-apple, circular movements, breasts, separation from the beloved, a mirror, full moon and beloved.

But a far greater task, perhaps the greatest challenge for the mimetic arts, is to express the inner life of a person in terms of moods and character values. *Vishnudharmottara Purana* shows that body movements can indicate persons of elevated, ordinary, or inferior character. For instance, an *uttama* is a person of noble character, while a *madhyama* is the average person, indicated by the facial features as uttama, except that the teeth show. Finally there is the *adhama*, or low character, indicated not only by the teeth showing, but also by loud and tearful laughter. Casting symbolic glances with a barely perceptible smile, without the teeth showing, can also signify the adhama.

These are but brief illustrations of the vast repertoire of body movements that cover every imaginable object, situation, event, mood, sentiment and moral quality of relevance to human beings. *Abhinaya Darpana* states:

Wherever the hands go, there the eyes should follow. Wherever the eyes go, there the mind. Wherever the mind goes, there the feeling. Wherever the feeling goes, there the mood (rasa) or flavour is found.
—**The Mirror of Gesture, Ananda Coomaraswamy**

The beauty in the art of dancing is centred in the body, but its perception transcends the body, achieving a spiritual statement of this beauty, submerging the material view in the abstract saundarya. From the earliest times man's deepest creative impulses, religious urges, emotions and sensibilities have found expression in the rhythms and movements of his body. In the Indian tradition, dance is a means of attaining liberation through *sadhana* or the discipline required to perfect it. And it is in this constant attempt to express the core of all human emotion, from joy and passion to anger and fury, through the gestures and movements of the human body, that offers the path to creative and spiritual fulfilment.

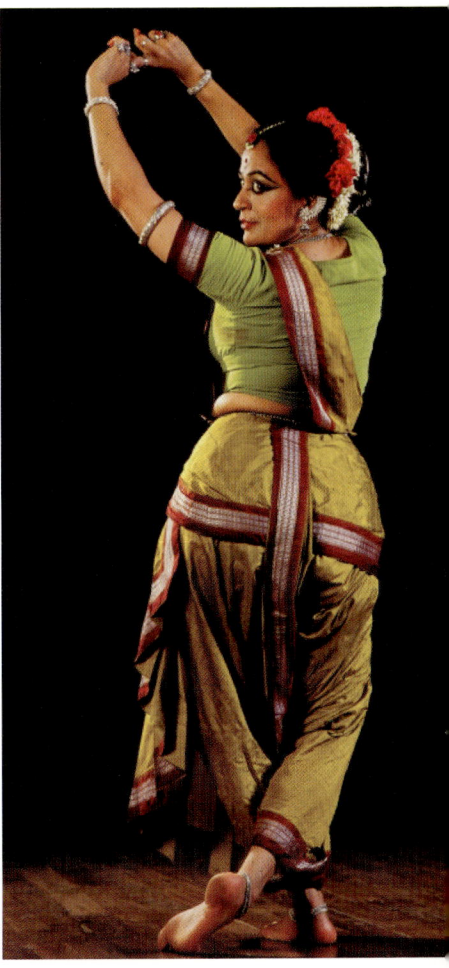

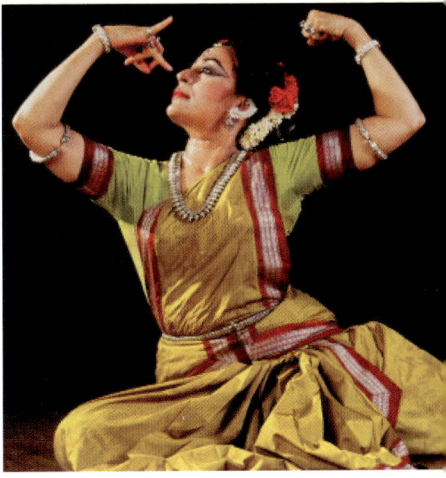

Dancer Sonal Mansingh, performing 'Abhinaya'

(Page 146) Sonal Mansingh, performing 'Nritya'

Nritya—joy in rhythm

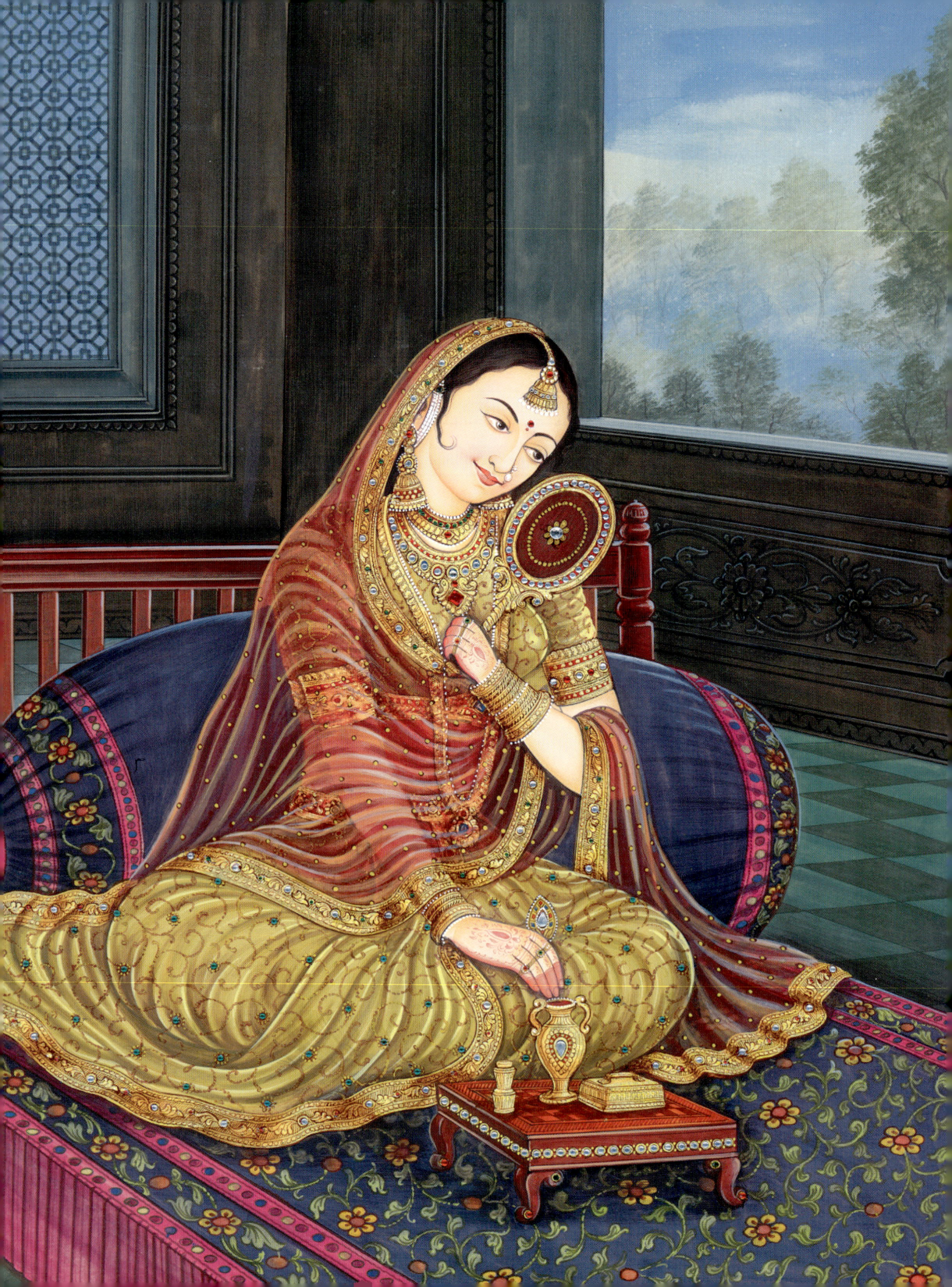

CHAPTER 10

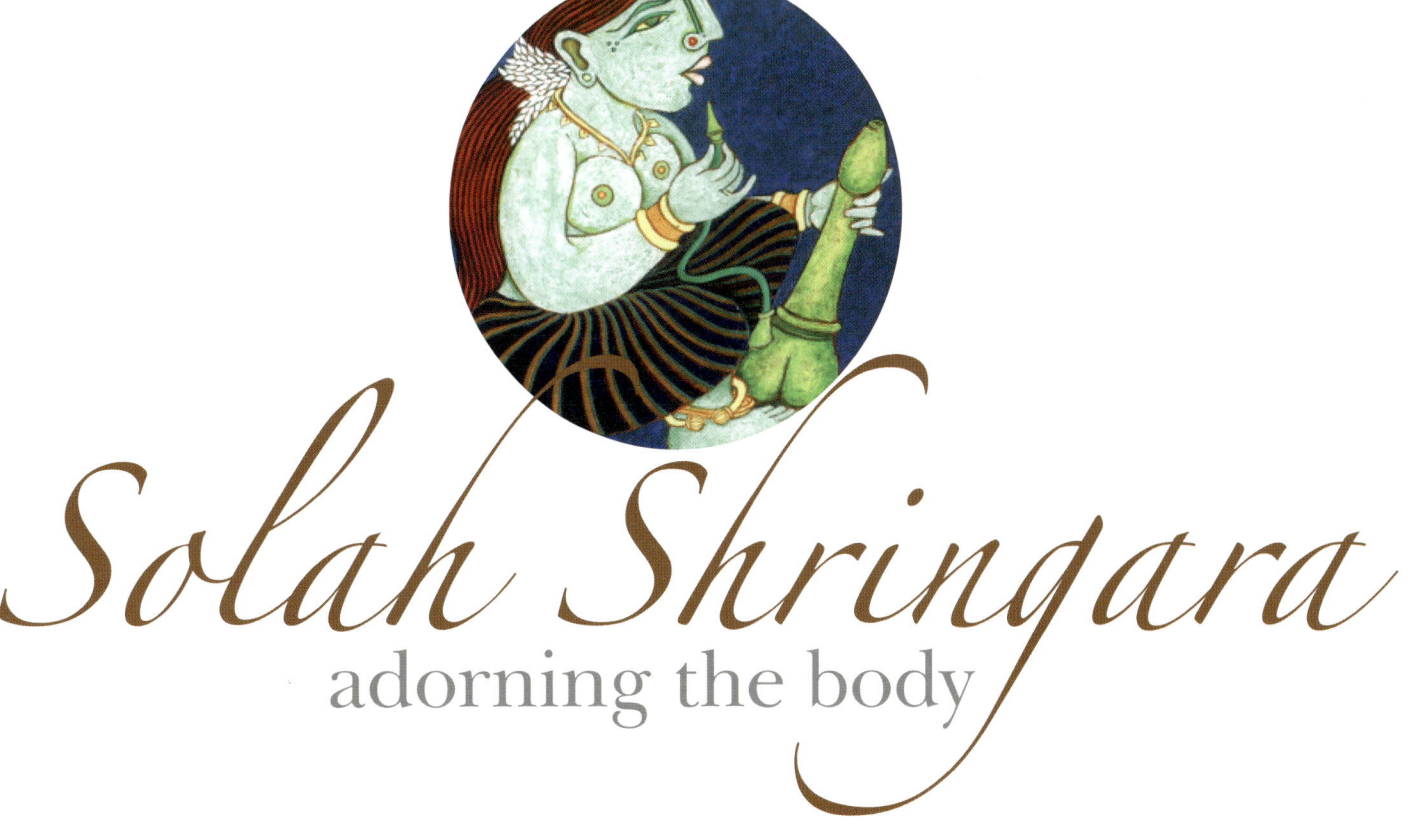

Solah Shringara
adorning the body

She appears like a flash of lightning:
Crowns of gold with rubies and diamonds set
And countless pearls,
Many a row of pearls is gleaming,
Many an anklet tinkling
Many a wreath of gems on her neck,
Diamonds and rubies threaded fair!
A slender waist is decked with bells,
Heart-ensnaring the ring in her nose!
Heavy tresses braided well
Where strings of jewels are woven in.
Beautiful rubies swing in her ears,
Bracelets yield delight:
Here there is worn a silken robe,
There are folds that make it fair.

ANONYMOUS, 8TH CENTURY AD

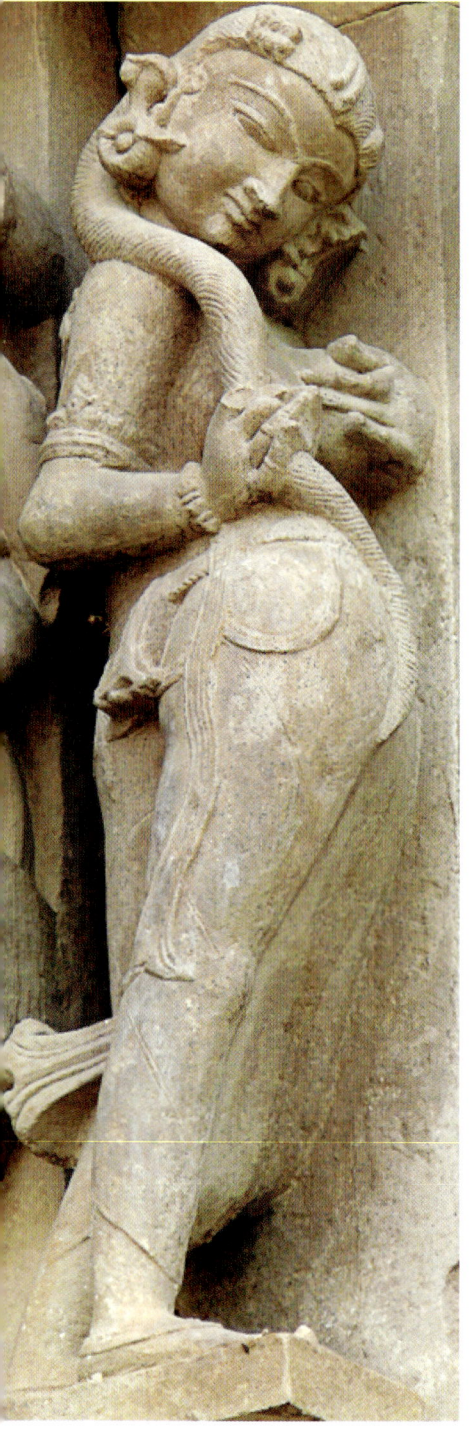

(Page 148)
Every detail of ornamentation

Woman adorning herself, Nandi Temple, Khajuraho

India is a land where beauty can be found in every shade of life. So innate is the concept of shringara and ornamentation in the lives of people, that there is hardly any ornament, embellishment or form of decoration, that does not have a deeper symbolism. Complementing this viewpoint is the conventional belief that the female form epitomizes the ideal beauty and mystery inherent in nature. The verb *alamkara*, which refers to adorning and decorating, literally means 'to make enough'; the simple appearance without ornaments is therefore 'not enough', and women must be careful not to undermine any aspect of their appearance.

Multiple Narratives

In keeping with this tradition, every piece of jewellery speaks a metaphorical language, communicating through its symbolism different meanings that travel between the wearer and the viewer. Jewellery and ornaments were initially born out of a cultural ethos where shringara takes centre stage and where each part of the body is associated with layered meanings. The ornaments express multiple narratives of desire, beauty, femininity and sensuality. Shringara and ornamentation also fulfil a more traditional purpose, which is to drive away all evil spirits through their symbolic power and designs and enhance the auspiciousness of each moment of life.

The process of adornment of the female form was canonized by categorizing it into sixteen different ornaments that covered the body from head to toe. This ornamentation was called the *solah shringara* and in Hindu philosophy, it corresponded with the sixteen phases of the life of the moon, which in turn was connected with a woman's menstrual cycle. This parallel is yet another indication of the deep connections that were believed to exist between the microcosm and the macrocosm, with the feminine physiognomy becoming a part of the larger and all-encompassing rhythm of nature. This chapter will elaborate on the solah shingara since its various facets explore every aspect of attire and adornment in Indian society.

Bindi (Dot on the Forehead)

The *bindi*, derived from the Sanskrit *bindu* (dot) is an ornamental dot placed at the centre of the forehead, slightly above the point between the eyes. This is believed to be the spot of the mystical third eye, supposed to endow a person with wisdom, intuition, and an insight into divine knowledge. While the two manifest eyes are capable of seeing the past and the present, the mystical third eye has the power to make the future appear before us through spiritual perception. Although many men can be seen with a *tilak* (an elongated version of the bindi) or a bindu

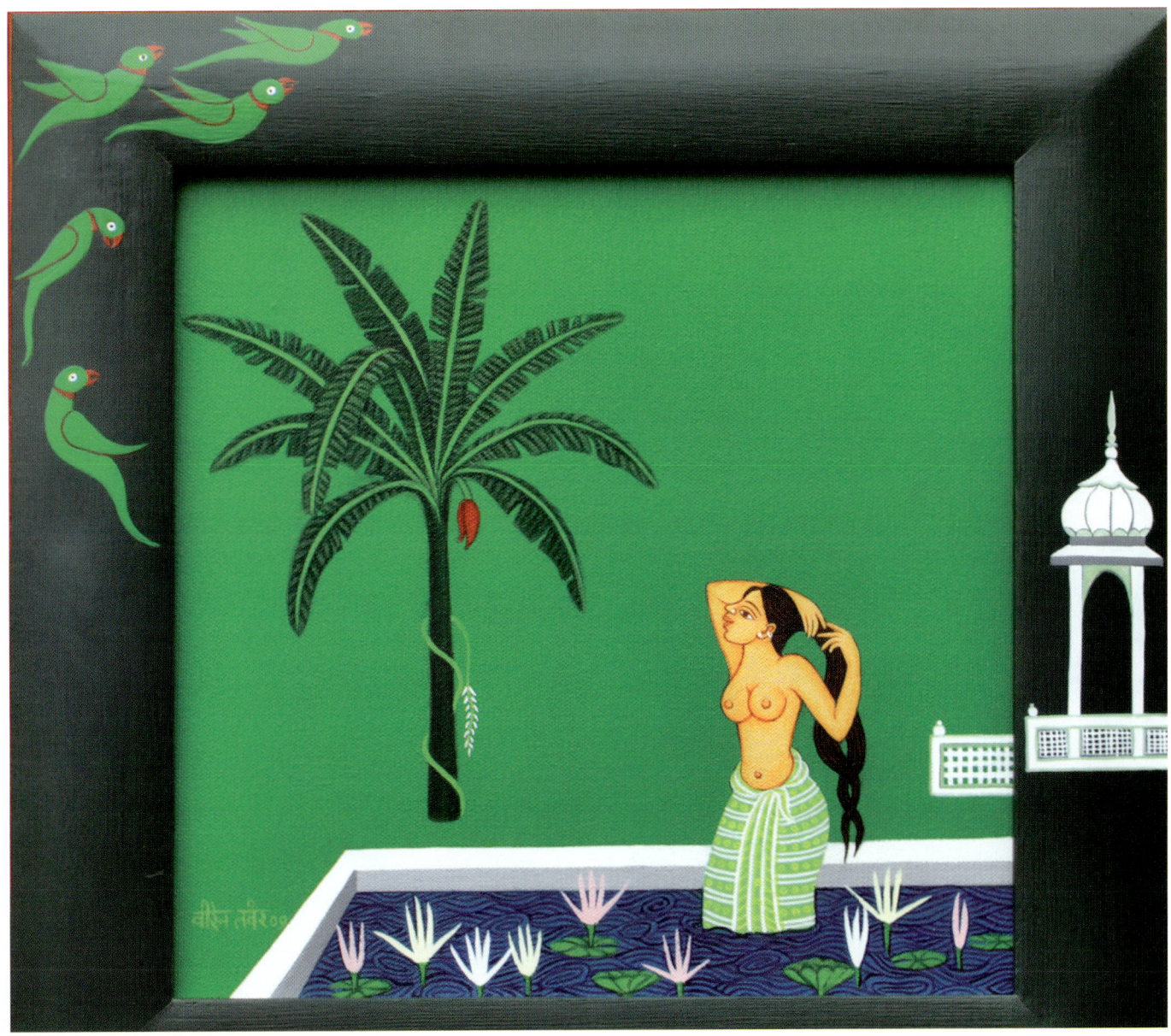

'Shringara', painting by Viren Tanwar, Essl Museum Collection, Austria

on their foreheads, it is essentially feminine. In recent times, bindis have moved past their earlier normative dot-like shape and have acquired various shapes, sizes and colours—all aimed at offsetting and complementing the rest of a woman's attire and her overall beauty.

Sindoor (Vermilion)

Sindoor or vermilion powder is traditionally applied by married Hindu women in the parting of the hair. It is one of the most obvious signs of marital status that sets a woman apart at first glance. The bright red colour is symbolic of a woman's procreative powers. Interestingly, it is also one of the several ingredients used in Hindu worship (*puja*) and is linked with purity. The concept of the pure is in turn associated with a married woman, who attains power through her loyalty to a single man. Her sindoor sets her apart from unmarried girls and also renders her out of bounds for other men.

Tika (Hair Ornament)

The *tika* is an ornament that is worn in the parting of the hair. Made up of a chain with a hook at one end, it bears a pendant that rests in the centre of the forehead. This particular spot is deeply relevant, as it is believed to be the location of the *ajna chakra*, the chakra of preservation. By wearing a tika a woman reinforces her position as the preserver of the human race. It is also interesting to note that the presiding deity of the ajna chakra is the androgynous Ardhanarishvara, a form of Lord Shiva as a hermaphrodite, representing a state where no dualities exist. This state of ultimate union becomes additionally relevant for young girls as they enter into matrimony, since it signifies a force strengthened by the coming together of male and female energies for creation and preservation.

Anjana (Kohl)

In India the black eye make-up or kohl is commonly known as *kajal*. It is used to accentuate the beauty of the eyes—an important facial feature that combines the power of the erotic and the emotional. Traditionally a silver pencil or a fine camel's hair brush was dipped in the kohl and then passed along the contours of the eye giving it an elongated almond-like shape, darkening the eyelashes and enhancing its luminosity. Also known as *anjana*, kohl is supposed to cleanse the eyes and make them more appealing through the play of the dark and the light.

Nath (Nose-ring)

The organ of smell, the nose is also a symbol associated with emotional responses related to sexual reflexes. In men, for instance, a large nose is taken to be the sign of a large sexual organ. In the Indian aesthetics of female adornment, the nose is decorated by a *nath* or nose-ring, that comes in various shapes and sizes, from tiny studs that just about catch the light as they sparkle, to more ornate gold hoops that cover a part of

Untitled, acrylic on canvas Board Collection, Viren Tanwar

(Page 153) Lady applying kohl, Parsvanath Temple, Khajuraho

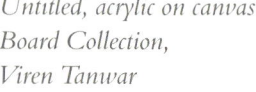

Sarpench is a bejewelled hair ornament, normally used on top of the pagri, a type of male headgear

Shringara—the many faces of Indian beauty

the face and add to the erotic symbolism by resting a pearl on the upper lip. So crucial is this particular ornament in the decoration of the woman, specially a bride, that the deflowering of a virgin is symbolically referred to as the removal of the nath. This analogy perhaps best exemplifies the erotic and sexually latent connotations of this ornament. An essential part of traditional bridal jewellery, many aristocratic families have a special nath brought out at weddings to be worn by the bride.

Haar (Necklace)

According to the occult, the neck is an important centre and necklaces are known to have occupied an important position amongst ornaments since time immemorial. To begin with, its proximity to the heart lent credence to the power of pendants that worked to protect, inspire emotion, bring luck and avert the evil eye. In many parts of the world necklaces were also considered protection against hypnotism, since it drew attention to itself.

In India, the beginnings of the necklace or *haar* can be found in flower garlands that have several references in literature and history. Garlands of certain flowers like champa were even more desirable since their fragrance added to the erotic appeal of the wearer. This is part of the reason why even today, despite necklaces being available in all possible materials, flower garlands are still used at marriages. Innocence, purity, youth, pleasure, and beauty are also some of the other qualities that are traditionally associated with flowers.

Karnaphool (Ear-flower)

Long ear lobes have traditionally been regarded as a sign of spiritual and intellectual advancement – as seen in Homer, Aristotle and the Buddha. On a more decorative level, all over the world, ear lobes are pierced for people to wear earrings. Not only does this add to a person's beauty; it is also supposed to offer protection from evil influences, with the ornaments serving as a talismanic deterrent.

Ear ornaments are, thus, an integral part of the overall female attire, especially for a married woman, in whose case the kind of ear ornament she wore was a reflection of her wealth and status.

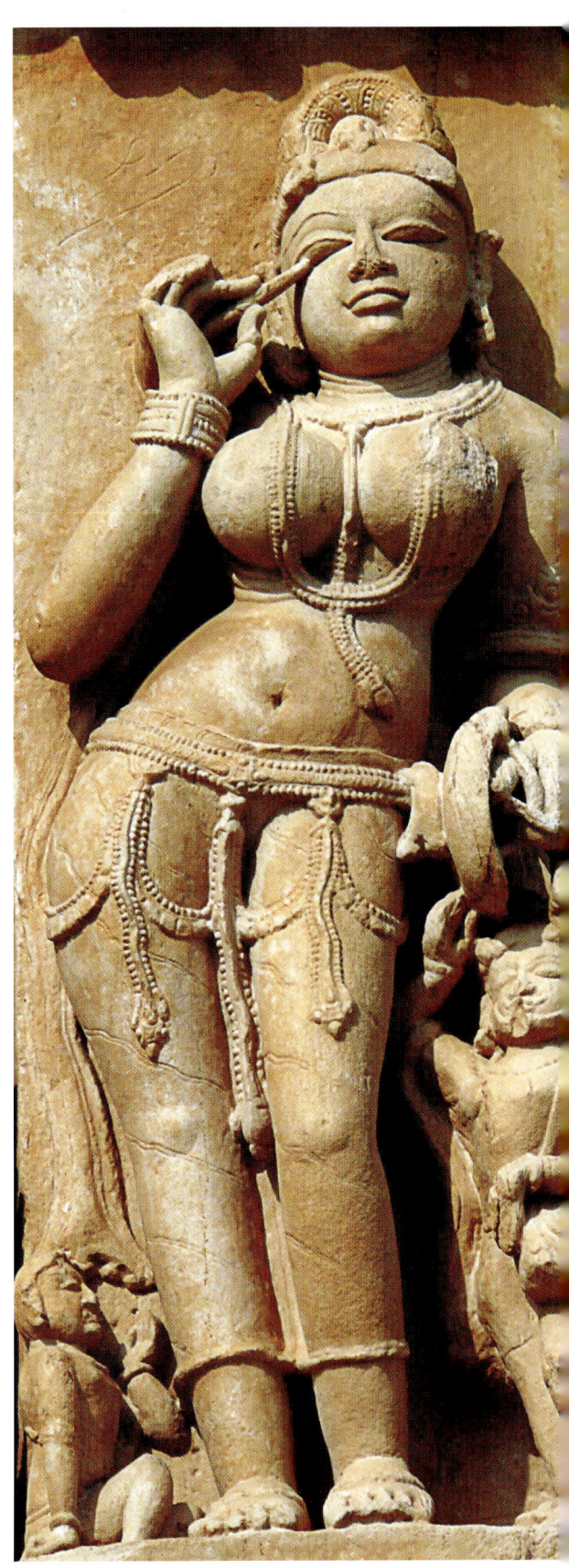

Solah Shringara—adorning the body

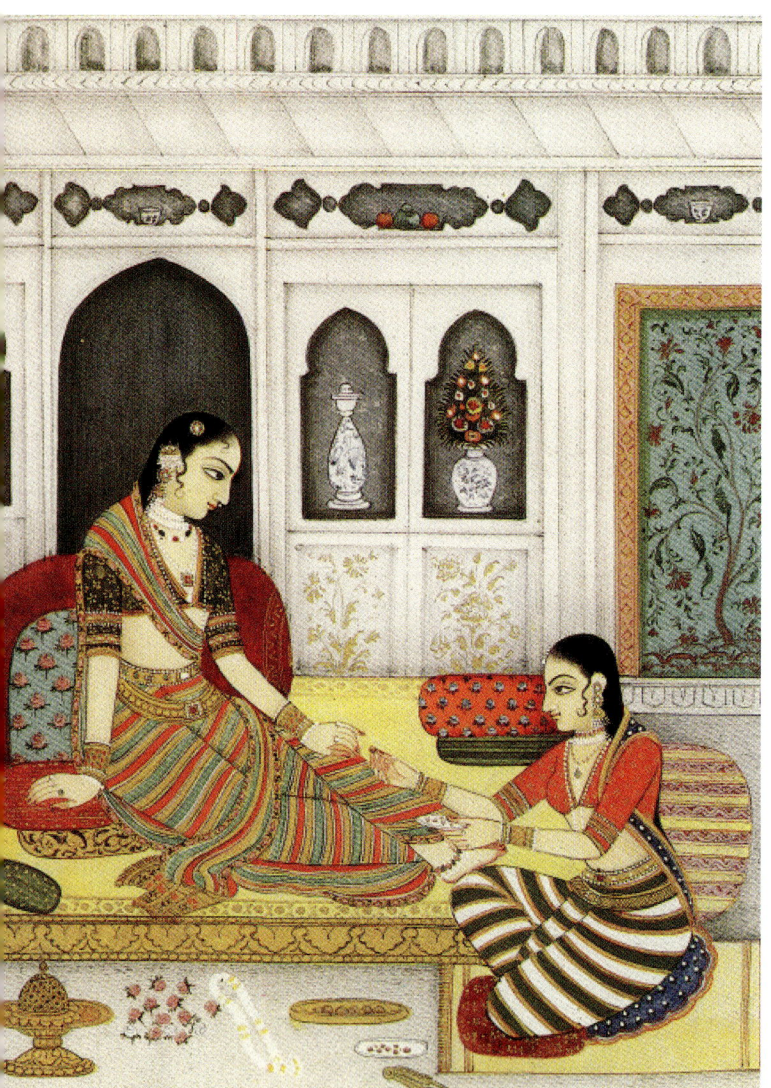

The karnaphool comprises bunches of metal flowers with a central stud at the back being the equivalent of a flower stem. The symbolism of the ornament runs deep. Apart from the erotic association based on the association with Kama, the god of love, flowers also hold within themselves the entire life cycle in a condensed form, moving from birth, life, death to rebirth and therefore become symbols of life and regeneration.

Mehndi (Henna)

When she puts henna on her hands
and dives in the river
One would think one saw fire twisting
and running in the water.

—Dilsoz, 18th century AD

Mehndi is a dye obtained from the paste of henna leaves that is used to create decorative patterns on the skin. The mehndi ritual has various levels of significance: to begin with it is supposed to be a talisman, keeping away all evil spirits from the wearer. Such protection is specially important when a woman is getting married since she is believed to be the most beautiful and vulnerable at that time.

Mehndi or henna is an organic colour used for making colourful and intricate patterns on the hands and feet. Here the nayika is being elegantly adorned by a maiden

In all Eastern wedding traditions the bride is decorated with mehndi on her hands and feet, often up to her knees and elbows. The deep red colour of the mehndi is also symbolic of fertility among both the Muslims and the Hindus. In fact, so crucial is the mehndi ritual to the bride that there is an entire night called *mehndi ki raat* (night of mehndi). During this night, the bride's female friends and relatives gather around her, singing, dancing and teasing her about the future.

The colour of the mehndi also signifies the strength of love and many believe that darker the colour, stronger the love and deeper the passion between husband and wife. In traditional societies, marriages are scheduled to coincide with ovulation and the dark red of the henna becomes symbolic of blood and the breaking of the hymen. After marriage, mehndi may be applied to a woman on any auspicious occasion, such as the birth or naming of a child.

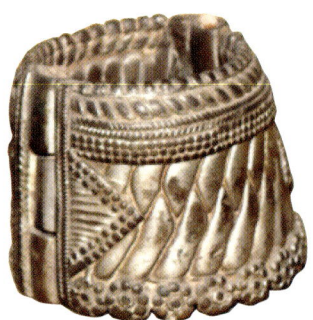

Silver armlet

Kangana (Wrist Ornament)

Bangle-sellers are we who bear
Our shining loads to the temple fair.
Who will buy these delicate,
bright rainbow-tinted circles of light?
Lustrous tokens of radiant lives
For happy daughters and happy wives.

—**Bangle Sellers** by Sarojini Naidu

Bangles and bracelets vary from state to state. Ornate and embossed, the gold 'kada' from Bengal seduces with its beauty

Bangles can be found adorning the hands of women in every region of India. Symbols of femininity and beauty, they symbolize the potent energy of the sun. They are made in a variety of materials ranging from terracotta, plastic, wood, stone and shell, to copper, bronze, silver or gold. In India the traditional bangle is made of glass and comes in various designs, embellished or plain.

The tinkling sound of glass bangles, as they move on the wrists of the woman, have been interpreted in a thousand ways, from expressing anger, resentment or impatience, to a wish for attention or desire. Certain colours like red or green are specially associated with marital status. Traditionally an Indian woman's hands are never supposed to be bare as long as she is a wife. This practice finds further reinforcement in the ritual of widows breaking their bangles when their husbands die.

Baajuband (Armband)

According to the principles of solah shringara, each part of the female body should be decorated, since the overall image of beauty can be created only in totality. The baajuband is tied to the upper arm and is often meant to work as an amulet and keep away the evil eye. It is also used for decorative reasons. A baajuband can be simple or ornate and, depending on the marital status of the woman and the region she belongs to, it can be a single piece or can even cover the entire upper arm.

Arsi (Thumb Ring with Mirror)

This special ring is made for the thumb and has a mirror set in its centre. This small mirror provides women, especially brides, an opportunity to check their appearance. The extent to which an arsi was popular can be judged by the frequent references made to it in paintings, poetry and even in songs.

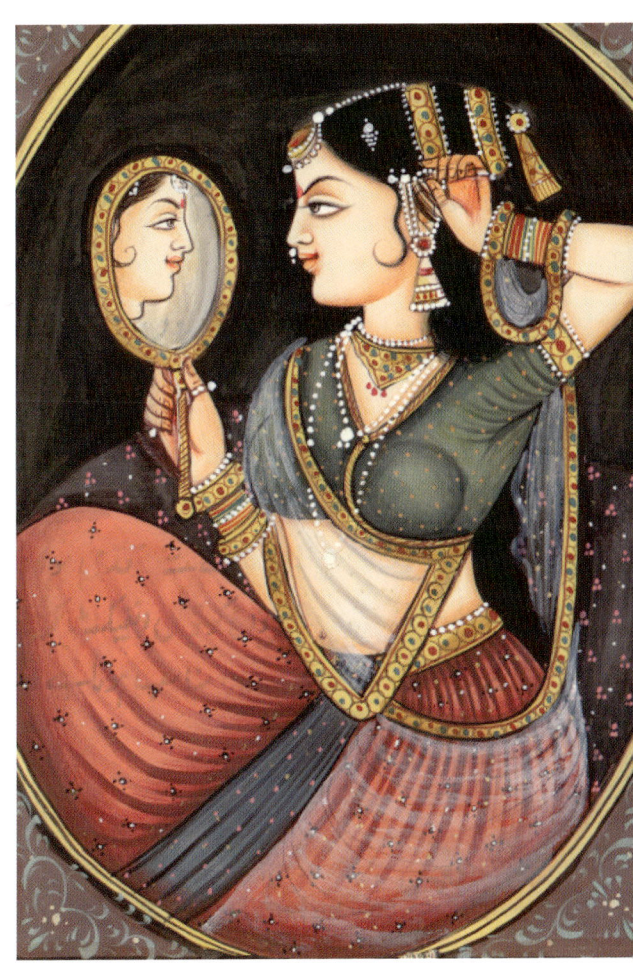

Rajasthan's miniature artists have their own way of depicting beauty. Here is a nayika setting her final piece of jewellery

Solah Shringara—adorning the body

Keshapasharachna (Coiffure)

Of all the visible parts of the human body, the hair occupy an unparalleled place. Hair have always been seen as a source of strength and magic and is supposed to exert special power in terms of attracting men. It was to curtail this temptation that women were required to visit temples with their hair covered so that devout men may not be distracted.

Regular oiling, combing, plaiting and adorning the hair are part of the daily rituals in most households. The hair was moistened, oiled and then curled over the forehead and across the head in ancient India. It was usually parted in the middle, although side partings, as shown in the sculptures of Sanchi, were evident as early as 2nd to 3rd century CE when the art of coiffure seems to have been at its peak.

The ideal coiffure is hair modelled to heighten the forehead with kumkum in the parting and flowers around the joora or bun. On festive occasions these were decorated with jewellery. Plaiting has special relevance among the Hindus since the three strands of hair are believed to represent the coming together of the three most venerated rivers: the Ganga, Yamuna and Saraswati; or the trinity of Brahma, Vishnu and Shiva. The 15th-century poet, Chandi Dasa, describes Radha's hair in the following words:

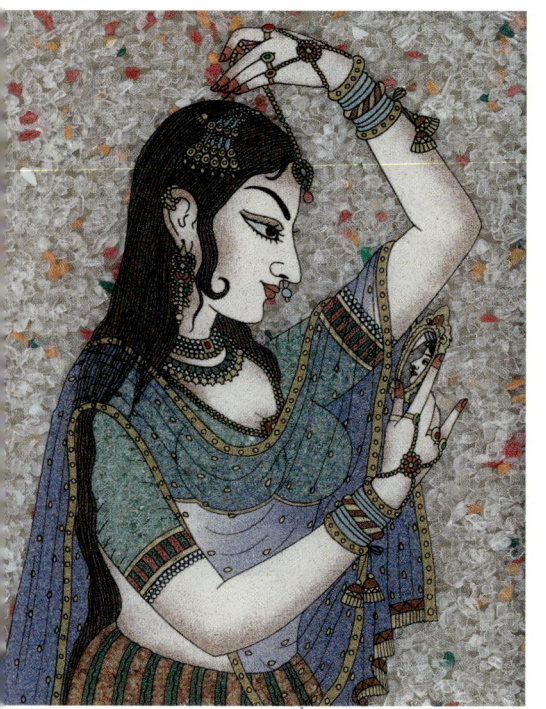

Long tresses were a yardstick of feminine beauty. To adorn and bejewel them was part of the daily makeup. Here the heroine is adding the final touches to her hairdo

*Like stilled lightning fair face
I saw her by the river.
Her hair dressed with jasmine,
Plaited like a coiled snake.*

Kamarband (Ornamental Girdle)

*So tender is her slender waist
It bends when a girdle of flowers is placed.*
— **Tirrukural (South India)**

The *kamarband*, derived from the Persian word *kamar* (waist) and *bandi* (band) is a waistband, particularly popular in northern India. The immense popularity of this ornament is evident in its portrayal in innumerable temple sculptures, frescoes and miniature paintings.

The bare female midriff has always been considered exceptionally

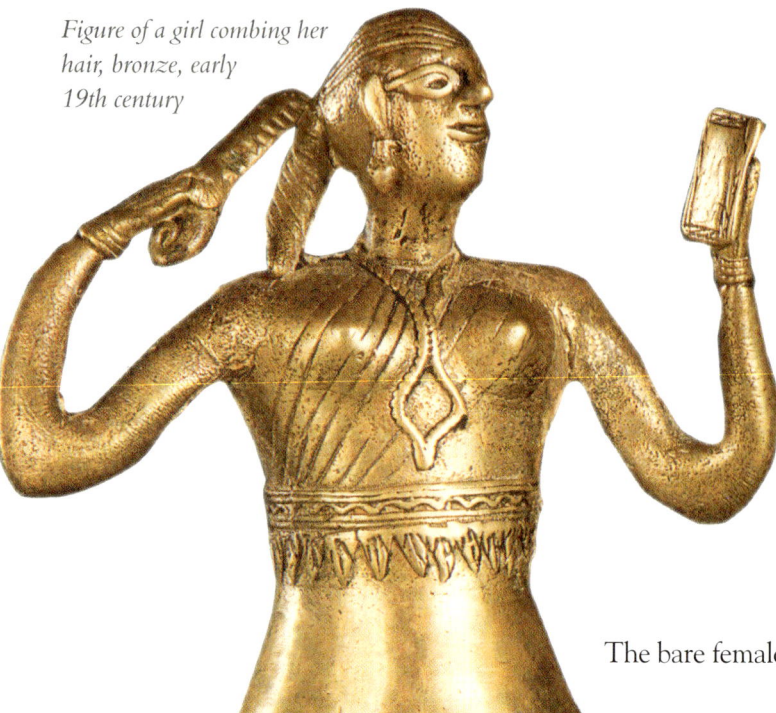

Figure of a girl combing her hair, bronze, early 19th century

attractive and erotic in India, and hence an apt embellishment of this particular part of the body is to be expected. The kamarband adds a decorative element to the waist while simultaneously fulfilling the utility of holding the lower garment, usually the folds of the sari, in place. It is also useful in holding the bunch of household keys, which signifies the assumption of a new position of authority by the bride or daughter-in-law.

Payal (Anklet) and Toe rings

*Hail to that foot of the lusty beloved
which hits the head of the lover, that foot which
is adorned with red paste and jingling anklets
is the banner of love and which is worthy
of adoration by inclining one's head.*
    —From the 5th-century drama, *Padataditakam*

Although the feet are considered to be important for the appearance, they are also considered the most impure and lowly. However, touching of feet or falling at someone's feet represents an act of humbling oneself and surrendering to the other completely. Indian aesthetic traditions, art and literature in particular, have several examples where a lover is shown falling at his beloved's feet, kissing them or admiring them in a state of complete submission.

*The hair of the lover, who has fallen at the
feet of his beloved, are entangled in her anklets,
which indicates that he has given up his pride.*
    —*Prakrit Pushkarini*

It was thus imperative for women to take as much care of their feet as they did of their faces, lavishing attention and ornamentation on them. One way of doing this was by decorating them with silver anklets (*payal*) embellished by tiny bells that made a tinkling sound as a woman moved.

In certain tribes, women wear anklets to frighten away snakes and insects when they walk outdoors, and also, in a less flattering sense, to enable their husbands to keep an eye on their whereabouts.

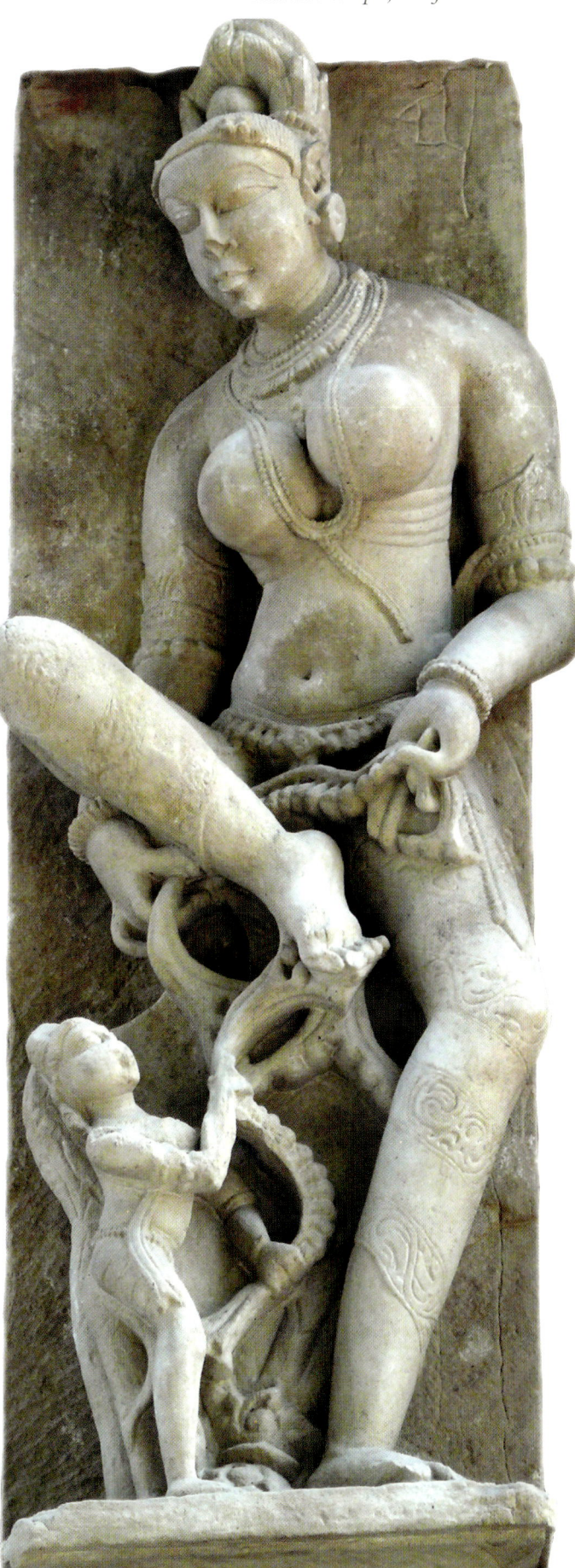

Adinath Temple, Khajuraho

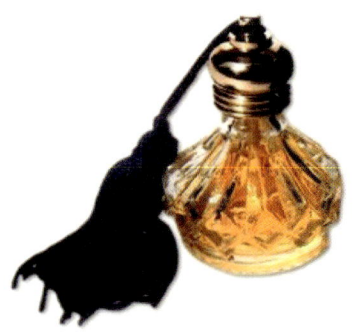

A vial of traditional 'itra'

An artist uses a peacock feather to decorate the nayika's feet with mehndi pattern

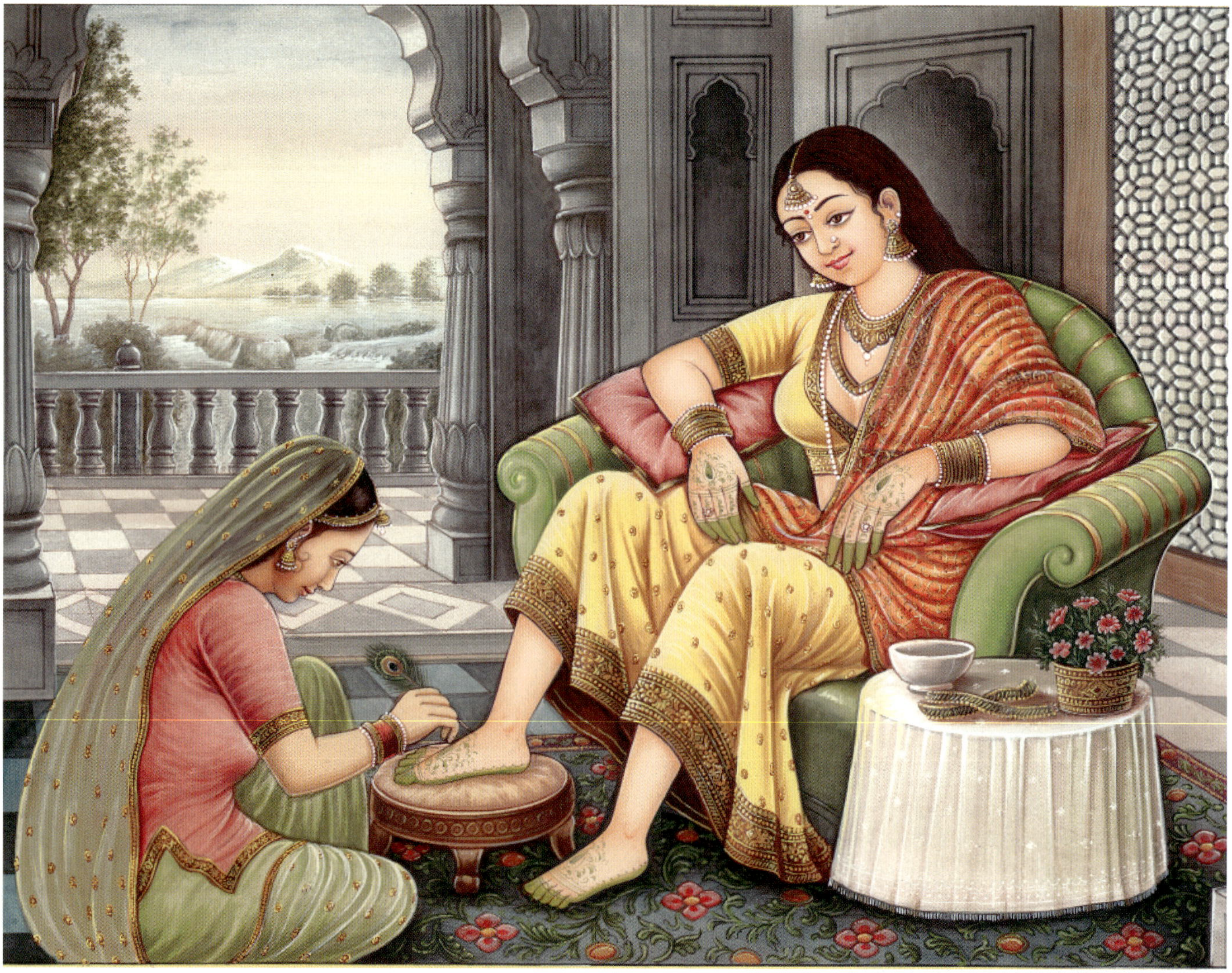

To enhance the decorative appeal, anklets are worn with toe-rings that are attached to them with delicate chains creating a web-like pattern. In most parts of the country, however, women do not wear gold anklets since the wearing of gold on one's feet is believed to be disrespectful of Lakshmi, the goddess of wealth.

Itra (Perfume)

Almost four centuries ago, Noor Jehan accidentally discovered the most expensive and erotic itra, the *Rooh-e-Gulab* when she spilled some oil into her rose-scented bath water. So began the tradition of flower-based perfumes. Different scents were used in different seasons and were used to enhance sensual appeal. Perfumes were also believed to work as aphrodisiacs. Certain scents like *khus* and *kewra* were also used in sweets and *kulfi*, and sprayed on fans to heighten freshness.

The Bridal Dress

The bride's shringara (toilette) includes cleansing of the body in medicated waters, perfuming it with scented oils, applying cosmetics, plaiting the hair and weaving it into patterns, decorating it with ornaments of gold and flowers, beautifying the parting with sindoor, adorning her hands and feet with henna, lining her eyes with kohl, and placing moles on the chin to keep away the evil eye.

Women were draped in flowing garments that fell from the hip to the ankles as evidenced in the sculptures of Sanchi, Amaravati, and Khajuraho. The tradition has continued in the sari of today. Bridal attire is almost always red in colour, largely because of its related sexual, fertility-based and auspicious connotations. Red also signifies the virginal status of the bride, as white does in the West.

Skin Care

The shastras came up with various formulae to guard against skin diseases, chief amongst which was a balanced diet. Face packs and lotions to cleanse and beautify the skin, protect it from the sun, smooth away wrinkles, and remove warts and moles have existed through the centuries. Soft pastes of *besan* (gram flour), white flour, oatmeal and other ingredients, usually mixed with a teaspoon of oil or cream are used as a cleanser. Mudpacks too have existed from ancient times—for example *gachni*, a kind of yellow clay, was coated on the skin to cool the body in the hot summer.

Similar treatments have been used for cleansing and softening the hands. The tradition of colouring the palms and fingertips with powered henna leaves dates back to the 4th century. After a simple manicure, henna paste was used to decorate the palms and myrrh was used to paint the nails. The shell of walnuts and the bark of walnut trees was used to redden the lips and to clean the teeth.

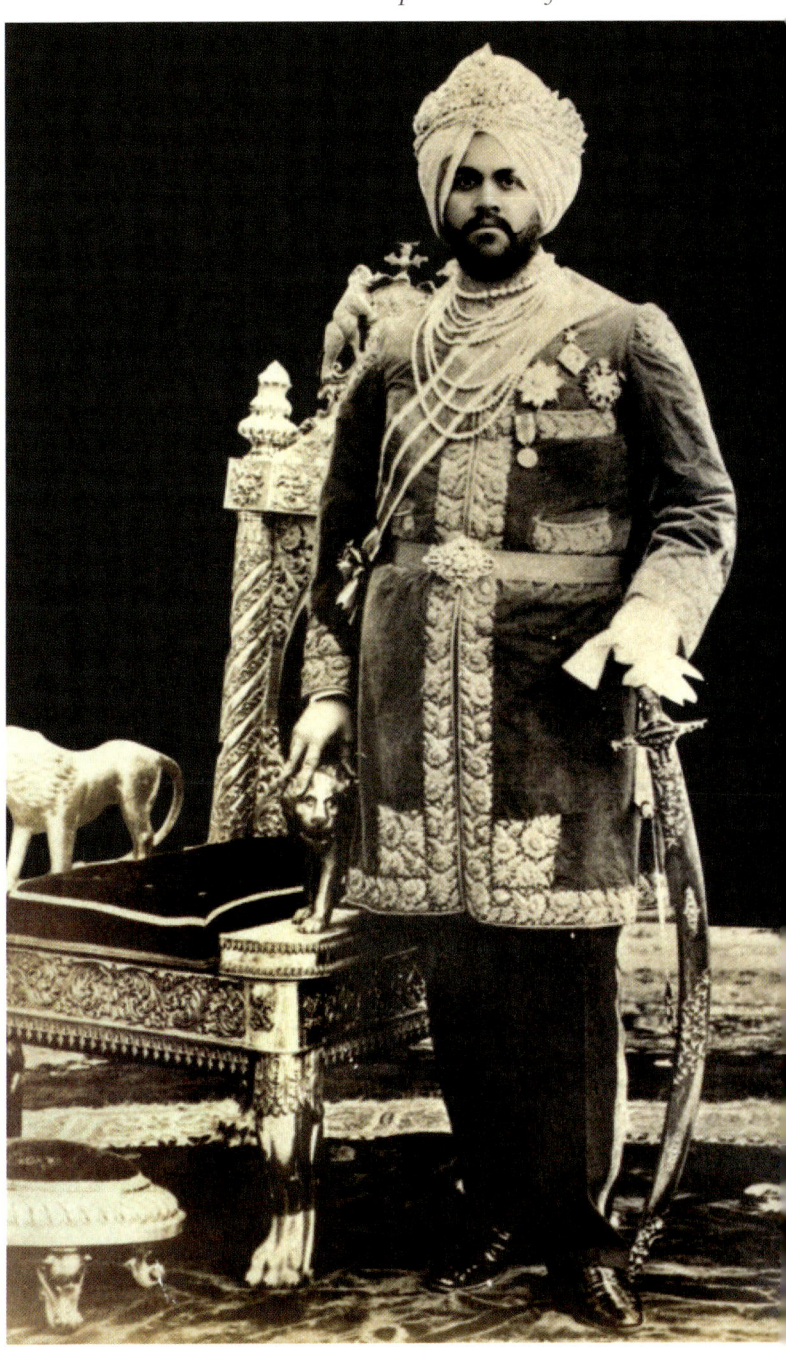

(Page 160)
Duladeo Temple, Khajuraho

(Page 161)
Dancer Sonal Mansingh gazes into the mirror while adorning herself

The Maharana of Mewar, resplendent in his formal attire

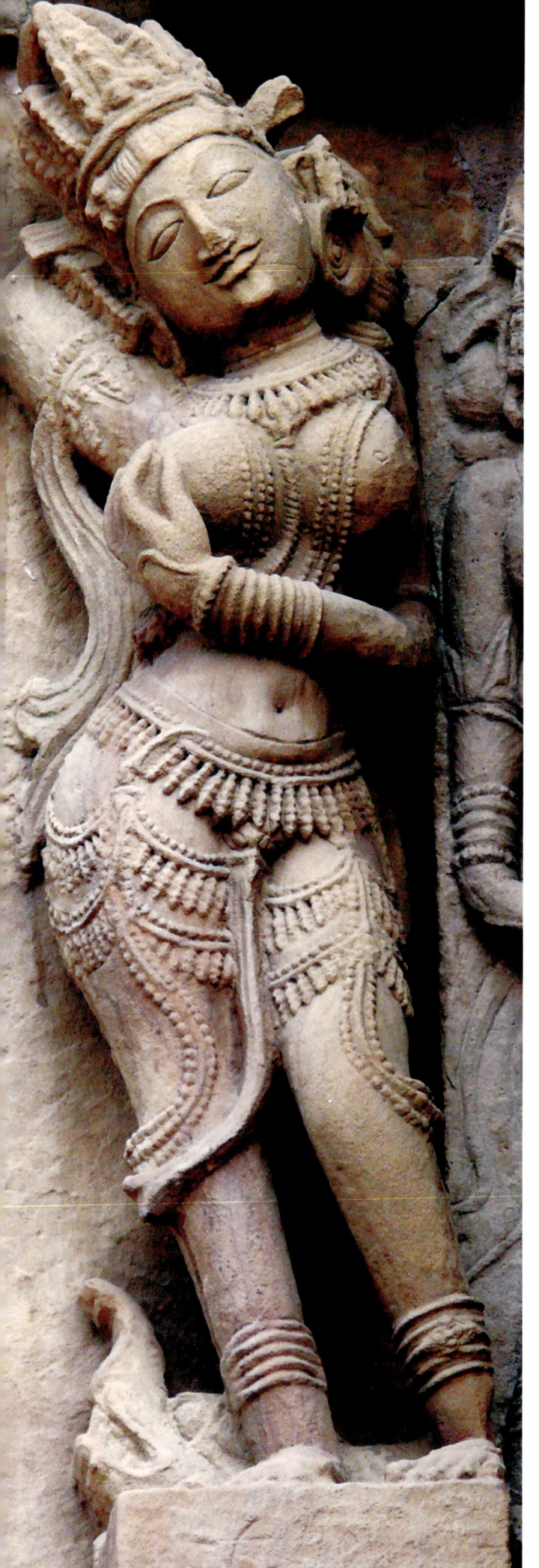

Traditional Attire

Well-fitted clothes, flowing drapes and colourful fabrics are all mentioned amongst the sixty-four fine arts listed by Vatsyayana in *Kamasutra*. There is little one can add to Kalidas's description of costumes to be worn in the different seasons, in his poem, *Ritusamhara*.

In summer:
> In the hot breathless summer the veil drops one
> By one, from the masses of dark hair, from
> the moving shoulders, the breasts and the thighs
> which were entangled, and now women's
> garments are mingled with fresh jasmine their
> Loins are held in gold.

In the rainy season:
> They brighten their ears with coloured blossom.
> They set new pearls about their nipples, and let fall
> their hair… a white garment strains their loins…

In autumn:
> … a young girl, close upon ripeness, has taken
> a thousand stars out of the jewel casket, and
> comes to us in a robe of stainless night.

With the coming of winter:
> … the time of the saffron unguents, of moon-bright garlands,
> has passed away. There are no more shell
> bracelets; and robes lie heavy upon breasts and
> loins… this is no time for coloured belts and
> gold cords and rings chiming like birdsong on
> feet as light as lilies.

And to celebrate the coming of spring:
> … life is in all things: pearls shake upon
> breasts, and the perfumed breath is shaken.
> Girdles are troubled upon the flanks of women.
> Tissues gilt with the sap of saffron lie upon
> Breasts, and loins fill a silk dyed
> with the red Kusumba…

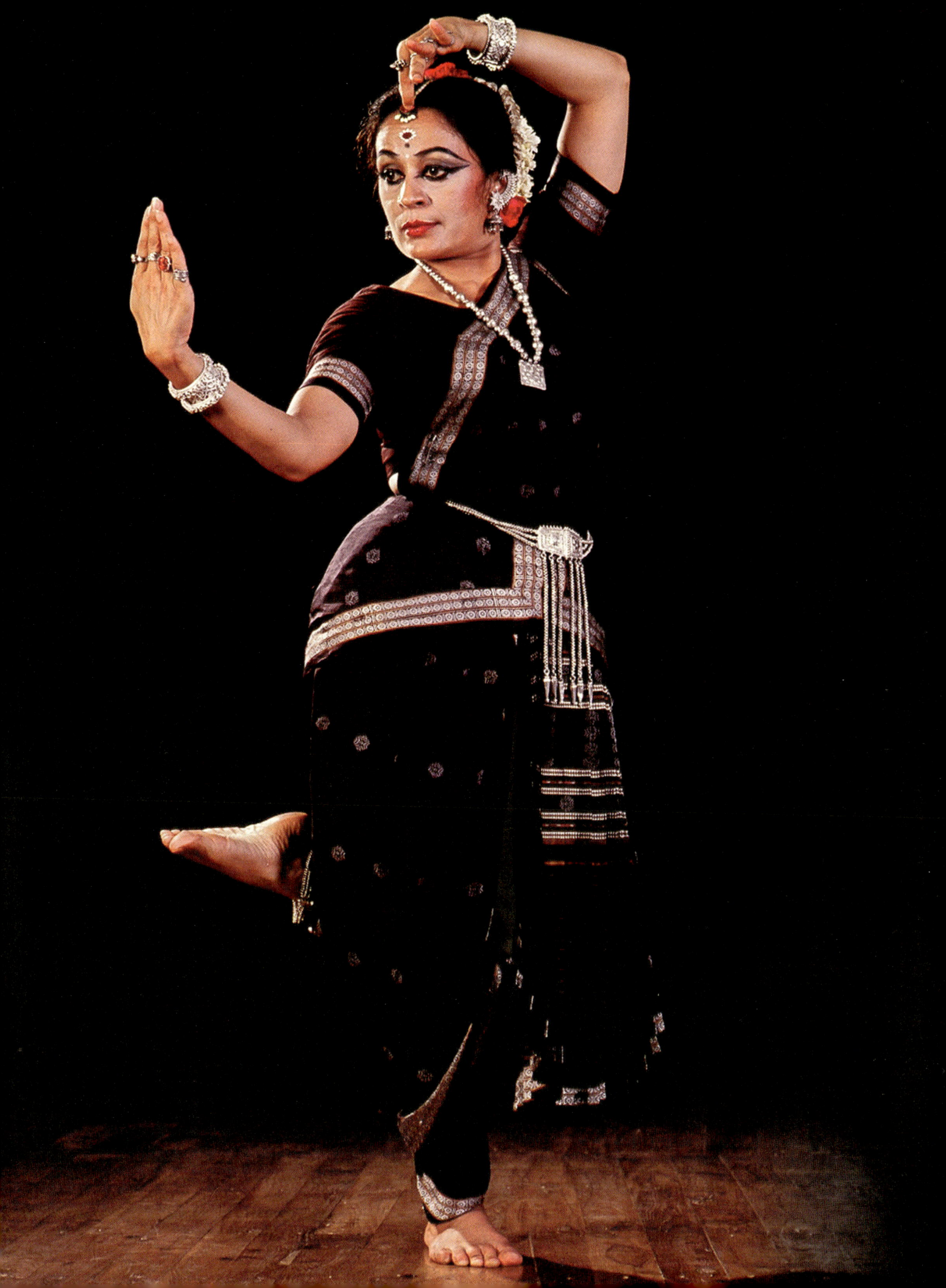

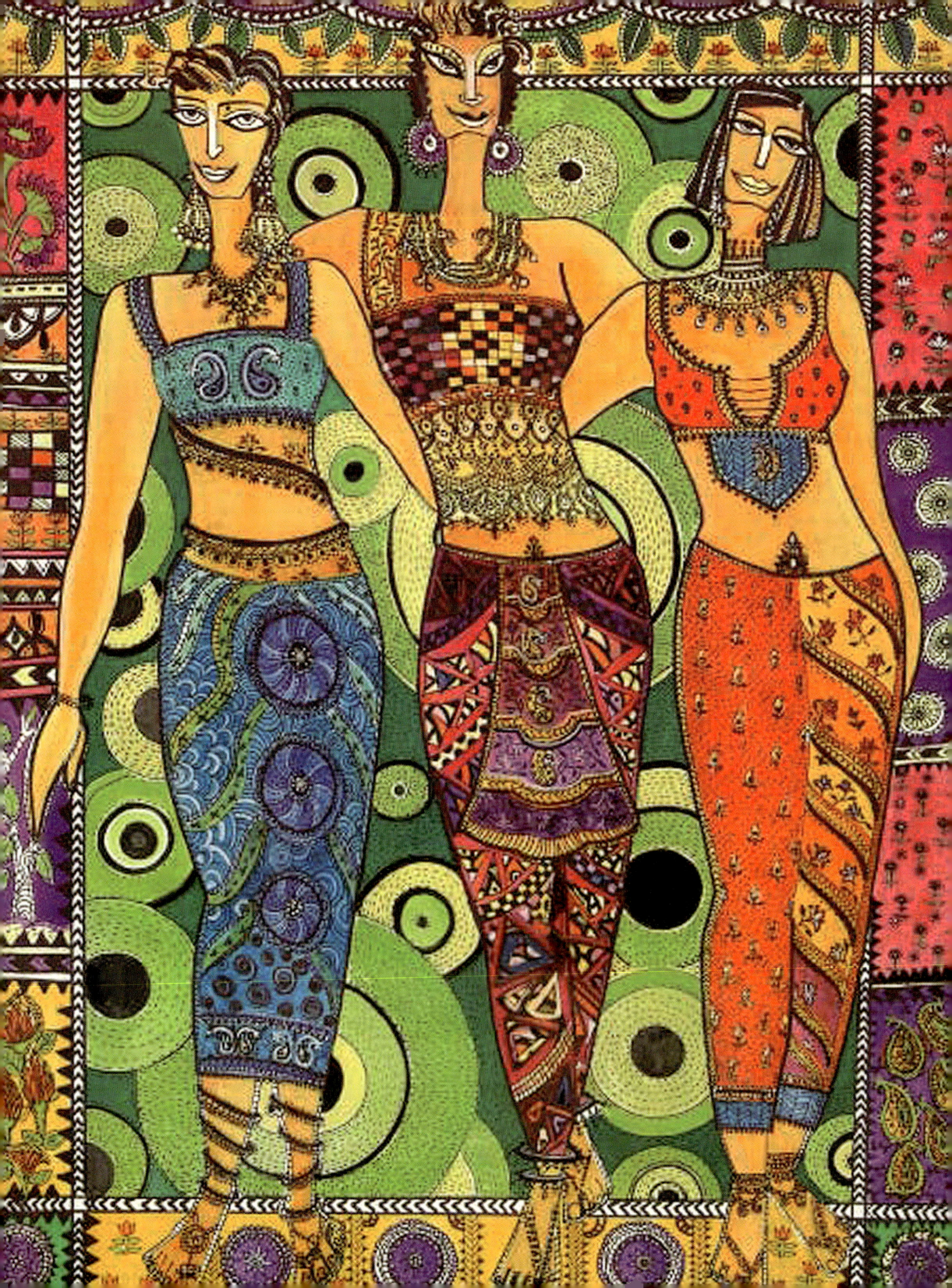

CHAPTER 11

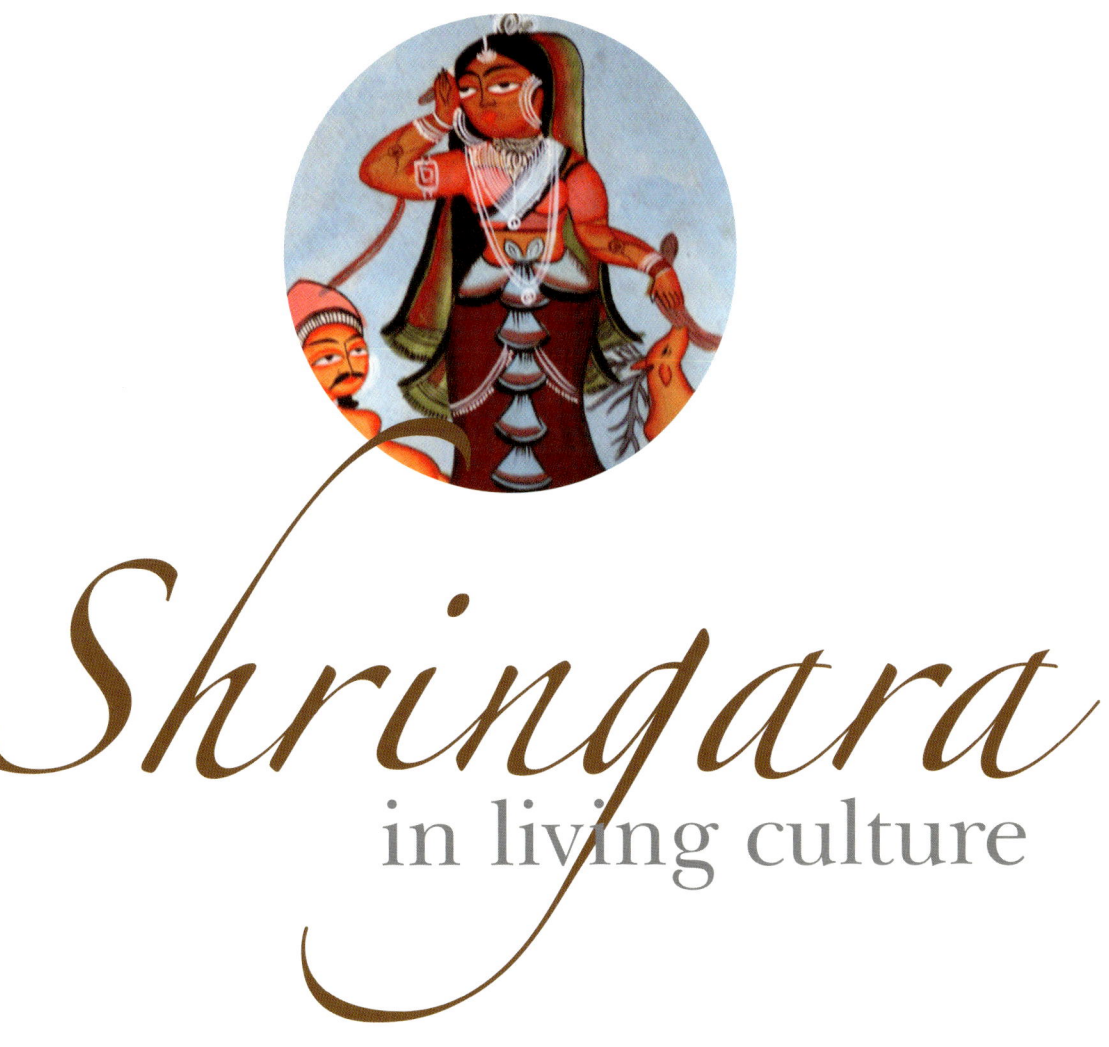

Shringara
in living culture

What then, in a nutshell is living culture? For a country as vast and diverse as India there can be no single absolute answer...

The Earthen Drum
Pupul Jayakar

*(Page 162)
Painting by Shelly Jyoti*

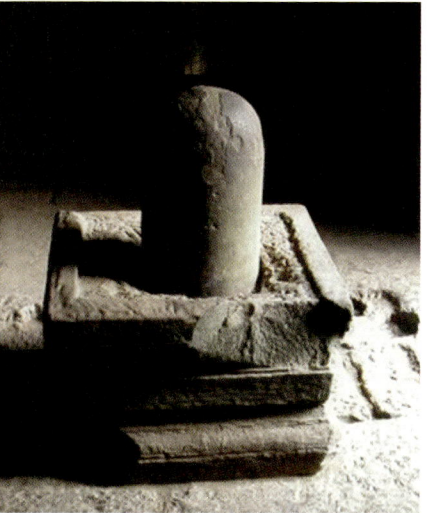

Shivalingam, a Tantric representation

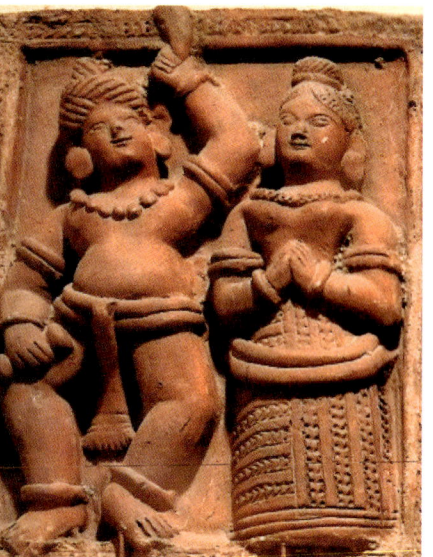

Shiva and Parvati, Terracotta, Bengal, Crafts Museum, New Delhi

The folk and tribal communities of India have traditionally been perceived as the non-visible communities of society. The situation today, however, is altering, with these communities becoming extremely visible in the economic, social and cultural milieu of the country. The lands they occupy are rich with forests, minerals and metals and because of the vast natural wealth of which these communities are the natural custodians, they have come into sharp focus. There has also been a far greater appreciation of their contribution to the artistic scene, with museums and art historians acknowledging their significance to the overall cultural ethos.

Pupul Jayakar was a pioneer in Indian culture with her pathbreaking work on the living cultures in India. She has written extensively and her thoughts are appropriate when she says: 'Rural arts are the arts of people living in forest and mountain, the ancient inheritors of this land, claiming to be the first-born of the earth.' She defines them as 'people with a remote past but with no recorded history; establishing kingdoms and ruling huge tracts of the heartlands of India and then disappearing into cave and mountain, hunting wild beasts, collecting wild products from the dark and pathless forests'.

She further adds in her iconic text that the indigenous people are those for whom religion gives every instant of their living a sense of mysterious sacredness. They are 'people with potent magic, with knowledge of incantation and ritual and with an intense sense of awareness born of man's earliest concern to combat and propitiate the terrible, the unseen'. At one level what keeps these cultures alive and vibrant is their very own personal laws. They are people with power over, and intimate kinship with, animals, with trees, with stones, and with water. Pupul Jayakar defines them as individuals 'with a central concern with fertility and with their ears close to the earth, who whisper to them her secrets so long as they do not wound her breasts with the plough. They who speak of themselves as *Har, Hara, Ho* and *Hora*—Man'.

Art of the People

It is, in fact, fascinating to see how so many tribal communities have managed to not only survive, but also preserve and continue with their ways, in the very midst of contemporary India. Art in these communities and societies is essentially the art of the people. In this situation, the distinction between the consumers and producers of art disappears, and creative representation becomes participatory. However, unlike the art forms of more hierarchical, structured societies, this art is characteristically impermanent and ephemeral, often a metaphor for their complex ritual and living traditions. Most of the art comes from the earth and returns to it without waste.

Ananda Coomaraswamy observes that art can be categorized as *desi* and *margi*. Art is termed desi (local) when it is more in tune with the worldly—the kind that lives out its validity with time. It is margi when it is sacred and goes beyond the 'limitedness' of time, generation or immediate contexts. Folk art is margi and combines within itself all the beauty and energy of imagination, mysticism, spirituality and creativity.

Folk and tribal communities have a way of life that links the organic relationship of man and god, nature and spirit—all believed to be fluid and flowing into each other within the larger scope of existence. The individual, in such a context, lives for more than himself, since his entire being is linked to the presence—physical or metaphysical—of ancestors, the larger community and the higher God.

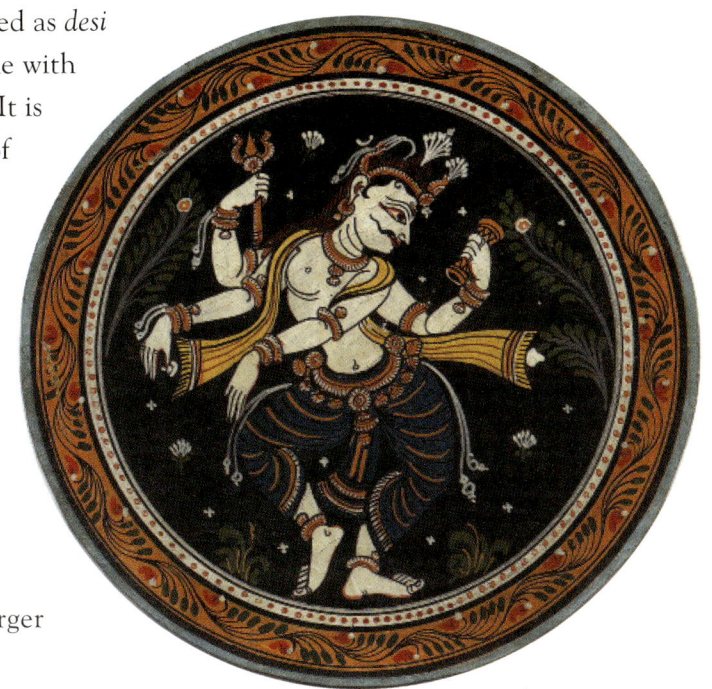

Patachitra, Orissa

'Significant symbols', an image of Parvati, Crafts Museum, New Delhi

The kind of culture in which shringara and saundarya serve a purpose greater than that of mere utility, is one that reflects the magnificence of living. It is a culture where connections between the immediate and the ultimate run deep—where the home is a temple, the tree a spirit to be worshipped, the jingle of bangles a sign of prosperity, and a shawl conjures up generations and ancestors long gone. What one witnesses here, as Jasleen Dhamija puts it, is the 'development of a certain style of creative expression that is closely linked to the beliefs of the people. This style transcends geo-climatic conditions, national boundaries and is incorporated within the larger concept, the cultural traditions and nuances of their beliefs and philosophical thought'.

Significant Symbols

According to experts in the field of cultural anthropology, thinking does not only consist of what happens in one's head, but also of several other symbols and their import. Margaret Mead calls them 'significant symbols' and, although they are mostly made up of words, they also include drawings, music, dance, and ornaments. Or rather, as Clifford Geetz describes as, 'Anything, in fact, that is disengaged from its mere actuality and is used to impose meaning upon experience.' Human beings see these signs around themselves from the time they are born, and it is this symbolic web that works as a reference point, helping them orient themselves in the socio-cultural world they inhabit.

Shringara—in living culture

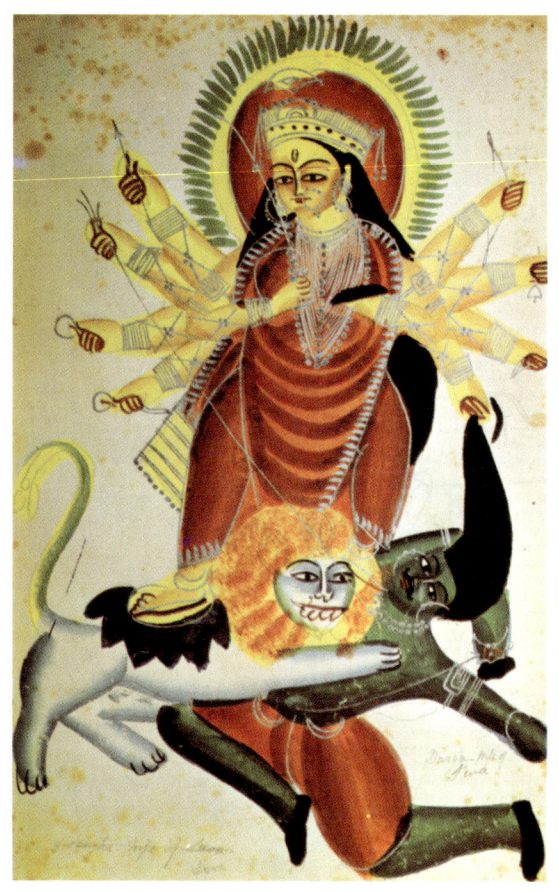

Kalighat painting, West Bengal

In 21st century India, while parts of the country are enveloped in the cross-currents of fast cars, fast food, fast returns and a fast life, there is another part that remains attached to the ways of its forefathers, rooted firmly in its cultural ethos—in its small and not-so-small customs and traditions. For those who live within this realm, culture is not something encountered in distanced ways. It is a reality, a tangible presence that finds reflection and representation in different facets of their lives—from the clothes they wear to the music they play, from the movements of their dances to the sounds they create. Their culture is as real as the air they breathe, as unique as their traditions, as alive as their very existence.

Unseen Communion

In many living cultures shringara takes on the form of narrative ritual, where the narrator and the listener are joined in an inexplicable communion of words, intonations and sounds. In such instances, the idea of beauty and pleasure connect to a form of multi-dimensional storytelling. They are also intertwined with the narrative itself, which develops into a multi-layered rendering of the sensory experience—be it live theatre, painting, song, puppetry, or the weaves that tell of entire worlds in their patterns. From the epics to folk tales, from the *phad* paintings of Rajasthan to the Bengali Kalighat art, from the leather puppets of Andhra Pradesh to the *pichhwais* of Nathdwara, the message is shrouded in layers of shringar that need to be decoded by the discerning eye of the aesthete before they can be understood and appreciated.

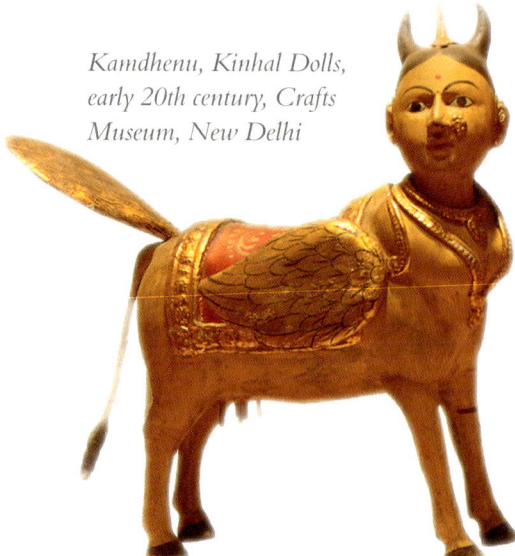

Kamdhenu, Kinhal Dolls, early 20th century, Crafts Museum, New Delhi

An example of this can be found in the painting traditions of Mithila in the Darbhanga district of Bihar. The Maithili community worships Shakti and Bhagvati Gauri is the *kula devata* of the tribe. The women of the community make paintings that, according to Pupul Jayakar, are 'elemental energy forms abstracted of all details. There is a stark austerity in the paintings, an unfolding energy and sense of magic that possibly has its source in tantric ritual and worship'. The women artists become the channels through which all inherited knowledge flows, constantly revisited and transcreated with symbols, idioms, themes and stylizations—all inherited from the timeless tradition (*parampara*) of the tribe's past. Similar pictographs can be seen in the Gonds of Mandla, Warlis of Maharashtra, Bhils of Gujarat, the Kalighat painters of Bengal, and other folk cultures throughout the country.

166   *Shringara*—the many faces of Indian beauty

The Circle of Life

Yet another example of this cultural ethos is the belief in the mandalas, a practice common to almost all the tribal communities in the country. The word mandala essentially means a circle. In almost all living cultures it symbolizes cosmic energy. Drawn on the earth, on rocks and stones, walls and floors, cloth or paper since time immemorial, the mandalas or magical drawings have been man's instinctive method of communicating meaning in non-verbal terms. Pupul Jayakar describes it most aptly when she says, 'It was born of ancient man's preconceptions of the cosmos and of the magical processes of birth, death, and existence, imponderables that can only be explained or revealed non-verbally through geometry and the mathematical abstractions of mathematical form.'

Man's primeval instinct to protect himself against unseen forces and evoke the auspicious, have led to the evolution of different tools in different cultures. The mandalas give visual form to this magical power that can be brought to life through incantation and ritual gesture. It may then generate and destroy, contain and repulse, attract and protect energy. Evidence of the belief in the mandalas has been found in the remains of the Indus Valley civilization and at the Beri Beri archaeological sites in Madhya Pradesh.

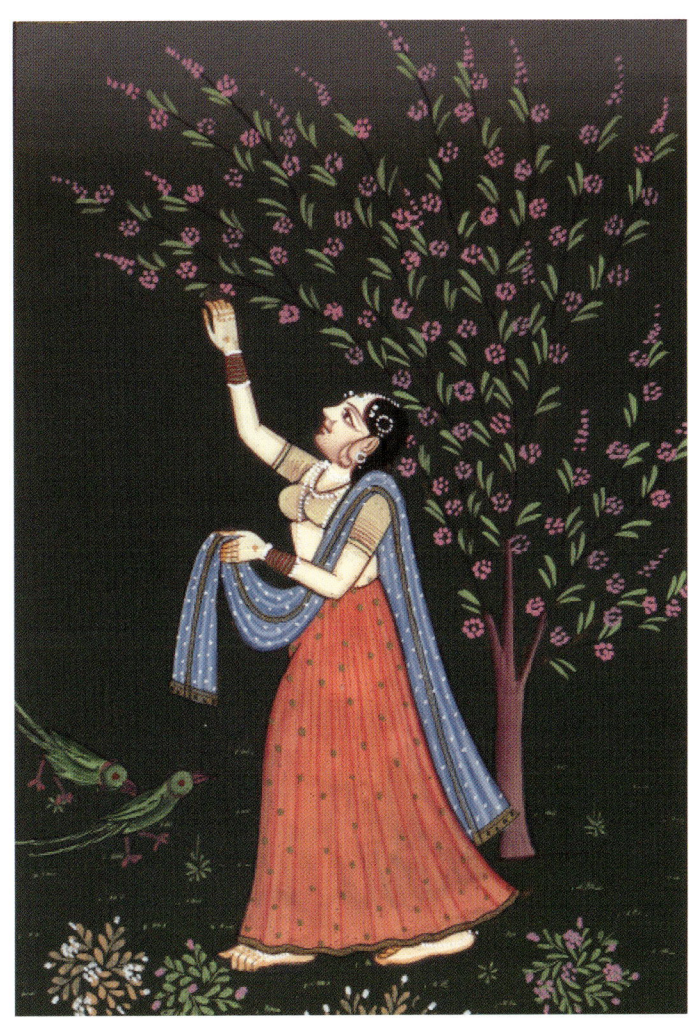

The female form is celebrated in Indian miniature painting. Here the heroine is seen gathering the flower blossoms in her 'odhni'

Some of the more common diagrams are the Chitra Bandha (a parallelogram with letters of the alphabet repeated on all sides), the Suryamandala (invoking the energy of the sun), the Ashtakona (eight-cornered diagram), Rasamandala (Krishna and Radha), Ashtadala (the eight-petalled cosmic lotus of energy at the heart of which is man), the shraddhamandalas (diagrams of the dead), Sarvobhadras (symbols of the virgin goddess and the rising sun) and the Vratamandalas (channels through which the energy of living things can be made operative in transformative rites).

Ritual, in fact, is the means whereby we seek to establish a connection between the microcosm and the macrocosm, between temporality and eternity, death and life. In most cultures, ritualized action, therefore, involves the use of several objects considered sacred and therefore beautiful. Due to the intermediary nature

Shringara—in living culture

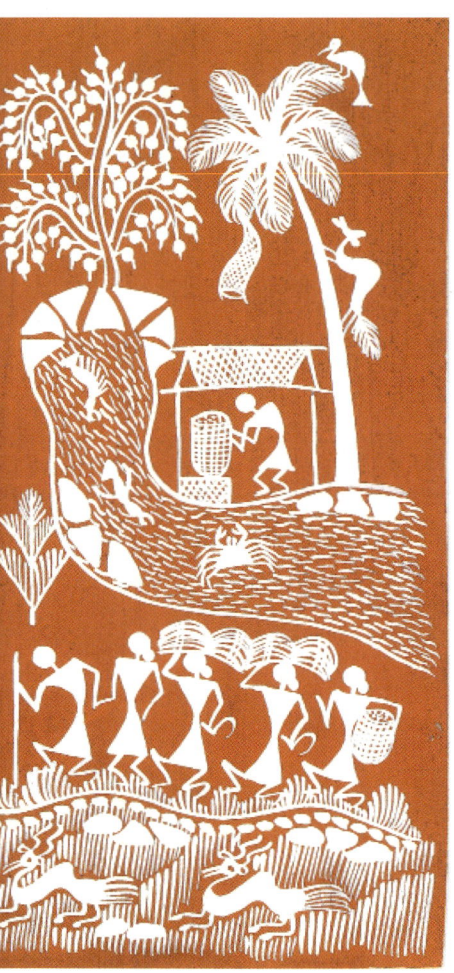

Warli painting, Maharashtra. Warli wall paintings use a very basic graphic vocabulary: a circle, a triangle and a square. The circle and triangle come from their observation of nature, the circle representing the sun and the moon, the triangle derived from mountains and pointed trees. The square apparently indicates a sacred enclosure or a piece of land

of such objects, ranging from a swastika drawn on a floor to the image of a tribal deity painted on the wall, they become visual prayers.

Marks of Distinction

Especially relevant are the tribal and folk cultures of the country. Every tribal community—be it the Bajanias, Bakaarwal Bangri, and Bedas, to name a few, has its own traditional jewellery and clothes through which they establish their identity, making one tribe distinct from the other. The women from the northern region are particularly fond of silver jewellery and wear strings of silver chains with intricately carved heavy pendants and large bell-shaped silver earnings.

For the married Hindu Kashmiri woman, the most important piece of jewellery is the *atteroo* and *dejharoo*, a pair of gold pendants hanging on a silk thread or gold chain passed through pierced ear lobes. This is the equivalent of *mangalsutra* worn as an indication of the married status by Hindu women in other parts of the country. Muslim women, on the other hand, wear heavy earrings supported by a thick silver chain. Additional ornamentation is provided by a variety of bracelets and necklaces, all of which combine to create an extremely aesthetic and shringara-enriched appearance. The *jhumar* is yet another ornament that is essential to complete the shringara of a married women. Worn on the hand, it adds sound as well as embellishment.

Shringara also includes clothing and handicrafts. In Kashmir hand embroidery, particularly of the *sozoni* style, is extremely popular, as is *zardozi* (gold thread embroidery) on saris, gowns and shawls. The *phiran*, a kind of loose knee-length coat worn by both men and women is usually made of wool and decorated with colourful floral motifs. The phirans that men wear are usually made of tweed or coarse wool. They also wear coats made of camel hair, cashmere and brocade.

The men of Ladakh wear long, grey, woollen gowns fringed with sheepskin and tied at the waist with girdles of blue. Multi-coloured velvet caps with black fur earflaps keep out the cold. The women's clothes are very colourful and a unique part of their attire is the *perak*, a scarf studded with turquoise, or decorated with broaches of semi-precious stones. Made of red cloth or goat-skin, it tapers from head to waist at the back. Bangles and earrings are used to embellish arms and ears.

Tribal Customs of Central India

In Central India one finds a number of small tribes—the Gonds, Murias, Koyas and Baigas. Despite the inroads made by 'development', the tribals in this area continue to follow an animistic way of life. The creative force of their art is

168   *Shringara—the many faces of Indian beauty*

mainly defined in terms of non-Hindu beliefs with carved figures and patterns that bear a resemblance to images of spirits and ancestors rather than to the more mainstream deities of the orthodox Brahmin religious fold.

The Gonds form the largest tribal group in Central India with more than 20 per cent of them living in the Bastar region of Chhattisgarh. The tribe has three major sub-castes—Maria, Muria and Dorla. Most of these communities have integrated the local language into their speech, Chhattisgarhi Hindi, and the younger people no longer speak pure Gondi.

The tribals worship a deity known variously as Persapen or Mahaprabhu. Both terms mean 'greatest of gods'. His shrine usually lies at a height on the clan's ancestral ground. Although many members of the various clans have become displaced over the years due to socio-economic reasons, they still live within a community framework. This serves as a permanent reference point governing all major decisions, regulating the areas of marriage, birth and death ceremonies.

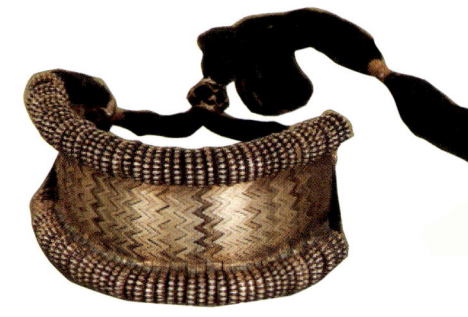

Baajubandh, silver and dyed cotton thread, early 20th century, National Handicrafts and Handlooms Museum, New Delhi

A Rajasthani beauty in all her splendour adorned from top to bottom

The School of Life

An integral and unique part of the living culture of the Marias is the *ghotul* system; its origin is linked to their goddess Lingopan. This is a mixed dormitory system in which young, unmarried boys and girls live together in a sort of clubhouse. Their days are strictly regulated—the daylight hours are devoted to cleaning the village streets, helping the old with chores such as fetching and storing water, repairing old houses, building new ones, and working in the fields.

This engenders a sense of responsibility to the community in the young, and at the same time, teaches them the rules that govern the clan or tribe. For example, they learn very early on, that marriage outside the clan is forbidden, that children, once they enter the ghotul at the age of seven or eight, belong to the whole village, not just to one set of parents, and that sex before marriage, although permitted, is not a passport to promiscuity.

Evenings at the ghotul are a time of relaxation after the food is cooked and eaten. There are discussions, group singing and dancing in preparation for a feast day. Music is played on the flute or the ektara and stories are told—that serve as both teaching aids for the young and repositories of the tribe's history

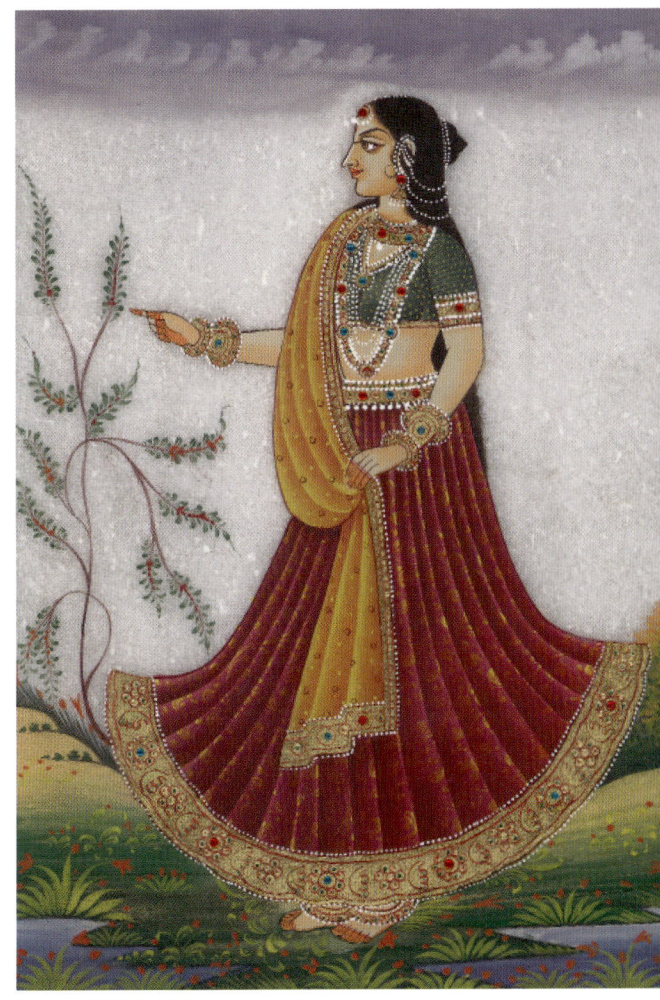

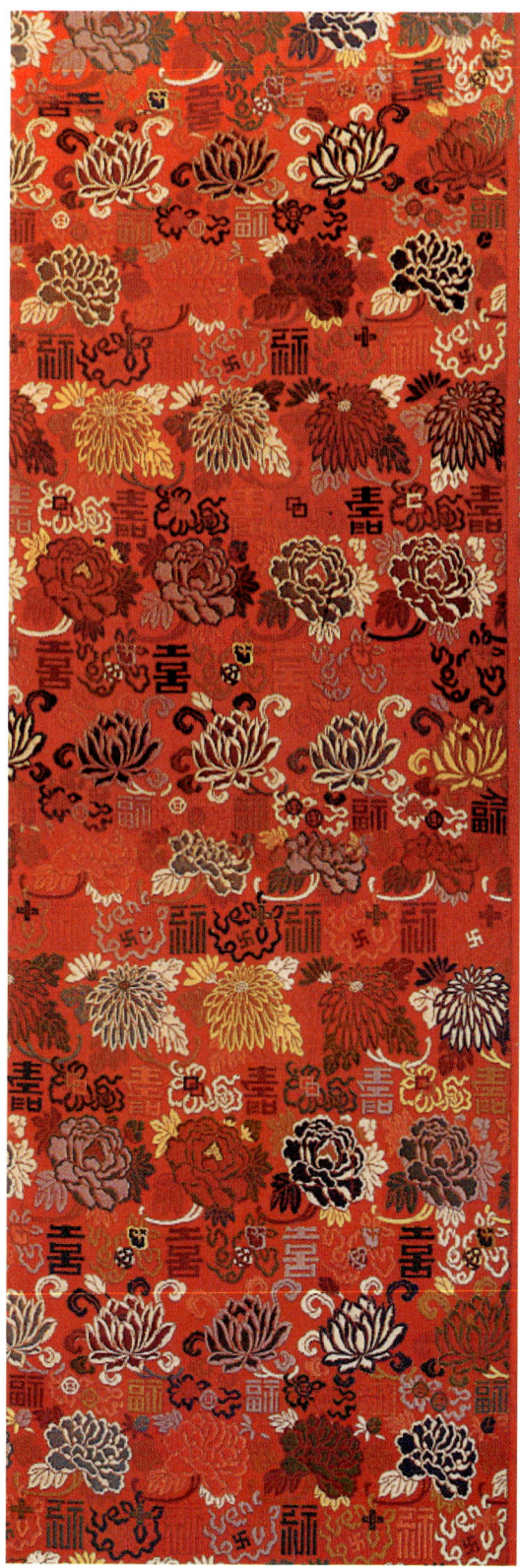

Buddhist wall panel, Varanasi

and religion. It is interesting to note that, although adults are strictly prohibited within the ghotul, the young do not run wild. They are brought up by their elders according to a strict code of values more stringent than in a boarding school.

Finery of the Marias

The Marias of Bastar have a distinct style of shringara. The girls spend hours massaging their skin with a paste made of turmeric and water that leaves the skin glowing gold and hairless. Their ornamentation is flowers—hibiscus in the hair, garlands of marigold around the waist, woven bands of coloured beads on the forehead and head, and rings on every finger. They wear a kind of mini sari tightly draped over the body and one shoulder, almost always white, that leaves the legs bare from knees downwards. The tribe is also known as the bison-horn Marias since the men who play the drums at weddings and festivals wear bison horns and a peacock feather headdress with a veil of cowrie shells.

Maria women make jewellery from indigenous materials like cane, glass, peacock feathers, wood, grass and beads. Often they adorn their long hair with wild flowers and leaves. In certain areas the women wear necklaces made of coins. A lot of jewellery is also made of metals like silver and bronze, crafted by the tribal metalsmith in elaborate and varied patterns, through techniques that have been passed down over generations. Jewellery is worn by both men and women, although different regions have their own unique styles and specifications. However, irrespective of the region it comes from, the ornaments are as distinctive as they are artistically creative.

The Beauty of the Banjaras

The western part of the country is home to a number of tribes among whom the Banjaras, a gypsy tribe, are known for their strong sense of community, freedom of spirit and rich folklore. Banjara women wear the *ghaghra*, a full-length skirt with bright borders embroidered with thick coloured thread. At the waist is a band decorated with traditional hand embroidery. The choli or blouse is also elaborately embroidered and decorated with mirrors and shells. The Banjara *odhni* or mantle traditionally used to cover the head is long enough to cascade over the shoulders and back until it almost touches the feet. A Banjara woman wears a profusion of ornaments—numerous bangles adorn her arms; her feet move to the sound of silver anklets; heavy earrings hang from her earlobes and shells and cowries find a place in her plaited hair. In addition there are necklaces, tikas for the forehead, tattoos and nose rings. She captures the very essence of shringara in all its throbbing, living vitality.

Telltale Tattoos

In Western India, the tattoo is a popular form of ornamentation amongst the Banjaras, Nath Yogis and Gadia Lohars of Rajasthan. Tattoos were believed to ward off evil spirits and it is interesting to see how, today, this form of body embellishment has lost its initial connotations and taken on an almost purely decorative value akin to mehndi. But amongst the tribal populations of the country, tatoos on the body are both ornamentation and symbols that represent the married state, the number of children and, of course, social status. For instance, a small mark on a boy's wrist, elbow or under the shoulder reveals his status as a milk-man.

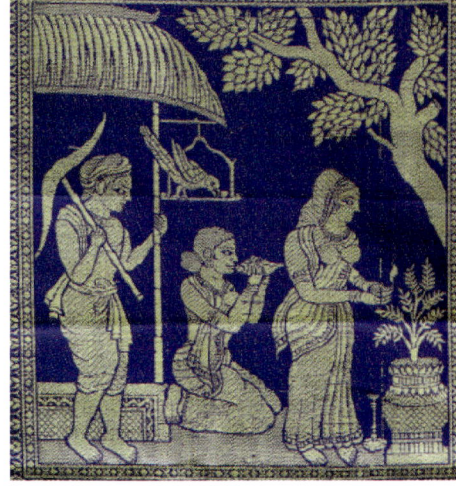

Baluchari sari, West Bengal. These usually depict scenes from the Ramayana

Until recently, Toda women in South India were tattooed in patterns of dots and circles as a sign of adulthood. Most Toda women also bear shoulder-to-shoulder girdles of tattoos in floral patterns that indicate the number of her husbands. As there are very few women amongst the Todas, a woman may have several husbands who are either real or clan brothers of the first man she marries. He is also the official father of all the children she bears.

Living Shringara

Ornaments, such as embellished hair combs, appear as love-tokens for the Juang tribe of Orissa. They also serve as symbols of marital status among the Muduvas of South India. Tribal costumes and ornaments are made from a wide range of materials like animal skin and fur, shells, cane, ivory, wood, and even monkey skulls. The latter are valuable for the power they are believed to possess and are worn only by a priest, a healer or perhaps a clan chief. Objects made of iron or cowrie shells are believed to protect the wearer from lightning and the evil eye. In earlier times, gold pendants with motifs of plants, rosettes and cowries were used even to decorate sacrificial buffalos.

A tribal tattoo design

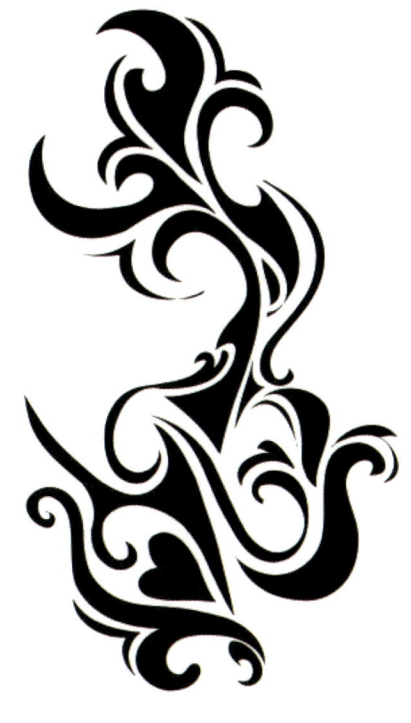

It is essentially in the lives of common people that one witnesses forms of unadulterated shringara as one sees how it is intertwined in the tribal ethos of the country. One realizes that it is in these spaces of 'living culture' that the 'real' notion of beauty operates intuitively, without ostentation or pretence—vibrant, real and with the mysterious simplicity to engage and enrich human existence.

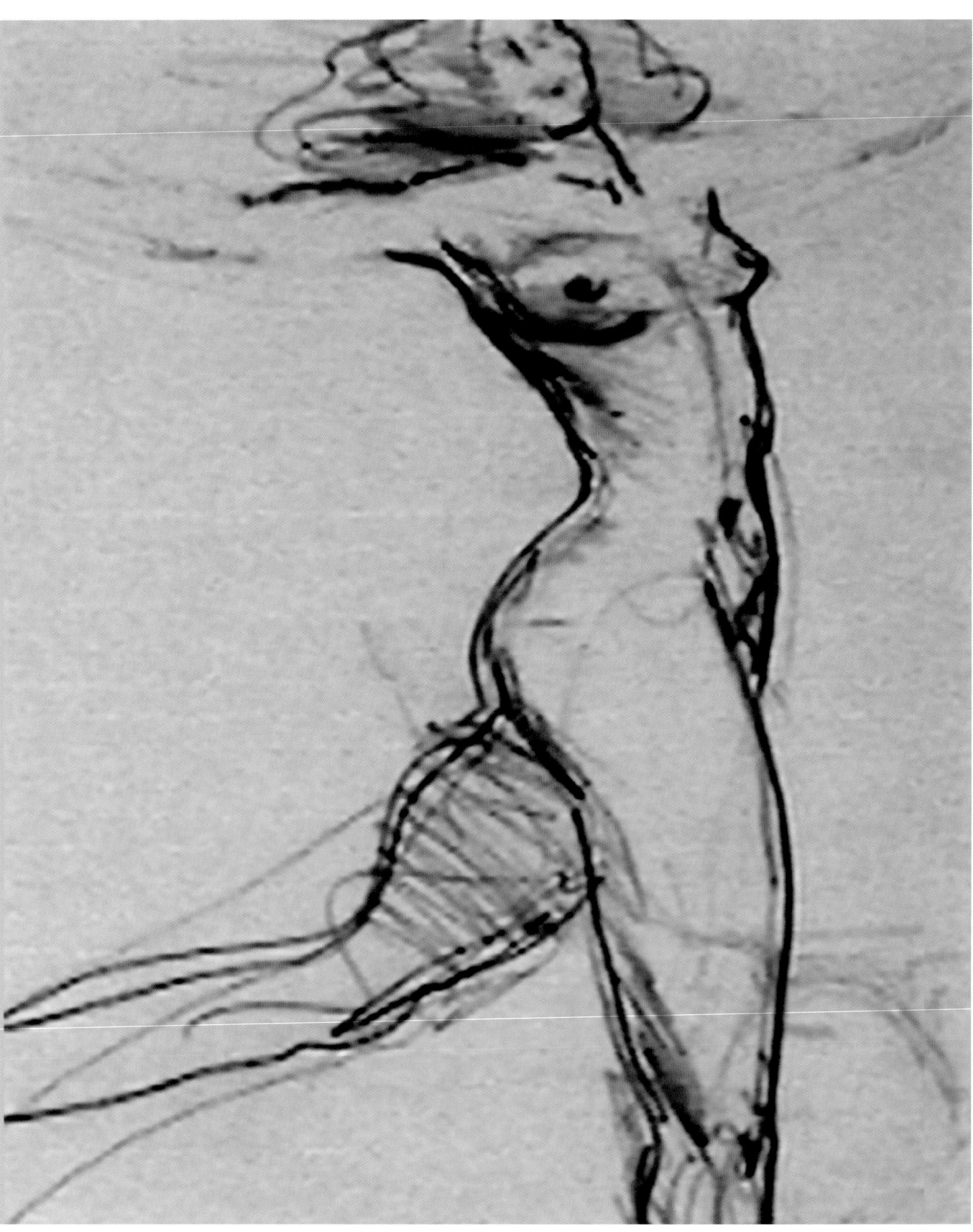

CHAPTER 12

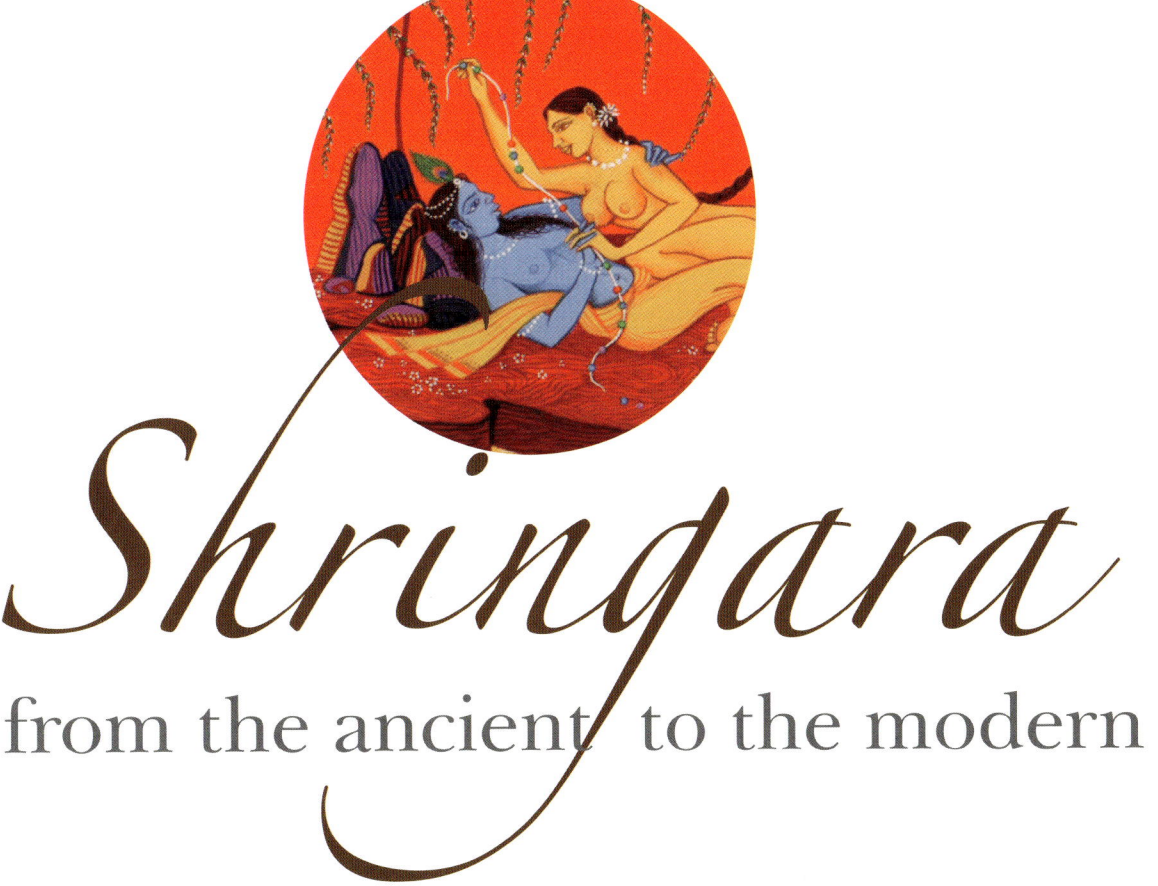

Shringara
from the ancient to the modern

*Beauty is not a need but an ecstasy
It is not a mouth thirsting nor an empty hand stretched forth.
But rather a heart enflamed and a soul enchanted
It is an image you see when you close your eyes
and a song you hear though you shut your ears.
It is not the sap within the furrowed bark
nor a wing attached to a claw.
But rather a garden forever in bloom
and a flock of angels in flight.
Beauty is life when life unveils her holy face
But you are life and you are the veil.
Beauty is eternity gazing at itself in a mirror
But you are eternity and you are the mirror.*

BEAUTY XXV, KHALIL GIBRAN

Nature and beauty share an extremely inclusive relationship, where one encompasses the other organically. However, over the years the patterns of beauty (saundarya, shringara) have evolved in tune with the modern concepts of physical and spiritual standards. It is the eye of the patron and the demands of society that have shaped the notions of beauty over the years. The evolution of art has followed the path of patronage, first received from the temple and village, to the court (durbar), and finally the artist as an individual following the dictates of the market.

The first patron of the arts was the temple. Beauty was worshipped in different forms—in dance performed to celebrate the gods and in rituals surrounding the daily routine of the deity. At the Jagannath Temple in Puri, for example, the tradition continues even today, although the temple dancers no longer dance for the gods.

Beauty Beyond the Physical

We have experienced how shringara goes beyond the physical. This is evident from the 10.8 cm-long bronze statue of the dancing girl from Mohenjodaro. The dancing girl has been a favourite of historians for her impeccable features and soulful expression and, most importantly, the confidence in her pose. The Harappans believed in the cult of the mother goddess, and the roots of the relationship between god and beauty can be traced from here.

The Kandariya Mahadev Temple at Khajuraho is an outstanding example of the beauty of representation, veracity, ardour and shringara. The spire is based on the metaphor of Mount Meru, the holy abode of Lord Shiva, and the exquisitely sculpted wall panels depict Lord Shiva and the apsaras. This is the height of idealized beauty, on the basis of which rest the canons of artistic representation.

Although the evolutionary thought processes of Eastern and Western philosophers and aestheticians share certain parameters of beauty, its representation in the West has notions of the sublime, of bliss, harmony, geometry and balance. In the Indian tradition, however, the definition of beauty is more complex because it has myriad manifestations: beauty as truth, as desire, as shringara or saundarya or as the union of the atma (soul) and parmatma (god).

Changing Patterns

The newer patrons of decorative fine arts and performing arts brought a change in the production and consumption of art. This was seen with the coming of the Central Asians and later, the establishment of the Mughal Empire. The advent

(Page 172)
Sketch by Shola Carletti

Mother Goddess from Mohenjodaro

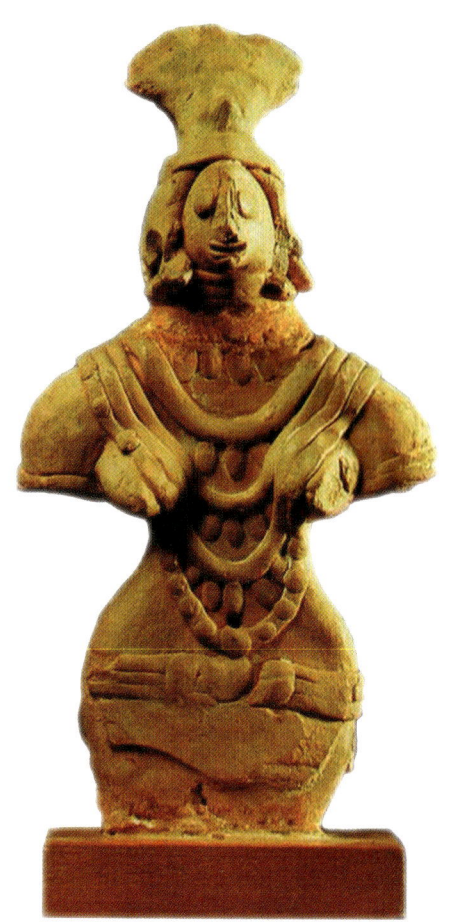

of Islam brought in a completely different insight of beauty, and shifted the focus from the idealized human figure to decorative symbols and forms. From the delicate *jalis* and *jharokhas* to the ornamented cloths studded with precious and semi-precious stones, the materials and forms started to undergo great change.

The cultural fabric became more challenging and dynamic as Islam settled into a primarily Hindu India. The 8th century saw the beginnings of a shared language that is reflected in literature, painting, sculpture, and costume. The synthesis of the Hindu and the Islamic is most evident in the architectural styles of the period. An especially charming example of this is the Adhai Din Ka Jhopda in Ajmer. Legend has it that the pavilion was built in two-and-a-half-days (*adhai din*). The relic of an old mosque and its ruined minarets blend perfectly with the building's screened façade, seven pointed arches and sculpted pillars.

Sketches of Life

The best example of Indo-Islamic architecture is perhaps Fatehpur Sikri, a city built by Emperor Akbar in the 16th century and representative of the tolerance and syncretism that typified that period of Indian history. The court encouraged painting and the miniature art form came into being. Important artists such as Basawan, Miskin and Mir Zafar created the most beautiful miniatures depicting animals, plants, court scenes, battles, and the life of women. Apart from being exquisitely beautiful in their execution, miniatures also give a vivid picture of the notions of beauty of the time, as they represent the patrons themselves, the kings and their subjects, local architecture, and different Islamic scripts.

The art of the miniature developed simultaneously in the courts of Rajasthan and slowly a fusion of the Mughal and indigenous styles of art and architecture began to be reflected in the palaces and paintings on the walls. Although the styles were similar, especially in painting, the content was vastly different: the Rajasthani schools of painting depicted a strong influence of the Hindu religious genre even when they dealt with the love play between Radha and Krishna.

Indian miniatures inspired the work of the Sri Lankan modernist painter George Keyt. He often paints nayikas in a simple unadorned style, very different from the painted women in the caves of Sigriya. The nayikas are romantic in the best sense of the term, not sentimental or cloying. They are delicate without being fragile. They represent all women in general and no woman in particular and bear witness to the traditions of shringara.

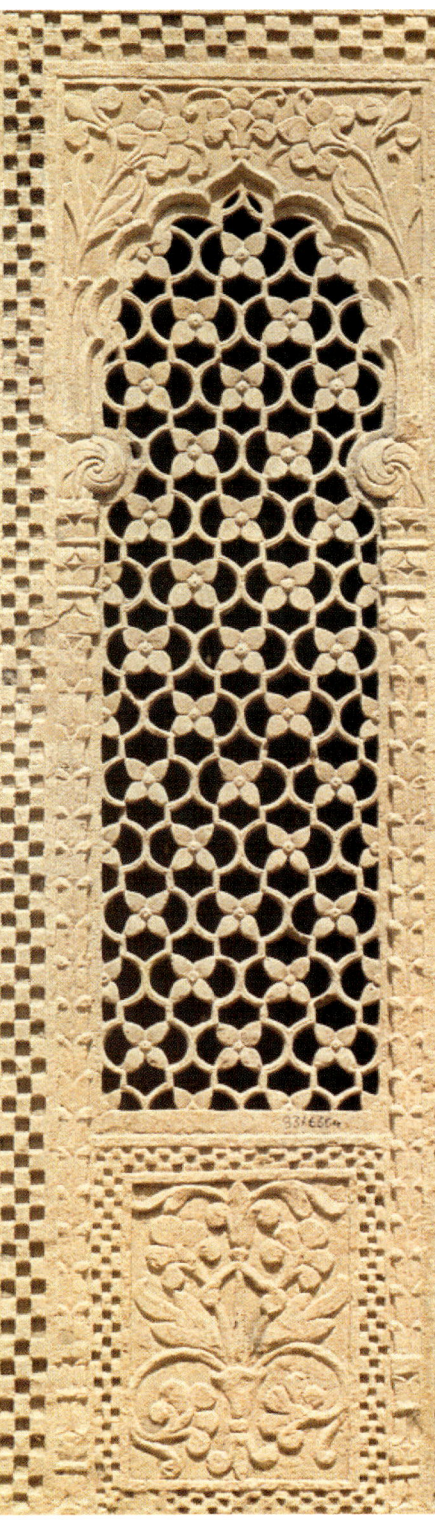

Sandstone jali, lattice work, 19th century, National Handicrafts and Handlooms Museum, New Delhi

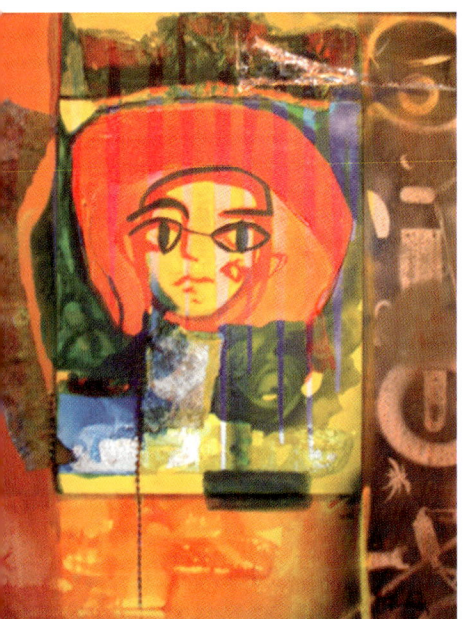

Painting by Brinda Miller

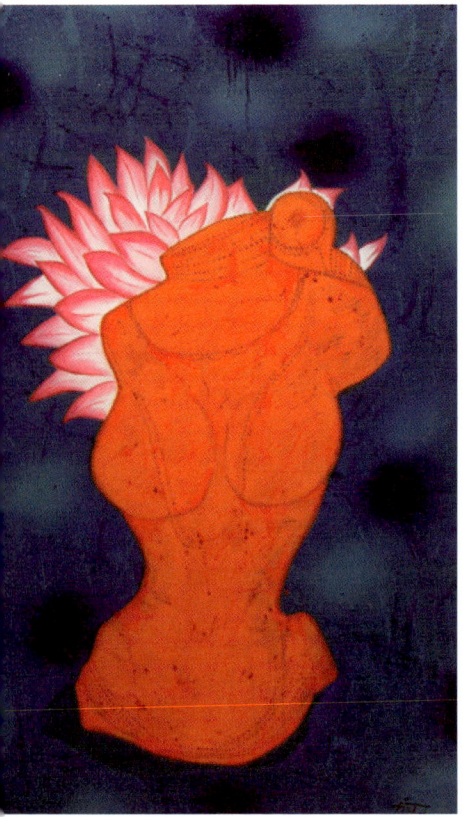

'Torso Allegro', painting by Kanchan Chander

The Pinnacle of Beauty

The Taj Mahal, considered the finest example of Mughal architecture, was built in a style that combined Indian, Persian and Turkish architecture. It exemplifies the fusion in art and architectural styles in the Mughal period, and the subsequent change in the perceptions of beauty and adornment. What sets the Taj apart is the element of romance the monument is associated with. While the white domed marble mausoleum is the most familiar part of the monument, the Taj Mahal displays myriad and complex design features: lotus decorations, shimmering walls of sheer white marble, intricate carvings and calligraphy, onion domes supported on cylindrical bases called drums, decorative sculpted panels (*dados*) lining the lower walls, *guldastas* or decorative spires, *chattris*, and arches… all of which combine to create an immortal beauty.

European Influence

The coming of the Europeans led to further changes. The first colonial settlement was established by the Portuguese in 1498 when Vasco da Gama discovered a new sea route and navigated his way into India. Soon the Portuguese made inroads into Goa. The Indian subcontinent, for the first time, saw churches and chapels. People were introduced to differently tailored attire. The Dutch who, arguably, created the first multinational company in the world followed the Portuguese, with the Dutch East India Company in Masulipatnam and the Malabar Coast. The French came later and their distinct influence continues to be seen in Pondicherry. With the Battle of Plassey in 1857, the British East India Company established its supremacy in the subcontinent. Thus the influence of baroque art was seen in Company art and in the architecture of churches and government buildings in Calcutta and Bombay.

Re-affirming Indian Ideals

With the growth of Indian nationalism the concepts of shringara became charged with its ideals based on the making of a new Indian identity. One of the first revolutionaries in Indian art, Rabindranath Tagore—poet, novelist, musician and playwright—reshaped Bengali literature and music in the late 19th and early 20th centuries He won the 1913 Nobel Prize for Literature for his *Gitanjali* – a song of offering.

In 1901, Rabindranath Tagore founded Shantiniketan where he started a school modelled on the ancient gurukul system. After he received the Nobel Prize the school was expanded into a university and renamed Visva Bharati, which, in the words of the founder, was 'where the world makes a home in a nest'. The aim of this educational institution was the quest for truth, blending the methods of learning of both the East and West. Tagore modernized Bengali art by turning away from rigid classical forms. His novels, stories, songs, dance-dramas and essays spoke of political and personal topics.

Among Tagore's best-known works are *Gitanjali*, *Gora* and *Ghare-Baire* (The Home and the World). His verse, short stories and novels were acclaimed for their lyricism, naturalism, and contemplation. Tagore also penned the national anthems of India and Bangladesh: *Jana Gana Mana* and *Amar Shonar Bangla*.

The Spirit of Freedom
After India's independence, the Progressive Art Group, led by F.N. Souza, S.H. Raza, M.F. Husain and Tyeb Mehta, among others, pioneered an important art movement. Human figuration once again became the central point of focus, and artistic independence gained fervour and momentum. The artists combined Indian subject matter with Post-Impressionist colours, Cubist forms and brusque Expressionistic styles. The group wished to encourage an Indian avant-garde, engaged at an international level. Their intention was to 'paint with absolute freedom for content and technique'. Although they worked under the umbrella of Western modernism, each of its members had uniquely different styles, from the Expressionism of Souza to specific Indian imagery and landscapes adopted by Mehta and Husain.

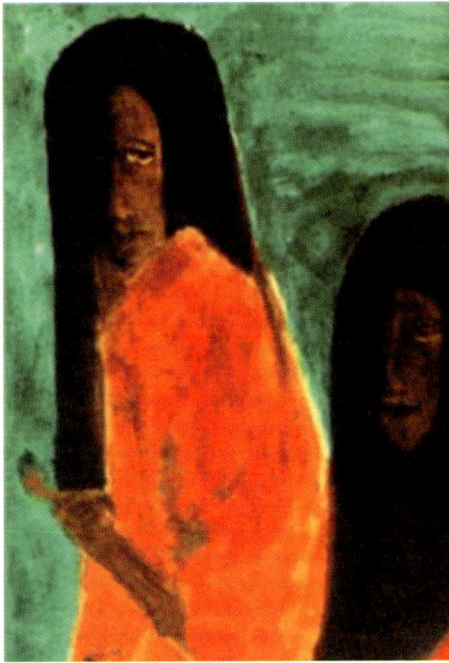

'Two women', ink and pastel, painting by Rabindranath Tagore

S.H. Raza ventured into spiritual abstraction, a move that was distinctly distant from figurative art. Raza's works are mainly abstracts in oil or acrylic, with a very rich use of colour, replete with icons from Indian cosmology as well as its philosophy. He was soon joined by J. Swaminathan and V.S. Gaitonde who experimented hugely with form and shape in his work. His wraith-like and multifaceted paintings invoke a concealed and obscure description of the real world. His paintings have the power to transform simple objects into spiritual elements. On the other hand, simplicity is the main feature of J. Swaminathan's paintings. The vivid imagery and bright colours are a celebration of the rise of the inner being over the commonplace. He was also influenced by tribal art, which led to the use of symbiology in his work.

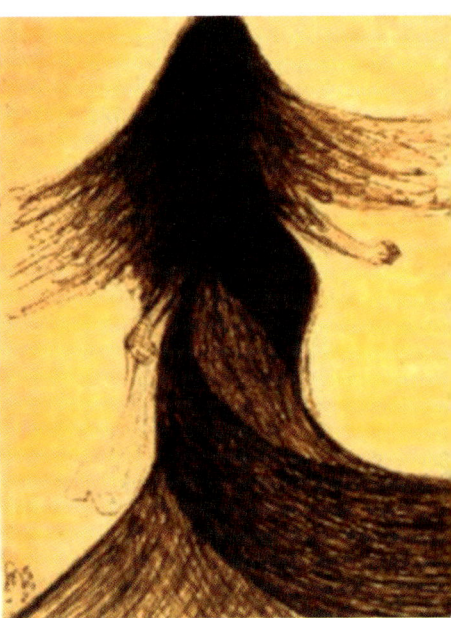

Painting by Rabindranath Tagore

The Modern Voices
Religious themes, love legends and tantra art soon gave way to societal, autobiographical, political and gendered themes in contemporary Indian art. The artists gained confidence as their views were accepted and applauded. This led to contemporary artists becoming conscious of their own cultural identity in the face of globalization, thus the subtle shifts in the progression of the representation of beauty. This is especially predominant in the works of Nilima Sheikh, who portrays the unsettling reality of contemporary life through

an amalgam of traditional idioms, and Rekha Rodwittiya and Anupam Sood who have consistently dealt with the problem of representing the female form in subtle and sensual ways. The late Meera Mukherjee, one of India's finest sculptors, documented the life of the common people, their music and dance.

Atul Dodiya's realistic works are subtly nuanced to provide a reflective medium to middle-class life, as well as political themes and issues of violence in contemporary India. Vivan Sundaram has been consistent in his pursuit of a politically-honed art, and Ravinder Reddy fuses the Hindu sculptural tradition with a contemporary pop sensibility. He also reflects the way young Indian women are recreating the feminine image, recognizing tradition while still being a part of the contemporary world. Subodh Gupta is known for incorporating everyday objects such as steel buckets, tiffin boxes and utensils. He uses these in his enormous sculptural work to reflect the economic changes in India and relates them to his own personal experiences. His partner, Bharti Kher, uses the bindi to adorn her art. Her work associates with identity through consumer culture, gender and race.

Digital Creations

Beauty is being encompassed through the mediums of video, photography and film. The digital media has brought its own aesthetics to art. From black and white to colour, from air brushing to Photoshop, digital art has reached a pinnacle in its journey of development. The journey includes the whole gamut from Lala Deen Dayal's photographic documentation of India's erstwhile royals in detailed portraiture, to Raghu Rai and Atul Bhalla's work depicting Indian social and political issues.

Veteran artist M.F. Husain has directed films such as *Gajagamini* and *Meenaxi: A Tale of Three Cities*. Both films have shared the screen with the more popular Bollywood films. These are but a few of the many manifestations and representations of beauty and its changing perceptions over the years.

The Performing Arts

The advent of modernism can be seen in the performing arts too. From their origins as temple dances, Bharatanatyam, Kathak and Odissi have adapted their art to perform for a secular audience.

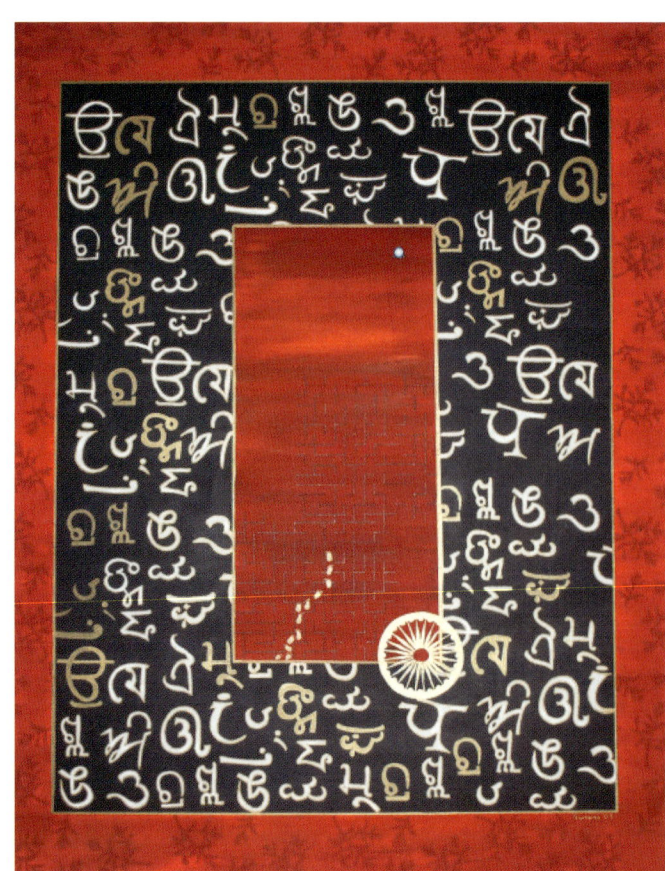

'Sighting', painting by Sunaina Bhalla

178 *Shringara*—the many faces of Indian beauty

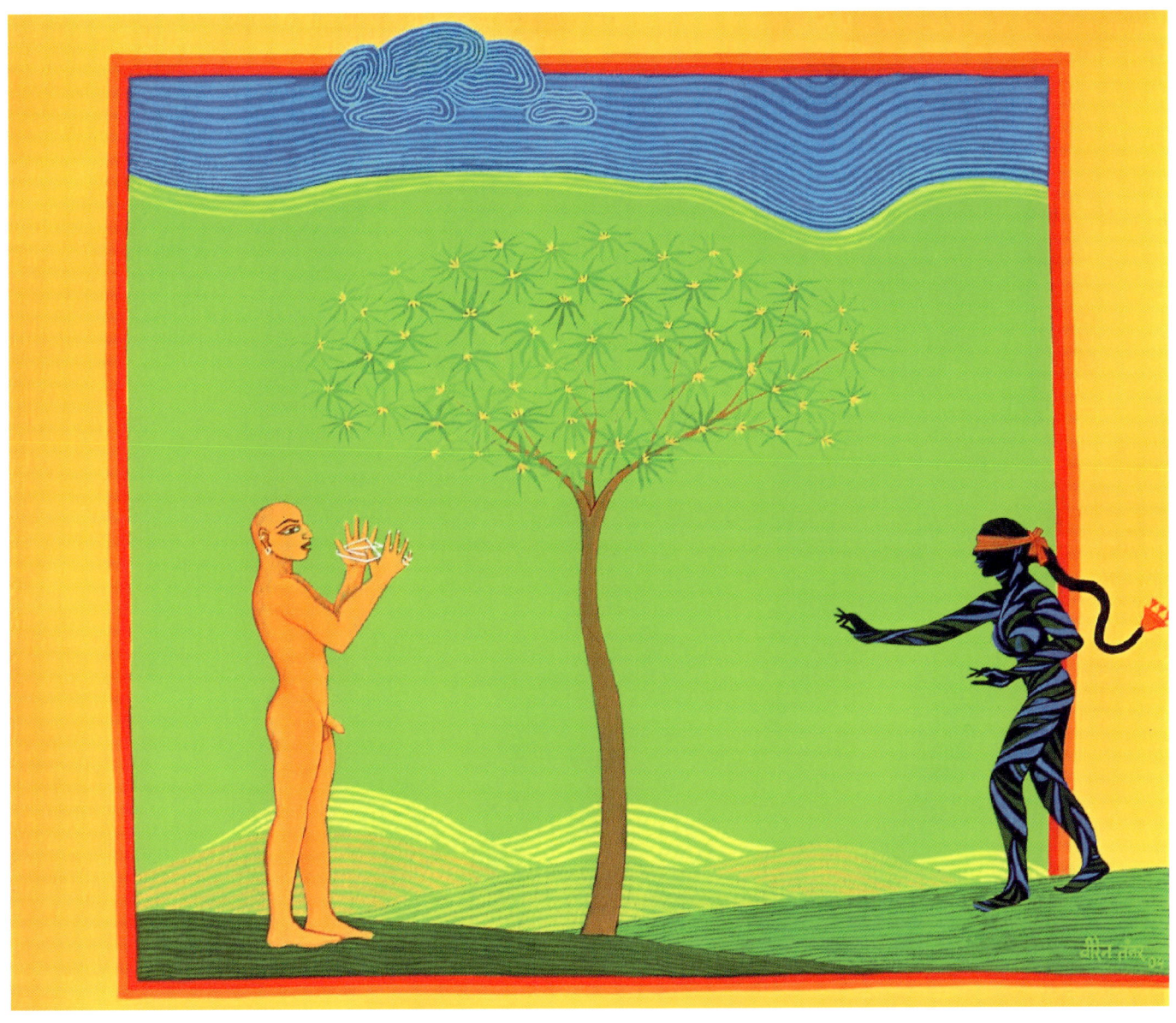

*'And We Played On',
painting by Viren Tanwar*

Today, the performances of courtesans or nautch girls have almost entirely disappeared from the stage, but classical dance performances draw full houses, continuing the traditions of the past into modern day India. The accompanying music too, vocal and instrumental, has evolved to keep pace with the dance. The classical dance we see today retains traces of temple and ritual dances and the influence of the Bhakti movement. However, accomplished dancers like Birju Maharaj, Keluchoran Mohapatra, Sanjukta Panigrahi, Leela Samson, Uma Sharma and Madhavi Mudgal have interpreted beauty in their own language. Dancers like Aditi Mangaldas and Daksha Sheth have experimented by combining Indian classical dance with Sufi thought and contemporary Western movements.

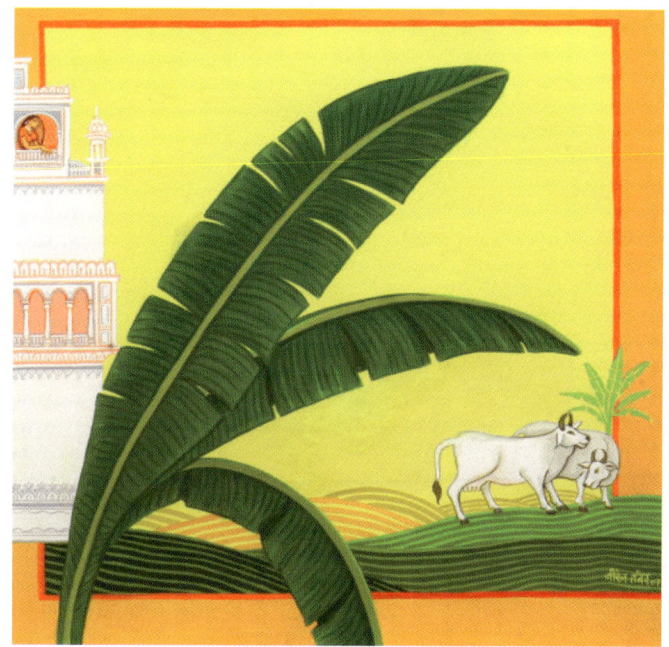
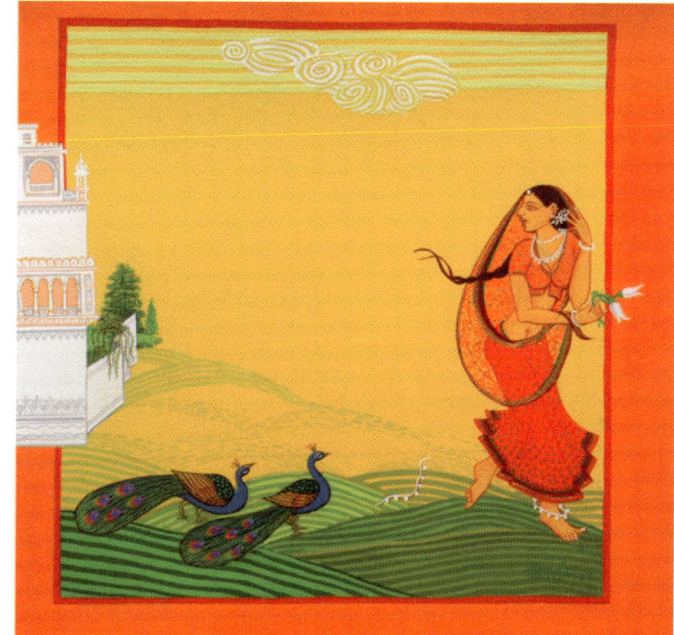

'The Eternal Wait', a series of paintings by Viren Tanwar

Indian classical music, Hindustani as well as Carnatic, has also evolved enormously. Traditional ragas have been combined with the works of contemporary Western composers to create the most beautiful fusion pieces. Pioneers in this 'new music' have been Pandit Ravi Shankar, jazz guitarist John McLaughlin, music composer Philip Glass, tabla maestro Zakir Hussain and the jazz composer Jan Garbarek. They have even experimented by merging cultural boundaries with artists like Nalini Malani who now focusses on video art, the painter Chitra Ganesh, and writers Vikram Seth and Salman Rushdie.

Shared Space

As opposed to the aesthetics discussed in *Natyashastra*, artistic expression in the contemporary world seems to be based on no fixed norms and, even those limited rules that can be said to exist, are consistently violated. Many artists have defied all known definitions and limits, branching out into new and brave areas of artistic exploration like the New Media that integrates digital technology, the Internet, and other traditionally-conflicting areas.

The Indian legacy of aesthetics, however, remains an invaluable resource and inspiration for all artists. In a world torn by the conflicting pulls of economic mergers and cultural exchanges, *Natyashastra*, with its emphasis on integrated experience, becomes all the more relevant. While there is always space for innovation, the simultaneous importance of shared aesthetics and holistic human experience should not be undermined.

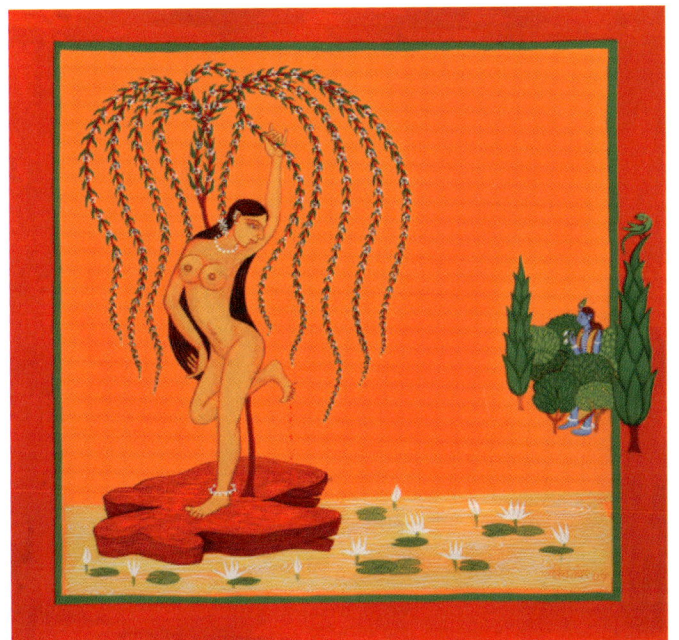 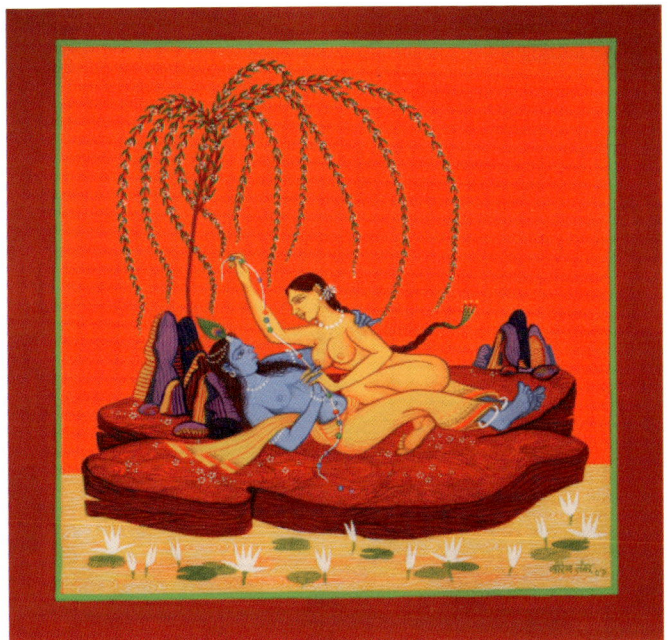

The flower children movement of the sixties also left a distinct mark on society, and many aspects of hippie culture have been assimilated into the mainstream. The religious and cultural diversity espoused by the hippies has gained widespread acceptance, and Eastern art and philosophy has reached a wider audience.

The New Language for Shringara

Today, the cultural diversity of India faces the pulls and pressures of tradition and modernity, rural and urban, folk and classical, and most importantly, local and global. Shringara, too, faces the challenges of perception where the beauty of adornment and the beauty of ugliness are two sides of the same coin. In fact, both these notions represent a tarnished mirror which will reflect the truth when polished. In his book *On Ugliness*, Umberto Eco asks: Just as Beauty lies in the eyes of the beholder, is repulsiveness, too, in the eyes of the beholder? Yet, in his analysis, the intentionally disharmonious can be anointed as a thing of beauty.

This is a time to ask important questions on the concept of beauty: Has the morphology of the old nayika been given up for more westernized perceptions? Has there been an Indian renaissance apart from the path-breaking initiatives of A.K. Coomaraswamy and Rabindranath Tagore? Who are the new patrons of Indian art? Is it the growing tribe of Indian art collectors within the country and abroad, the Indian media and larger public, or the growing number of private museums, that are the vibrant art market for contemporary Indian art? And finally, will our local and ancient traditions survive the onslaught of globalization? Do we simply venerate shringara as a holy relic of the past? Or will we have the courage to establish a new language for shringara?

Glossary

abhinaya	acting	*navina*	new/ later
advaita	oneness/ non-duality	*nayika*	heroine/ beloved
alekhya	indefinable	*niras*	devoid of emotions
ananda(m)	beatitude/ joy	*padma*	lotus
anantam	infinite	*paramatma*	supreme soul
anumana	thoughtful inference	*parampara*	tradition
arpana	offering	*prakriti*	nature
artha	material means	*pratibha*	creativity/ talent
atma(n)	being/ self	*pratyaksha*	contemplative perception
besan	gram flour	*prayojana*	goal
bhajan	devotional songs	*prem*	love
bhakti	worship/ devotion	*purusha*	being
bhava	emotional state of being	*purushartha*	aim of life
chakra	revolving wheel	*rachna*	texture
chamatkara	miracle	*rang*	colour
chitra	painted image	*rasa*	taste/ flavour/ emotive juice
dampati	married couple	*rasavadana*	tasting of flavour
dharma	religious duties	*rekha*	line
dholaka	drum	*rishi*	seer
dhvani	poetic resonance/ sound	*rupa*	form
durbar	court	*sahridaya*	similar heart
ektara	single stringed instrument	*sahridayata*	selfless sympathy
garbhini	pregnant woman	*sangha*	union
ghungroo	ankle bells	*sangita*	music
goti	footwork in dance	*santam*	silence
guldasta	decorative spires	*sants*	poetic saints
guru	teacher	*sat*	truth
hamsa	swan	*saundarya*	beauty
haveli	palace	*sawan*	rainy season
hridaya	heart	*shabda*	sound
kama	desire	*shadanga*	six canons
kamar	waist	*shakti*	power
karuna	pathos	*shilpi*	sculpture
kausala	skill	*shunyata*	emptiness
kavya	poetry/ literature	*sivam*	goodness
khadaun	wooden slippers	*sukha*	happiness
khartal	wooden cymbals with strings	*sundaram*	beauty
kunda	altar-hearth	*svara*	tone
langala	spade	*tala*	beat
lavanya	grace	*tantric*	ritualistic
laya	rhythm	*vastu*	architecture
lingam	phallus	*yoni*	female sexual organ
lokachara	public morality		
mahasukha	great happiness		
maithuna	sexual act		
maya	illusion		
moksha	final liberation/ salvation		
mudra	hand gestures		
muni	seer		
nada	sound		
natya	dance/ drama		

Bibliography

General

- *Academic American Encyclopedia By Grolier Incorporated*, USA: Grolier Incorporated, 1994.
- Barlingay, S.S. *A Modern Introduction to Indian Aesthetic Theory: The Development from Bharata to Jagannatha*, New Delhi: D.K. Printworld, 2007.
- Board of Scholars. *The Natya Shastra of Bharatamuni*, New Delhi: Sri Satguru Publications, 2000.
- Bharatamuni. Second revised edition, in Manmohan Ghosh (tr.) *Natyashastra*, Baroda: G.O.S., 1956.
- Chākyār, Māni Mādhava. *Nātyakalpadrumam*, New Delhi: Sangeet Natak Academi, 1975.
- Danielou, Alain. *Virtue, Success, Pleasure & Liberation*, Vermont, USA: Inner Traditions / Bear & Company, 1993.
- Doniger W. *Splitting the Difference: Gender and Myth in Ancient Greece and India Hindu Myths:* A Sourcebook Translated from the Sanskrit, Chicago: University of Chicago Press, 1999.
- Doniger O'Flaherty, Wendy. *Karma and Rebirth in Classical Indian traditions*, Berkeley: University of California Press, 1980.
- Gandhi, M.K. *Hind Swaraj*, Ahmedabad: Navjivan, 1998.
- Gupta, Shyamala. *Art, Beauty and Creativity: Indian and Western Aesthetics*, New Delhi: D.K. Printworld, 1999.
- Hegel. *Hegel's Introduction to 'Aesthetics'*, USA: Oxford University Press, 1979.
- Hegel. *Philosophy of Art*, New York: Prometheus Books; Reprint edition, 1990.
- Hiriyana, M. *Art Experience*, Mysore: Kaivalya Publicaions, 1954.
- Hiriyanna, M. *The Essentials of Indian Philosophy*, London: Diamond Books, 1996.
- Hospers, John. *The Sense Of Beauty: Introductory Readings in Aesthetics*, University of Southern California: The Free Press New York, 1969.
- Nandy, Ashis. 'Cultural Frames for Social Intervention: A Personal Credo', *Indian Philosophical Quarterly*, 11 (4): 411–421, October 1984.
- Nanyadev. *Bharat Bhashsya*, Khairagarh Edition.
- Rao, Raja. *The Meaning of India*, New Delhi: Vision Books, 1997.
- Rege, M.P. 'Svaraj in Ideas and Hind Swaraj Reconsidered', *New Quest*, 143: 65-91, January–March, 2001.

- Shah, Ramesh Chandra. *Ancestral Voices: Four Lectures Towards a Philosophy of Imagination*, London: The Temenos Academy, 2001.
- Subhāshitāvali. *An Anthology of Comic, Erotic and Other Verse*, India: Penguin Books India, 2007.
- Randacharya, Adya. *The Natyasastra, English Translation with Critical Notes*, New Delhi: Munishiram Manoharlal Publishers Pvt Ltd, 1996.
- V. Raghavan. (ed.). *Bhoja's Sringara Prakasa*, Chennai: The Theosophical Society, 1966.
- Wangu, Madhu Bazaz. *Images of Indian Goddesses: Myths, Meanings and Models*, Pune: Abhinav Publications, 2003.

Kavya—beauty in verse
- Basham, A.L. *The Wonder that was India: A Study of the History and Culture of the Indian Sub-continent Before the Coming of the Muslims*, UK: Hawthorn Books, 1963.
- Bhatnagar, Ved. *Shringar the Rasraj: A Classical Indian View*, Pune: Abhinav Publications, 2004.
- Bhatnagar, M.K. *The Poetry of A.K. Ramanujan*, New Delhi: Atlantic Publications, 2002.
- Desai, Rakesh. *W.H. Auden's Poetry: The Quest for Love*, New Delhi: Atlantic Publications, 2004.
- Herman, A.L. *An Introduction to Indian Thought*, New Jersey: Prentice-Hall, 1976.
- Joshi, Natwar Lal. *Poetry Creativity and Aesthetic Experience (Sanskrit Poetics and Literary Criticism)*, New Delhi: Eastern Book Linkers, 1994.
- Kapoor, Subodh. *An Introduction to Classical Indian Literature*, New Delhi: Cosmo, 2003.
- Kinsley, David R. *The Sword and the Flute: Kali & Krsna: Dark Visions of the Terrible and the Sublime in Hindu Mythology*, New Delhi: Motilal Banarsidass, 1995.
- Mittapalli, Rajeshwar and Piciucco, Pier Paolo. *Kamala Das: A Critical Spectrum*, New Delhi: Atlantic Publications, 2001.
- Rahman, Anisur. *Expressive Form in the Poetry of Kamala Das*, Pune: Abhinav Publications, 1987.
- Sahu, Nandini. *Recollection as Redemption: A Study in the Poetry of Jayanta Mahapatra, A.K. Ramanujan, R. Parthasarathy and Kamala Das*, New Delhi: Authors Press, 2004.
- Sadarangani, Neeti M. *Bhakti Poetry in Medieval India: Its Inception, Cultural Encounter and Impact*, New Delhi: Sarup and Sons, 2004.

- Sharma, Raghu Nath. *Bhakti in the Vaisnava Rasa-sastra*, New Delhi: Pratibha Prakashan, 1996.
- Thielemann, Selina. *Rasalila: A Musical Study of Religious Drama in Vraja*, New Delhi: APH Publishing, 1998.
- Warder, A.K. *Indian Kavya Literature : Vol. III. The Early Medieval Period (Sudraka to Visakhadatta)*, (Reprint), New Delhi: Motilal Banarsidass, 1990.

Kama—the erotic

- Anand, Mulk Raj & Dane, Lance (eds). *Kama Sutra of Vatsayana*, Ukraine: Aspect Publications, 1991.
- Anand, Mulk Raj. *Kama Kala: Some Notes on the Philosophical Basis of Hindu Erotic Sculpture*, New York: Lyle Stuart, 1962.
- Basu, M. *Kama Sutra Knowledge For Men Wisdom For Women*, New Delhi: Roli Books, 2005.
- Bose, Brinda and Bhattacharya, Subhabrata. (ed.). *The Phobic and the Erotic—The Politics of Sexualities in Contemporary India*, London: Seagull Books, 2007.
- Bhattacharyya, N.N. *History of Indian Erotic Literature*, New Delhi: Munshiram Manoharlal Publishers, 1975.
- Chopra, Tarun. *Kamasutra: World's Oldest Treatise On Sex*, New Delhi: Prakash Publications, 2006.
- Chopra, D. *Kama Sutra*, USA: Virgin Books, 2006.
- Dane, Lance. *The Complete Illustrated Kama Sutra*, Vermont: Inner Traditions. 2003.
- Daniélou, A. *The Complete Kama Sutra: The First Unabridged Modern Translation of the Classic Indian Text*, Vermont: Inner Traditions. 1993.
- Doniger O'Flaherty, Wendy. *Asceticism and Eroticism in the Mythology of Siva*, USA: Oxford University Press, 1973.
- Ellis, Albert. *The Folklore of Sex*, New York: Grove Press, 1961.
- Ferrero, Carlo Scipione. *Eros: An Erotic Journey through the Senses*, New York: Crescent Books, 1988.
- Hooper, Anne. *The Kama Sutra*, India: Dorling Kindersley Publishers Ltd, 2000.
- Kakar, S. *Ecstasy and The Ascetic of Desire*, New Delhi: Viking-Penguin, 2001.
- Kulshreshtha S. *Erotics in Sanskrit & English Literature-I Kalidasa & Shakespeare*, New Delhi: Eastern Books, 1997.
- Kulshreshtha, Sushma. *Kumarasambhava-Kamakelisati: Enjoyment of Bliss in Kumarasambhava: Erotica India*, New Delhi: Sanjay Prakashan, 2007.

- McConnachie, J. *The Book Of Love: In Search of the Kamasutra*, New Delhi: Atlantic Books, 2007.
- Mishra, Prafulla K. *Ethics, Erotics and Aesthetics*, New Delhi: Pratibha Prakashan, 2004.
- Mulchandani, S. *Erotic Literature of Ancient India: Kama Sutra, Koka Shastra, Gita Govindam, Ananga Ranga*, New Delhi: Roli Books, 2006.
- Mulchandani, S. *Kama Sutra For Women*, New Delhi: Roli Books, 2004.
- Norton, B. (ed.). *The Kama Sutra: The Erotic Essence of India*, Israel: Astrolog Publishing House, 2001.
- Pande, A. *Indian Erotica*, New Delhi: Roli Books, 2001.
- Pande, A. *The New Age Kama Sutra for Women,* Noida: Brijbasi Art Press, 2006.
- Pinkney, Andrea Marion. *The Kama Sutra Illuminated: Erotic Art of India*, New York: Harry N. Abrams, 2002.
- Saili, G. *Kama Sutra Feminine Pleasures*, New Delhi: Roli Books, 2006.
- Sinha, Indra. *The Love Teachings of Kama Sutra: With Extracts from Koka Shastra, Ananga Ranga and Other Famous Indian Works on Love by Vātsyāyana*, Castlewood: Hamlyn, 1980. Original from the University of Michigan.
- Varma, Pavan K & Mulchandani, S. *Love and Lust—An Anthology of Erotic Literature from Ancient and Medieval India*, New Delhi: Harper Collins, 2004.
- Doniger, W., Kakar, S. (tr.). Vatsyayana, M. *Kamasutra*, USA: Oxford University Press, 2002.
- Sinha, Indra. (Tr.) Vātsyāyana. *The Love Teachings of Kama Sutra: With Extracts from Koka Shastra, Ananga Ranga and Other Famous Indian Works on Love*, Castlewood: Hamlyn, 1980.

Chitra—lines of pleasure
- Behl, Benoy K. *The Ajanta Caves: Ancient Paintings of Buddhist India*, New York: Thames and Hudson; 2005.
- Kamboj, B.P. *Early Wall Painting of Garhwal*, New Delhi: Indus, 2003.
- Sivaramamurti, C. *Chitrasalas, Ancient Indian Art Galleries*, Triveni Vol VII No. 2.
- Sivaramamurti, C. 'Note on the Paintings at Tirumalaipuram', *Journal of the Indian Society of Oriental Art.*
- Sivaramamurti, C. *Vijayanagar Paintings from Temple at Lepakshi*, Madras.
- Coomaraswamy, Ananda K. *Nagara Painting*, Rupam, 1929.
- Coomaraswamy, Ananda K. *Arts of Transitional India, 20th Century*, Maharashtra: Popular Prakashan, 1988.

- Dehejia, Harsha. *Parvatidarpana: An Exposition of Kasmir Saivism through the Images of Siva and Parvati*, New Delhi: Motilal Banarasidass, 1977.
- Dwivedi, Prem Shankar. *Durga—Theme in Varanasi Wall Paintngs*, New Delhi: Vedam Books, 1993.
- Mukhopadhyay, Amit (ed.). *A. Ramachandran: Portfolio Prints*, New Delhi: Lalit Kala Akademi, 2002.
- Grunwedel, Albert. *Buddhist Art in India* (Reprint), New Delhi: Asian Educational Services, 1999.
- Goetz, H. *The Neglected Aspects of Ajanta Art*, Mumbai: Marg, Vol II.
- Burgess, J. *Notes on the Buddha Rock Temples of Ajanta, their paintings and sculptures and on the paintings on the Bagh Caves*, Bombay: Archaeological Survey of India, 1879.
- Jerath, Ashok. *Dogra Legends of Art and Culture*, New Delhi: Vedam Books, 1998.
- K.H. Vakil. *At Ajanta*, Bombay, 1929.
- Srinivasan, K.R. *South Indian Paintings, Proceedings of the Indian Historical Congress*, 1944.
- Lal, B.B. *Rock Paintings of Central India Archaeology in India*, New Delhi, 1950.
- Mookerjee, Ajit. *Indian Primitive Art*, Oxford Book and Stationery Co., 1959.
- Ghosh, M. *Rock Paintings and other antiquities of pre-historic and later times Memoirs of the Archaeological Survey of India*, Govt. of India Central Publication Branch, 1932.
- Agarwal, O.P. and Rashmi Pathak. *Examination and Conservation of Wall Paintings: A Manual*, New Delhi: Sundeep Prakashan, 2001.
- Pathy, Dinanath. *Essence of Orrisan Paintings*, New Delhi: Harman Publishing House, 2001.
- Rawson, Philip S. *Indian Painting*, Paris: P. Tisne, 1961.
- Singh, Kishore. *Shekhawati: Painted Townships*, New Delhi: Cross Section Publications, 1995.
- Soulie, Bernard. *Tantra: Erotic Figures in Indian Art*, London: Miller Graphics, 1982.
- Tagore, Abanindranath. *Sadanga or Six Limbs of Painting Modern Review*, Calcutta: Indian Society of Oriental Art, 1921.

Shilpa Shastra—adornment in stone
- Begde, Prabhakar V. *Living Sculpure: Classical Indian Culture as Depicted in Sculpture & Literature*, New Delhi: Sagar Publications, 1996.
- Berkson, Carmel. *Life of Form in the Indian Sculpture*, New Delhi: Abhinav Publications, 2000.

- Berkson, Carmel. *Ellora,* New Delhi: Abhinav Publication, 1992.
- Boner, Alice. *Principles of Composition of Hindu Sculpture,* E.J. South Asia Books; First edition, 1990.
- Elisofon, Eliot and Alan Watts. *The Temple of Konarak: Erotic Spirituality,* London: Thames and Hudson, 1971.
- Kramrisch, Stella. *The Hindu Temple,* Calcutta: University of Calcutta, vols. I and II., 1946.
- Kramrisch, Stella. 'The Temple as Puruṣa', *Studies in Indian Temple Architecture,* ed. Pramod Chandra, Banaras: American Institute of Indian Studies, 1975.
- Morley, Grace. *Indian Sculptures,* New Delhi: Roli Books, 2005.
- Mitchell, George. *The Hindu Temple,* Chicago and London: The University of Chicago Press, 1988.
- Ohri, Vishwa. *Sculpture of Western Himalayas,* New Delhi: Agam Kala Prakashan, 1991.
- Randhava, Mohinder. *Indian Sculptures,* Vzkil Feffers And Simons Ltd. 1985.
- Rawson, Philip, David James and Richard Lane. *Erotic Art of the East: The Sexual Theme in Oriental Painting and Sculpture,* London: Minerva, 1973.
- Rawson, Philip, *Indian Sculpture,* New York: E.P. Dutton & Co., 1966.
- Varadpande, M.L. *Woman in Indian Sculpture,* New Delhi: Abhinav Publication, 2006.

Sangeet—food for the soul
- Balasubramaniam, K. *Rig-a Two-in-One Marvel: (Raga Identification/Pancharatna Kritis),* Chennai: K. Balasubramaniam, 2005.
- Brahaspati, Dr. K C Dev. *Bharat ka Sangeet Siddhant,* Lucknow: Publishing Division, 1959.
- Bahadur, Krishna P. *Mira Bai and her Padas/Translated into English verse,* 1998.
- Devi, Ratan and Ananda K. Coomaraswamy. *Thirty Songs from the Panjab and Kashmir.* Revised new edition/edited by Premlata Sharma, 1994.
- Dey, Ananya Kumar. *Nyasa in Raga: The Pleasant Pause in Hindustani Music,* New Delhi: Kanishka Publishers, 2008.
- Dey, Suresh Chandra. *Quest for Music Divine,* New Delhi: APH Publishers, 1990.
- Mahajan, Anupam. *Ragas in Hindustani Music: Conceptual Aspects,* New Delhi: Gyan, 2001.
- Misra, Susheela. *Among Contemporary Musicians,* New Delhi: Harman Publishing House, 2001.

- Nadkarni, Mohan. *Music to Thy Ears: Great Masters of Hindustani Instrumental Music*, New Delhi: Somaiya Publication, 2002.
- Kuppuswamy, Gowri and M. Hariharan. *Great Composers/edited*. Reprint, Nagercoil: CBH Publications, 2005.
- Goswami, Saurabh and Selina Thielemann. *Music and Fine Arts in the Devotional Traditions of India Worship Through Beauty*, New Delhi: A.P.H. Publishers, 2005.
- Mansur, Mallikarjun. *Rasa Yatra : My Journey in Music*, Rajshekhar Mansur (tr.), New Delhi: Roli Books, 2005.
- Mukherjee, Bimal and Sunil Kothari. *Rasa: The Indian Performing Arts in the Last Twenty-five Years*, Kolkata: Anamika Kala Sangam Research and Publications, 1995.
- Prakashan, Sanjay *The Importance of Tone, Tune and Text in Indian Music*, New Delhi: Debashree Bhattacharya, 2007.
- Shanker, Ravi. *Bharthrihan's Vairagya and Shringar Shatams*, New Delhi: Bharatiya Vidya Bhavan, 2000.
- Nithya, Raj. *Gana Saraswathi: D.K. Pattammal: Dimensions of a Divine Songster*, Mumbai: Bharatiya Vidhya Bhavan, 2007.
- Ray, Sukumar. *Music of Eastern India: Vocal Music in Bengali, Oriya, Assamese and Manipuri With Special Emphasis on Bengali*, (Reprint), Calcutta: Firma KLM, 1985.
- Sambamurthy, P. *The Teaching of Music*, (Fourth Edition), Chennai: The Indian Music Publishing House, 1998.
- Shankar, Vidya. *The Art and Science of Carnatic Music*, (Reprint), Chennai: Parampara, 1983.
- Sharma, Manorama. *Tradition of Hindustani Music*, New Delhi: A.P.H. Publishers, 2006.
- Suresh, Vidya Bhavani. *What is Carnatic Music?*, Chennai: Skanda Publications, 2002.
- Thielemann, Selina. *Rasalila: A Musical Study of Religious Drama in Vraja*, New Delhi: A.P.H. Publishers, 1998.
- Vijaylakshmi, M. *Indian Music: Its Origin, History and Characteristics*, Delhi: 2004.

Nritya—joy in rhythm
- Gaston, Anne Marie. *Bharatanatyam: From Temple to Theatre*, New York: Oxford University Press, 1996.
- Coomaraswamy, Ananda K. *The Dance of Shiva: Fourteen Indian Essays*, Bombay: Asia Publishing House, 1952.
- Coomaraswamy, Ananda. *The Mirror of Gesture*, New York: E. Weyhe, 1936.

- Dehejia, Harsha V. *A Celebration of Love: The Romantic Heroine in the Indian Arts*, New Delhi: Roli Books, 2004.
- Gaston, Anne-Marie. *Bharata Natyam: From Temple to Theatre*, New Delhi: Manohar Publishers & Distributors, 1996.
- Kashyap, Tripura. *My Body, My Wisdom: A Handbook of Creative Dance Therapy*, New Delhi: Penguin, 2005.
- Meduri, Avanthi. *Rukmini Devi Arundale (1904-1986): A Visionary Architect of Indian Culture and the Performing Arts*, New Delhi: Motilal Banarsidass, 2005.
- Narayan, Shovana. *Folk Dance Traditions of India*, Gurgaon: Shubhi Publications, 2004.
- Kulkarni, R.P. *The Theatre According to the Natyasastra of Bharata*, (Reprint), New Delhi: Kanishka Publishers, 2008.
- Sindhoor, Aparna. *Dance Teachings in Cambridge*, MA: August 1999- July 2000.
- Schweig, Graham M. *Dance of Divine Love: The Rasa Lila of Krishna from the Bhagavata Purana, India's Classic Sacred Love Story*, New Delhi: Motilal Banarsidass, 2007.
- Triveni Dance Studio, *Dance Teachings in Brookline*, MA: September 2000- February 2001.
- Venkataraman, L. and A. Pasricha. *Indian Classical Dance: Tradition in Transition*, New Delhi: Roli Books, 2002.
- V. Raghavan. *Splendours of Indian Dance (Forms-Theory-Practice)*, Chennai: Dr. V. Raghavan Centre for Performing Arts, 2004.

Solah Shringara—adorning the body
- Dhanamjaya. *The Dasarupa: A Treatise on Hindu Dramaturgy*, first translated from the Sanskrit with the text and an introduction and notes, New York: Columbia University Press, 1912.
- Hill, Jeff. *India Love Poems: Selected and with an Essay on Woman in India by Tambimuttu*, New York: Peter Pauper Press, 1954.
- Mehta, Nandini. *Vidyadharas in Ancient Indian Art*, New Delhi: Harman Publishing House, 2004.
- Shukla, K.S. *Pura Sri: Beauty and Wealth of Ancient India*, New Delhi: B.R. Publishing, 2008.

Shringara—in living culture
- Cooper, Ilay and John Gillow. *Arts and Crafts of India*, New York: Thames and Hudson, 1996.

- Dalmiya, Yashodhara. *The Painted World of the Warlis*, New Delhi: Lalit Kala Academy, 1988.
- Dube, S.C. *Tribal Heritage Of India*, New Delhi: Vikas Publishing House, 1987.
- Elwin, Verrier and Geoffrey Cumberlege. *Tribal Art Of Middle India*, USA: Oxford University Press, 1951.
- Jain, Jyotindra and Ganga Devi. *Tradition and Expression in Mithila Painting*, Ahmedabad, India: Mapin Publishing Pvt Ltd., in association with The Mithila Museum, Niigata, Japan, 1997.
- Jain, Jyotindra. *Painted Myths of Creation: Art and Ritual of an Indian Tribe*, New Delhi: Lalit Kala Akademi, 1984.
- Anand, Mulk Raj. *Madhubani Painting*, New Delhi: Publications Division, Ministry of Information and Broadcasting, Government of India, 1984.
- Mulvey, Laura. 'Visual Pleasure and Narrative Cinema' in *Screen*, 1975.
- Ohri, Chander Vishwa. *The Technique of Pahari Painting: An Inquiry into Aspects of Materials, Methods and History*, New Delhi: Aryan Books, 2001.
- Roy C. Craven. *A Concise History of Indian Art*, London: Thames and Hudson; New York: Praeger, 1976.
- Stallabrass, J. *High Art Lite: British Art in the 1990s*, London: Verso, 1999.
- Warr, T. and A. Jones. *The Artist's Body*, London: Phaidon, 2000.
- Wheeler, Monroe. (ed.) Jayakar, Pupul and John Irwin. *Textiles and Ornaments of India*, New York: The Museum of Modern Art, Simon and Schuster, 1956.
- Youngblood, G. *Expanded Cinema*, New York: E P Dutton, 1970.

Photo Credits

Amit Mehra
126, 127, 144

Arpana Kaur
99

Asmita Theatre Group
14, 15

Avinash Pasricha
16, 17, 22, 23, 24, 25, 26, 124, 128, 134, 142, 146, 147(top, bottom), 160

Brinda Miller
176

Chandigarh Museum
35, 38, 47, 54

Cylla
71

Dhara Mehrotra
XX

Kalpana Shah
78

Kanchan Chander
43, 60, 89, 176(bottom)

Katherine Virgils
XXIII(top)

Madhura Mukherjee
VIII, IX, XII, XVI, XXII, XXIII(bottom), 2, 5, 6, 7, 8, 9, 10, 12, 13, 18, 20, 21, 27, 31, 32(bottom), 46, 50, 51, 53, 56, 57, 63, 64, 65, 69, 73, 75, 76, 79, 85, 87, 90, 91, 94, 95, 96, 97, 98, 100, 102(top), 102-103(panel)105, 106, 107, 108, 109, 110, 111, 112, 113, 114, 115, 116, 117, 118, 121, 123, 125, 130, 131, 132, 136, 143, 145, 150, 153, 157, 161, 164(bottom), 165(bottom), 166(bottom), 167, 170, 171(top).

N.C. Mehta Collection
28, 34, 37, 40-41, 42, 48, 49, 58, 59, 66, 67, 68, 72, 82, 84, 86, 92-93, 95, 120, 138-139

Navin Sakhuja
137

Pramod K.G.
159

Rajita Schade
80-81

Rupa Collection
X, 4, 11, 30(top, bottom), 32(top), 33, 36, 39, 44, 52, 55, 70, 74, 88(top, bottom), 90, 104, 122, 133, 140(top, bottom), 141, 148, 154(top), 155, 156, 158, 169(bottom)

Shelly Jyoti
XXIV, 162

Shola Carletti
XXI, 172

Sidharth
XV

Sunaina Bhalla
178

Viren Tanwar
XVII, 151, 152(top), 179, 180-181

Index

Abhayagiriya Dagaba, 112
Abhijnana Shakuntalam, 8
Abhinavabharati, 4
Abhinavagupta, xx, xxi, 4, 7, 17, 20
Abhinaya Darpana, 147
Adhai Din Ka Jhopda, 175
Adi Granth, 127
Adi Shankara, xix
Aesthetic beauty and philosophical beauty, xvi
Aesthetic experience, xiv, xvi, xvii, xx, 5–6, 8–9, 11–13, 15, 20–21, 26, 35, 62, 121
Aesthetics of Ugliness, xxiv
Aesthetics
    keystones of, 11–13
    legacy of, 180–181
Aham poetry, 30, 74
Ajanta and Ellora, 84, 112, 115
Akbar, 98, 175
Akbarnama, 98
Alamkara-shastras, 4
Alvars and Nayanmars, 74
Amarusataka, 87
Amaravati stupa, 112
Ananda, state of (bliss), xix, xx, 30, 46
Anandavardhana, 4, 7
Anang Ranga, 30, 73, *see also* Kalayanmalla
Appreciation of beauty, xvi
Appreciation process, 11
Apsara (celestial nymph), 64
Ardhanarishvara, 152, *see also* Shiva
Aristotle, xviii, 153
Arjan Dev, Guru 127
Art of the People, 164–165
Art theory, Indian, 21
Art
    definitions of, 5
    evolution of 174
Aryan ritualism, 76
Ashokan Pillar, 112
Ashoka's conversion to the Buddhist faith, 85
Ashtachap, 131
Ashvaghosha, 62
Ashvamedha yajna, 48
Atharva Veda, 32, 46
Atman or soul of art, 8
Aurangzeb, 98
Avalokiteshvara, 27

Bana, 50, 102, 145

Barahmasa songs, 128
Basawan, 175
Beauty Beyond the Physical, 174
    dancing girl, Mohenjodaro, 174
    Kandariya Mahadev Temple, Khajuraho, 174
    Mount Meru, metaphor of, 174
Beauty in Ugliness, xxiii
Beauty of the Banjaras, 170–171
Beauty of the Devil, xxiii
Beauty, philosophy of, 5
Bengali Kalighat art, 166
Beri Beri archaeological sites, 167
Bhagavata Purana, 13, 39, 75, 80, 87
Bhagvad Gita, 32, 46
Bhakti (devotional religion), literature of 73
Bhakti cult, 99, 131–132
Bhakti era, poetry of the 30
Bhakti literature, 74, 76–77
Bhakti movement, 39, 74, 77, 132, 179
Bhakti path, 39
Bhakti poetry, 42
Bhakti rasa, 122, 132
Bhakti shringara, romantic tradition of, 75
Bhakti songs, 74
Bhaktikavya, 70, 74
Bhalla, Atul, 178
Bhamaha, 16
Bharata Muni, 4, 15, 140
Bharata Natyam, 137
Bharatanatyam, 137, 140, 144, 179
Bhartrihari, 63, 68
Bhatta, Bhushana, 50
Bhimbetka caves, 84
Bhujra Patra—earliest Buddhist manuscripts, 85
Bilhana, 50, 76, 84
Birju Maharaj, 179
Bison-horn Marias, 170
Blissful state of *ananda* (*anandaghana*), 35
Bodhisattva, 27
Buddhism, 34, 59, 110, 112
Bulleh Shah, 77, 127
Bundi painting, 35, 95
Bundi School of Rajput painting, 88
Burton, Sir Richard, 31

Cage, John, 43
Celestial virgins, 57
Chaitanya, Sri, 39

Chand, Ghamand, 88
Chandayan, 128
Chandragupta II, 50
Chatuhshashthi-kala, (sixty-four arts), 12
Chaurpanchasika, 50, 76, *see also* Bilhana
Chitra Bandha, 167
Chitra Ganesh, 180
Chitra, 83–99
    Ajanta and Ellora, 84
        cave and temple paintings from, 84
        Konark and Khajuraho, 85
    ancient canons of art, 97
        Jayamangalatika, 97
        Kamasutra, 97
        Vishnudharmottara Purana, 97–98
    beginnings of the miniature form, 84
    Bhimbetaka caves, paintings, 84
    Bhujra Patra—earliest Buddhist manuscripts, 85
    Bundi School of Rajput painting, 88
    celebrating spring, 94
        Bundi paintings, 95
        Raga Vasanta paintings, 95
        Ragamala painting, 96
    complex tapestry, 96
        Barahmasa series, 97
    Eternal Nayika, 88
    Kangra paintings, 88
    Kangra School in the Punjab hills, 87
    local flora and fauna, depiction of, 94
    miniature's magic, 87
    musical moods, 90
    Nitya-Lalita
        divine enchantress, 85
        female principle of, 87
        pahari tradition, 87
    Prudery to Plain-Spoken, 98
        Akbarnama, 98
        bhakti cult, 99
        Hamzanama, 98
        Mughal School of miniature painting, 98
        Pahari School of art, 98
        Rajput and Pahari Schools of painting, 99
        Tutinama, 98
        Tuzuk-i-Jahangiri, 98
        victorian prudery, 99
    Radha and Krishna, love between, 87
    Ragamala paintings, 90, 94
    Rajput schools of painting, 87
    unbroken tradition, 84
Circle of Life, 167

Classical culture, amalgamated 50
Clothing and handicrafts, 168
    phiran, 168
    sozoni style (Kashmir hand embroidery), 168
    zardozi (gold thread embroidery), 168
Coomaraswamy, A.K., xx, 147, 165, 181
Cosmic beauty, perception of 11
Courtesans, 81, 125, 145, 179
Cult of Desire, 110
Cultural fabric, 30, 175

Da Gama, Vasco 176
Daksha Sheth, 179
Damodaragupta, 81
Dance of Siva: Fourteen Indian Essays, xx
Dancing girl from Mohenjodaro, 174
Danielou, 33–34
Dard, 77
Das, G.N., 75
Das, Jatin, 99
Dasa, Chandi, 156
Daud, Mulla, 128
Deccan School, 88
Desire and delight, 31
Devadasi, 144–145, *see also* Temple dancers
Devatmaya rupa, 94
Dhamija, Jasleen, 165
Dhrupad, 123, 131
Digital creations, 178
Divinity, 15
Dodiyas, Atul, 178
Dutch East India Company, 176

Ear ornaments, 153
East India Company, 125, 176
Eco, Umberto, 181
Egyptian pyramids, 112
Ellora caves, 107
Emotion, integrity of 15
Erotic love, 50, *see also* Kama – the erotic
Erotic metaphors, 54, 67
Erotic symbolism, 30, 153
Erotica, 30, 48, 54, 85, 99, 102, 114, 116
European Influence, 176

Fatehpur Sikri, 175
Feminine beauty, ideals of 65
Fifth Veda, *see Natyashastra*
Finery of the Marias, 170
First patron of the arts, 174
Folk and tribal communities, 165
Foreplay, 65

Four stages of life, 46
Freud, Sigmund, 22
Funeral pyres, 59

Gaitonde, V.S., 177
Gandhara School of art, 110
Ganikas or courtesans, 81
Garbarek, Jan, 180
Gaston, Anne-Marie, 137, 144
Geetz, Clifford, 165
Ghare-Baire (The Home and the World), 177, see also Tagore, Rabindranath
Ghazal *gayaki*, 125
Ghungroos, 140
Gita Govinda, 34, 42, 67, 69, 85, 131, see also Jayadeva
Gitanjali, 176–177, see also Tagore, Rabindranath
Glass, Philip, 180
Gods of Love and Ecstasy, 33
Gora, 177, see also Tagore, Rabindranath
Graeco Roman influence, 110
Gupta, Subodh, 178

Haider, Ali, 127
Hamzanama, 98
Harivamsha, 13, 39
Harshavardhan, 12
Harshvardhan, King, 50
Haveli sangeet, 131
Heer-Ranja, 77
Hegel, George Wilhelm Friedrich, xviii
Hinayana and Mahayana phases, 110
Hindu cosmology, 32
Hindu sculptural tradition, 178
Hinduism, 46, 50, 59, 62, 70, 104, 131
Hoysala temples, 113
Human emotion, hierarchal structure of 16
Hume, David, xviii
Husain, M.F., 99, 177–178
Hussain, Zakir, 180

Indian Culture, Golden Age of 50
Indo-Greek literature, 30
Indo-Islamic architecture, 175
Indus Valley Civilization, 50, 102, 167
Islam, advent of, 175
Islamic culture, elements of 70
Islamic mysticism, 77

Jagannath temple, 174
Jagannatha, 4
Jagdambi temple, 115

Jainism, 59
Jalis and jharokhas, 175
Jayadeva, 34, 42, 69–70, 78, 85, 131
Jayakar, Pupul, 164, 166–167
Jayasi, Malik Muhammad, 77
Jhumar, 168
Juang tribe, 171

Kabir, 39, 74–75, 131, see also Bhakti path
Kadambari, 12, 50, see also Banabhatta
Kailashanath temple, Ellora, 113
Kalayanmalla, 73
Kaleka, Ranbir, 116
Kalidasa, 8, 30, 50, 67–68, 102, 126, 131
Kalinga, battle of, 112
Kama – the erotic, 45–59
    Act of Creation, 52
    Ajanta, 57
    alasya kanyas, 57
    auto-eroticism to homo-eroticism, 59
    Brahmas directive to, 55
    cosmic and physical reality of creation, 47
    Divine Union, 46
    erotic metaphors, 54
    kama shastra, 50
    Khajuraho's visual art 57
    Krishna and Radha, eternal love of, 48
    Marriage of, 55
    phallus, 53
    principal ingredient in, 32
    sacred tradition, 50
    sensual element, 46
    sex worship, 48
    sexual union and ecstasy, visualization of, 52
    Shiva and his consort, Parvati, 48
    tantric worship, 48
    Victorian morality, 46
Kamadeva, 30
Kamasutra, 13, 30–32, 56–57, 64–67, 73, 85, 97, 114, see also Vatsyayana
Kandariya Mahadeo temple, 115, 174
Kangra art, 36
Kangra paintings, 88
Kangra School in the Punjab hills, 87
Kangra School of miniature, 36
Kant, Immanuel, xvii, xix
Kashmiri Shaivism, xxi, 4
Kashyapashilpa, 102
Kathak, 140, 179
Kathakali, 140
Kaushitaki Upanishad, 98

Kavya, 61–81
    different strands, 70
    ecstatic devotion, 74
    epitome of shringara, 78
        courtesans, opposed the activities of 81
        ganikas or courtesans, 81
        Kandukuri Viresalingam, 81
        Keshavdas, 79
        Kuttanimata, 81
        Radha and Krishna, love play between, 81
        Radha-Krishna poetry, devotional, 78
        Rasikapriya, 79
        riti poetry, 79
        Ritikavya, 78
        Vallabhacharya, 80
        Victorian morality, 80
    King of Love Poetry, 69
    literary genres, kinds of, 63
    lovemaking, lessons in, 62
    metaphors from nature, 67
    Sufi tradition, 77
        Amir Khusrau, 77
        Bulleh Shah, 77
        Dard, 77
        ghazal in Urdu poetry, 77
        Heer-Ranja, 77
        Laila-Majnu, 77
        Mahmud-Ayaz, 77
        Malik Muhammad Jayasi, 77
        Mir Taqi Mir, 77
        Punjabi *kafi*, 77
        Radha-Krishna tradition of bhakti, 77
        Raskhan and Rahim, 77
        Sauda, 77
        Shah Laatif, 77
        Shirin-Farhad, 77
        Sohni-Mahiwal, 77
        Yusuf-Zulaikha, 77
Kavyalamkara, 16, *see also* Bhamaha
Kavyalamkarasutra, xix, *see also* Vamana
Keat, John, xx
Keshavadas, 36, 78–79, 88, 99
Keyt, George, 175
Khajuraho, 8–9, 11–13, 30–32, 56–57, 85, 114–115, 152, 159
Khayal sangeet, 123
Kher, Bharti, 178
Khusrau, Amir, 77, 125
Kokashastra, 30, 73
Konark, 85, 115
Krishna and Radha, eternal love of 48
Krishna Bhakti, 39, 74, 80

Kuchipudi, 140
Kukkoka, Pandit, 73
Kumarasambhava, 50, 67, 131, *see also* Kalidasa
Kuntaka, 4, 17

Laatif, Shah, 77
Laila-Majnu, 77
Living Shringara, 171
Lochana, xx, *see also* Abhinavagupta
Lollata, Bhatta, 4
Love
    rati or love between man and woman, 68
    vatsalya or love between mother and child, 68
    bhakti or devotion towards god, 68

Mahabharata, 25, 33, 50, 59
Mahendravarman I, King 104
Mahimabhatta, 4
Mahmud-Ayaz, 77
Maithili community, 166
Maithuna (sexual act), 30
Malani, Nalini, 180
Mammata, 4
Mangaldas, Aditi, 179
Mangalsutra, 168
Mango blossoms, 36
Manipuri, 140
Manmatha, 30
Manual for marriage, *see* Anang Ranga
Marks of Distinction, 168
Mathura and the Gandhara Schools of art, 109
Mathura School, 109–110
Mauryan dynasty, 50
Mayamata, 102
McLaughlin, John, 180
Mead, Margaret, 165
Medieval Bhakti poetry, 43
Medieval Hindi literature, golden age of 39
Meghadutam, 8, 68, 102
Mehndi ki raat (night of mehndi), 154
Mehta, Tyeb, 177
Mir, Mir Taqi, 77
Mirabai, 22, 39, 74, 178
Miskin, 175
Modern Voices, 177–178
Modernism, advent of, 178
Mohapatra, Kelucharan, 179
Mohiniattam, 140
Moksha, 7, 13, 16, 31–32, 46, 59
Mount Meru, metaphor of 174

Mudgal, Madhavi, 179
Mughal Empire, 98, 174
Mughal period, 73, 99, 176
Mughal School of miniature painting, 98
Mughal School, characteristics of the 88
Mukherjee, Meera, 178
Musical composition, essence of a 21
Musical Moods, 90

Nadamaya rupa, 94
Nanak Dev, Guru 127
Narrative ritual, form of 166
Nationalism, growth of, 176
Natyashastra, 4–5, 7–9, 11–17, 20, 53, 62–63, 102, 120, 140, 145, 180, *see also* Bharata Muni
Natya-shastras, 4
Navina School, 4, 9
Nayaka, Bhatta, 4, 7
New Language for Shringara, 181
Nimmat Nama, 30
Nine rasas, or the *Navarasas*, 8
Noor Jehan, 158
Nritya, 135–147
    abhinaya, 145
   beginning and end of performance, 143
   Bharatanatyam, 137
   erotic dance, 145
   facial gestures *rasadrishtis*, 144
   footwork or goti, 143
   gesture of reverence, 143
   Kathak, 140
   Kathakali, 140
   Kuchipudi, 140
   Manipuri, 140
   Mohiniattam, 140
   mudra, meaning of, 143
   Odissi, 140
   origins of, 137
   standing posture, 143
   Tandava, 137
   theory of dance, 140
   Traditional training, 144
Nymphs, 57

Odissi, 140, 179
On Ugliness, 181

Pahari tradition, 87
Painting traditions, 98
Pancham veda, 16
Panchivedas, 73
Panigrahi, Sanjukta, 179
Parekh, Manu, 116
Patterns of beauty, 174
Performing Arts, 178–180
Phad paintings of Rajasthan, 166
Photoshop, 178
Pinnacle of Beauty, 176, *see also* Taj Mahal
Plassey, Battle of, 176
Plato, xvii
Poetics, 5
Polygamous lifestyles, 48
Pratiharenduraja, 4
Pravara-lalita, 53
Pritam, Amrita, 127
Progressive Art Group, 177
Pushti Sangeet style, 131

Qawwali, 132

Raas lila of Lord Krishna, 76
Radha and Krishna, legend of 35
Radha and Krishna, love between 70, 74, 85, 87
Radha-Krishna poetry, devotional 78
Radha-Krishna tradition of bhakti, 77
Raga Vasanta paintings, 95
Raga Vasanta, 94–95
Ragamala paintings, 36, 90, 94, 96–97, 122, 129
Rai, Raghu, 178
Rajasthani schools of painting, 175
Rajput and Pahari Schools of painting, 99
Rajput schools of painting, 87
Rama and Krishna cults, 131
Ramacharitmanas, 74, *see also* Tulsidass
Ramayana, 25, 50, 87
Rasa theory, 4–5, 13, 120, 140
Rasa, Cradle of, 8–11
Rasamanjari, 70, 99
Rasamanjari, Bhanudattas, 99
Rasas, Spectrum of, 21–27
   adbhuta, or the sentiment of wonder, 27
   bhayanaka or the sentiment of fear, 25–26
   bibhatsa, 26
   hasya or the comic sentiment, 21
   karuna or pathos, 22
   raudra (furious), 22, 25
   shanta, peace or inner serenity, 27
   shringara rasa, 21
   vira or the heroic sentiment, 25
   visual and performance arts, 27
Rasikapriya, 35, 43, 79, 87–88, 99, *see also* Keshavadas
Raskhan and Rahim, 77
Rati Rahasya, 73

Ratnakar, Sarangadevas Sangita, 145
Raza, S.H., 177
Re-affirming Indian Ideals, 176
Reddy, Ravinder, 178
Religious and secular literature, 64
Representational beauty, ingredients of xxii
Rig Veda, 46, 62
Riti poetry, 79
Ritikavya, 70, 78
Ritual sacrifice, 48
Ritusamhara (garland of seasons), 30, 67–68, 126, 160, *see also* Kalidasa
Rodwittiya, Rekha, 178
Romantic aspects of interaction, 64
Rousseau, xviii
Rudrata, Kashmiri poet, xix, 11, 17
Rushdie, Salman, 180
Ruskin, John, xvii

Sacrificial ritual, 33, 47
Sahitya Darpana, xx
Samaranganasutradhara, 16
Samson, Leela, 179
Sanchi stupa, 112
Sangeet, 119–132
    Antar Bhakti – Bahir Shringar, 131
        Ashtachap, 131
        bhakti cult, 131–132
        bhakti movement, 132
        bhakti rasa, 132
        bheda-abheda, nuances of, 132
        Haveli sangeet, 131
        Pushti Sangeet, 131
        qawwali, 132
        Rama and Krishna cults, 131
    concept of rasa, 121
    divine art form, 121
    eternal couple, 129
        parakiya shringara or illicit love, 129
        romantic couple, Radha and Krishna, 131
    face of joy, 126
    Goddess Saraswati, 121
    Lord Krishna, 121
    Lord Shiva, 121
    Natyashastra with rasa theory, 120
    pathos of separation, 128
        barahmasa songs, 128
        Sanskrit shadritu poetry, 128
    romantic forms, 123
        courtesans, 125
        ghazal *gayaki*, 125
        Hindustani music, 123
        thumri, 125
    seasonal songs, 126
        Raga Tukhari, 127
        Shadrituvarnan, 126
    stepping stones, 121
        Asawari, 122
        Bhairavi, 122
        bhakti rasa, 122
        Brihaddeshi, 121
        decoration of a composition, 123
        dhrupad, 123
        evoking the mood, 122
        Kafi, 122
        khayal sangeet, 123
        shabdapradhan, 123
        swaradevata, 122
        Todi, 122
        vadi swara, 122
        vivadi swara, 122
    sthayi and *sanchari*, 120
    unravelling layers, 129
        manifestation of the cosmic leela, 129
        Ragamala paintings, 129
Sangita-shastras, 4
Sankuka, Sri, 4
Sansar Chand, 88
Sanskrit shadritu poetry, 128
Sarnath stupa, 112
Satyam, Shivam, Sundaram, xx–xxiii, xx
Sauda, 77
Saundarya —Indian Approach, xix–xx, xix
Saundarya Shastra, xiv, xxiv
Saundarya, closest interpretation of, xxii
Saundaryalahari, xix, *see also* Adi Shankara
School of Life, 169–170
Selfless sympathy (*sahridayata*), 6
Seth, Vikram, 180
Sex worship, 48
Sexual force, importance of 33, 53
Sexuality, 30, 65
Shabdapradhan, 123
Shah, Wajid Ali, 123
Shaiva Siddhanta tradition, 33
Shankar, Pandit Ravi, 180
Shantiniketan, 176, *see also* Tagore, Rabindranath
Sharma, Uma, 179
Sheikh, Nilima, 177–178
Shilpa Ratna, 16
Shilpa Shastra, 101–116
    buddha in stone, 109
    eternal image, 116
    faces of Shiva, 107
        Ardhanarishvara, 107
        Ellora caves, 107

Gandhara School of art, 109–110
Graeco Roman influence, 110
Hinayana and Mahayana phases, 110
Holy Trinity, manifestations of, 104
    Dhaka museum, 106
    Lakshmi bathed by the elephant, 106
    Mandagapattu inscription, 104
    Vishnus first avatar, 106
Indus Valley Civilization, 102
Mathura school, 109–110
Monasteries and Stupas, 110–113
    Abhayagiriya Dagaba, 112
    Ajanta and Ellora caves, 112
    Amravati stupa, 112
    ancient cave monasteries, 112
    Ashokan Pillar, 112
    Buddhist architectural forms, 112
    Kailashanath temple, 113
    Kalinga battle, 112
    Sanchi stupa, 112
    Sarnath stupa, 112
pinnacle of adornment, 115
    Jagdambi temple, 115
    Kandariya Mahadev temple, 115
    Khajuraho's architectural style, 115
    Vishvanath temple, 115
Sex as Sacred, 114
    Aihole, 115
    Ajanta and Ellora, 115
    architecture, 114
    graphic stone carvings, 114
    Kanchipuram, 115
    Khajuraho, 114–115
    Konark, 115
    public arena, 115
    Ramgarh (Rajasthan), 115
    scantily-clad women, Ajanta, 114
symbols of significance, 107
    erotic desire, 109
    multiple arms of deities,
representation of, 109
tantric rites, 116
    tantric iconography of sexual union, 116
temple art, 113
    Dravida or southern style, 113
    granite, use of, 114
    Hoysala temples, 113
    ivory and sandalwood, use of, 114
    Nagara or northern style, 113
    Pallava temples, 114
    Vesara or hybrid style, 113
terracotta seal, 102
Vedic Pantheon, 103
shivalingam, 103
Surya and Indra at the Bhaja caves, 103
vedic deities, 103
Shilpa Shastras, 4, 13, 16
Shirin-Farhad, 77
Shiva Purana, 34, 54–55
Shiva, 22, 25, 32, 34, 48, 50, 52–55, 67, 87, 102–104, 106–107, 115–116, 121, 131, 137, 152, 156, 174
Shringara—Rasaraja, 29
    Ananda—the Ultimate Pleasure, 33–35
    Divine Ecstasy, 39–43
        Bhakti movement, 39
        Bhakti path, 39
        Bhakti poetry, 42
        Krishna Bhakti, 39
        medieval Bhakti poetry, 43
        shringara-bhakti, romantic tradition of, 39
    Flowering of the Nayika, 35
        Bundi painting, 35
        erotic paintings of Guler, 36
        folk songs, 36
        Kamoda Ragini, 35
        Kangra art, 36
        Kangra School of miniature, 36
        mango blossoms, 36
        Ragamala paintings, 36
    kama in the scriptures, 32–33
Shringara – Supreme Rasa, 13–16
Shuddhavaita school of Vaishnavism, 74
Shukraniti, 7
Sixteen rituals or samskaras, 46
Sixty-four arts, 97, 145, 160
Socrates, xviii
Sohni-Mahiwal, 77
Solah Shringara, 149–160
    Anjana (Kohl)—*Kajal*, 152
    Arsi (Thumb Ring with Mirror), 155
    Baajuband (Armband), 155
    Bindi (Dot on the Forehead), 150–151
    Bridal Dress, 159
    Haar (Necklace), 153
    Itra (Perfume), 158
    Kamarband (Ornamental Girdle), 156–157
    Kangana (Wrist Ornament), 155
    Karnaphool (Ear-flower), 153–154
    Keshapasharachna (Coiffure), 156
    Mehndi (Henna), 154
    Multiple Narratives, 150
    Nath (Nose-ring), 152–153
    Payal (Anklet) and Toe-rings, 157–158

Rooh-e-Gulab, 158
Sindoor (Vermilion), 151–152
skin care, 159
    cleansing and softening the hands, 159
    face packs, 159
    mudpacks, 159
Tika (Hair Ornament), 152
Traditional Attire, 160
Sood, Anupam, 178
Souza, F.N., 99, 177
Spirit of Freedom, 177
Spiritual fervour, 7
Sufi thought, classical dance with 179
Superconsciousness, state of, 9
Sur Sagar, 74, 80, 132
Surasundari (musical beauty) or, 64
Surdas, 74, 80, 132
Swaminathan, J., 177
Symposium, xvii, see also Plato

Tagore, Rabindranath, 13, 75, 176, 181
Taittriya Upanishad, 32, 46
Taj Mahal, 176
Tales, metaphors and symbols, 31
Tandava, 137
Tantra school of worship, 48
Tantra yoga, 48
Tantraloka, 4
Tantras, 48
Tantric Worship, 48
Tantrism, 48
Tasting of flavour or *rasavadana*, 8
Tasting, degrees of, 20
Tawaif or courtesan, 123
Telltale Tattoos, 171
Temple dancers, 144
Thumri, 123, 125
Traditional sculpture, 64
Transcending the Divide, 20–21
Tribal communities, 164, 167
Tribal customs of Central India, 168–169
True function of art, 12
Tulsidas, 74
Tutinama, 98
Tuzuk-i-Jahangiri, 98
Twelve sargams or songs of *Gita Govinda*, 70

Unseen Communion, 166

Vaishnavism, 80
Vallabhacharya, Shri, 131
Vamana, xix, 8, 17

Vastu-shastras, 4
Vatsyayana, 13, 31, 65, 97, 160
Vedanta School, 7
Victorian morality, 46, 80
Vidyeshvara Samhita, 34
Vilasam bhava, 30, 46
Vinay Patrika, 74, *see also* Tulsidas
Vishnu Purana, 13
Vishnudharmottara Purana, 7, 16, 97, 102, 147
Vishvakarma, the Divine Architect, xv
Vishvanath temple, 115
Vishwanath, Kaviraj, xx
Vishwanatha, 11
Visva Bharati, *see* Shantiniketan
Vivan Sundaram, 178

Way of Aesthetics, 4–8
Ways of Perceiving Beauty, xv–xvii, xv
    beauty through narrative, xv
    beauty through participation, xv
    beauty through ritual, xv
    beauty through shringara, xvi
    non-verbal attributes of beauty, xvi
    performing arts, xvi
Western aesthetic model, xxiii
Western Theories on Beauty, xvii–xix, xvii
Women, classification of, 73

Yajur Veda, 32, 34, 54
Yama, the god of death, 22
Yashodhara, 8, 97
Yezirah, Sefer, 53
Yusuf-Zulaikha, 77

Zafar, Mir, 175

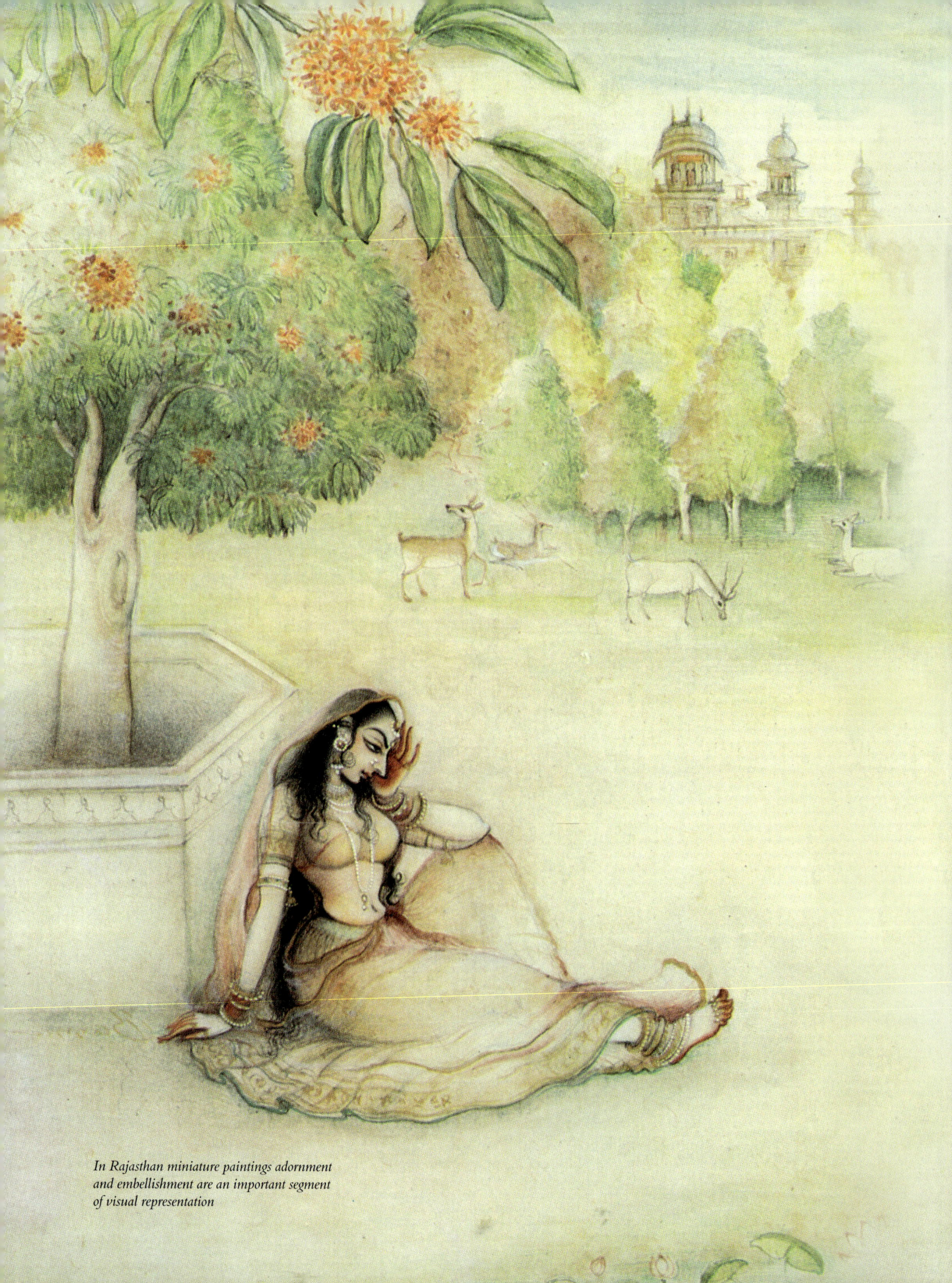

In Rajasthan miniature paintings adornment and embellishment are an important segment of visual representation